Handbook of Breast Cancer Treatments

Handbook of Breast Cancer Treatments

Editor: Brianna Peralta

AMERICAN
MEDICAL PUBLISHERS
www.americanmedicalpublishers.com

AMERICAN
MEDICAL PUBLISHERS
www.americanmedicalpublishers.com

Cataloging-in-Publication Data

Handbook of breast cancer treatments / edited by Brianna Peralta.
p. cm.
Includes bibliographical references and index.
ISBN 978-1-63927-606-6
1. Breast--Cancer. 2. Breast--Cancer--Treatment. 3. Breast--Cancer--Diagnosis. I. Peralta, Brianna.
RC280.B8 H36 2023
616.994 49--dc23

American Medical Publishers,
41 Flatbush Avenue,
1st Floor, New York,
NY 11217, USA

ISBN 978-1-63927-606-6 (Hardback)

Contents

Preface

Every book is a source of knowledge and this one is no exception. The idea that led to the conceptualization of this book was the fact that the world is advancing rapidly; which makes it crucial to document the progress in every field. I am aware that a lot of data is already available, yet, there is a lot more to learn. Hence, I accepted the responsibility of editing this book and contributing my knowledge to the community.

Breast cancer refers to a type of cancer that develops in the breast cells. Invasive lobular carcinoma and invasive ductal carcinoma are the two most common types of breast cancer. There are various symptoms and signs associated with this type of cancer, such as a newly inverted nipple, a breast lump, pitting or redness of the skin above the breast, changes in the size, appearance or shape of a breast, etc. Some of the major risk factors linked to breast cancer include a family history of breast cancer, obesity, drinking alcohol and radiation exposure. There are different ways to diagnose it, such as through ultrasonography, magnetic resonance imaging (MRI), mammogram and positron emission tomography (PET) scanning. Immunotherapy, radiation therapy, surgery, targeted drug therapy, chemotherapy and hormone therapy are some of the techniques used to treat this disease. This book is compiled in such a manner, that it will provide in-depth knowledge about the diverse treatment strategies for breast cancer. A number of latest researches have been included to keep the readers up-to-date with the various aspects of this medical condition and treatment procedures.

While editing this book, I had multiple visions for it. Then I finally narrowed down to make every chapter a sole standing text explaining a particular topic, so that they can be used independently. However, the umbrella subject sinews them into a common theme. This makes the book a unique platform of knowledge.

I would like to give the major credit of this book to the experts from every corner of the world, who took the time to share their expertise with us. Also, I owe the completion of this book to the never-ending support of my family, who supported me throughout the project.

Editor

1

Reduction of Serum Concentrations and Synergy between Retinol, β-Carotene and Zinc According to Cancer Staging and Different Treatment Modalities Prior to Radiation Therapy in Women with Breast Cancer

Cintia Rosa [1,*], Carlos Franca [1,2,3,4], Sérgio Lanes Vieira [2,3], Antônio Carvalho [4], Antônio Penna [2,3], Carla Nogueira [1], Suzane Lessa [1] and Andrea Ramalho [1]

1 Social Applied Nutrition Department, Micronutrients Research Center (NPqM), Federal University of Rio de Janeiro, Rio de Janeiro 21.941-902, Brazil; cfendlich@gmail.com (C.F.); carlafrancanut@yahoo.com.br (C.N.); suzane.laura@gmail.com (S.L.); aramalho.rj@gmail.com (A.R.)
2 Department of Radiation Oncology, Ingá Radiotherapy Clinic (CRI), Brazilian Institute of Oncology (IBO), Federal University of Rio de Janeiro, Niterói 24.210-470, Brazil; cringa@cringa.com.br (S.L.V.); antoniopcringa@cringa.com.br (A.P.)
3 Department of Radiation Oncology, Pontifical Catholic University of Rio de Janeiro, Rio de Janeiro 22.451-900, Brazil
4 Department of Radiology, Clementino Fraga Filho University Hospital, Federal University of Rio de Janeiro, Rio de Janeiro 21.941-902, Brazil; antoniocars@gmail.com
* Correspondence: cintialeticia2005@yahoo.com.br

Abstract: The procedures used for breast cancer treatment are able to increase the level of oxidative stress and cause depletion of antioxidants. Objectives: To investigate the relationship between serum concentrations of retinol, β-carotene, and zinc, according to breast cancer staging, considering different treatment modalities prior to radiation therapy and the synergistic action between these micronutrients. Methods: This is a cross-sectional observational study comprising a cohort of patients with breast cancer which was carried out prior to radiation therapy. Patients were divided into 3 groups: G1 comprised women who had undergone breast-conserving surgery, G2 comprised those who had undergone chemotherapy, and G3 those who had undergone breast-conserving surgery and chemotherapy. Serum concentrations of retinol, β-carotene, and zinc were quantified. Breast cancer staging was based on the TNM (Tumor, Node, Metastasis) classification of malignant tumors, a type of staging tool for different cancers. Results: A total of 230 patients were assessed. A decrease of the serum concentrations of the micronutrients assessed as the staging level of the disease increased was observed. Surgery alone had a greater negative impact on serum concentrations of retinol. Considering the treatments prior to radiotherapy, patients undergoing surgery alone and chemotherapy associated with surgery had higher percentages of deficiency of β-carotene and retinol. There was a positive correlation between the concentrations of zinc, retinol, and β-carotene, showing a synergy between these micronutrients. Conclusion: A significant reduction in the serum concentrations of the assessed micronutrients was observed, according to the increase in breast cancer staging. The synergy between the micronutrients must be considered in order to maximize the benefits and minimize the adverse effects of irradiation to normal cells.

Keywords: radiotherapy; antioxidants; toxicity; chemotherapy; conservative surgery; breast cancer

1. Introduction

Breast cancer is one of the most occurring malignant tumors in women. According to the Global Cancer Statistics (GLOBOCAN), worldwide, there will be about 2.1 million newly diagnosed female breast cancer cases in 2018, with 626,679 related deaths, accounting for almost 1 in 4 cancer cases among women [1].

Despite being considered a cancer with a relative favorable prognosis if diagnosed and treated properly, mortality rates for breast cancer are still high in Brazil [2]. However, survival rates are different when the disease is restricted to the organ where it started and when it spreads to other organs. Its classification in stages [3] is an important tool for evaluating the prognosis of these patients [4].

Cancer treatment aims to cure the disease, but when this is not possible, efforts focus on controlling the disease to extend life and preserve its quality. To achieve this goal, treatment protocols are proposed involving surgery, radiation therapy, chemotherapy, or a combination of these [5,6]. Treatments for this disease are able to generate free radicals, reduce intrinsic antioxidants, worsen pre-existing cancer comorbidities, or cause them to emerge as a result of the treatment itself [7].

Recently, the literature has been pointing out a relationship between nutrients with antioxidant function and cancer therapy. Among the antioxidants studied, some have been highlighted, such as vitamin A due to its role in cancer therapy, given its chemoprotective and antioxidant role, which is able to decrease, in the short and long term, the harmful effects of cancer treatment [8–10].

Zinc has an important antioxidant action, acts in the immune system and induces apoptosis in tumor cells [11]. In addition, this mineral is required for hepatic synthesis and secretion of retinol-binding proteins (RBP), and, in situations of deficiency, RBP synthesis may be impaired, resulting in a secondary vitamin A deficiency [12].

Despite the available knowledge, the use of these micronutrients in clinical practice is still controversial, and few scientific studies address this topic. In this context, the aim of this study is to investigate the relationship between serum concentrations of retinol, β-carotene, and zinc, according to the stage of breast cancer considering different treatment modalities prior to radiation therapy and the synergistic action between these micronutrients.

2. Methods

This is an observational and cross-sectional study in a cohort of free admission of patients with breast cancer prior to radiation therapy conducted in a private clinic in Rio de Janeiro state in the period from October 2011 to December 2012.

Patients were divided into 3 groups comprising those who had undergone breast-conserving surgery (G1)alone, chemotherapy alone(G2), and a combination of breast-conserving surgery and chemotherapy (G3). These treatment modalities were performed between 7 and 14 days prior to radiation therapy.

For biochemical analysis, an aliquot of blood was collected for dosage of vitamin A (retinol and β-carotene) and mineral zinc after at least 8 h of fasting. The samples were protected against oxidation and sent immediately to the laboratory to be analyzed.

The method for quantification of retinol and β-carotene used was high performance liquid chromatography by ultraviolet detector (HPLC-UV). The cut-off point used to detect retinol deficiency was <1.05 μmol/L and <50 μg/L to detect β-carotene [13]. The method used for quantification of zinc was atomic absorption spectrophotometry. The cut-off point used to indicate zinc deficiency was <587 mcg/L [14].

The study comprised women aged ≥20 years who had been diagnosed with breast cancer and its staging (TI-III N0 M0) based on the classification of malignant tumors proposed by the Union for International Cancer Control (UICC) [15], which was confirmed by histopathological reports and indication of external radiation therapy after breast-conserving surgery and/or chemotherapy.

Patients who showed disabsorptive syndromes, liver diseases, kidney diseases, diabetes mellitus, patients using, or who had used in the past 6 months a supplement containing vitamin A (retinol or β-carotene) or zinc were excluded from the study. Additionally, patients were excluded who had not had a regular clinical control after treatment, patients who died of a non-neoplastic disease-related death, and patients with missing data in their medical records.

Quantitative variables were expressed as mean and standard deviation, and qualitative variables were expressed as percentages. The Kolmogorov–Smirnov test was used to test the normality of continuous variables. The Mann–Whitney test was used to compare two groups, and the Friedman test was used to compare three groups. The Chi-square test was used to evaluate the association between categorical variables. Spearman's correlation was used for correlation analysis. The significance level adopted was 5% ($p < 0.05$). The analyses were carried out with the Statistical Package for Social Sciences (SPSS) Program version 15.0.

This study was approved by the Ethics and Research Committee of Hospital Universitário Clementino Fraga Filho (CEP_HUCFF UFRJ 19109), and an informed consent form was signed by all the participants.

3. Results

A total of 230 women with mean age of 63.6 years (SD+9.3) were assessed. Age difference between the groups was not significant ($p = 0.28$) (Table 1).

Table 1. General characteristics of the sample.

Variables	Mean	SD	N
Age (years)			
G1	61.9	7.7	52
G2	64.6	9.2	51
G3	64.0	9.2	127
p-value	0.06		
Stage	I (%)	II (%)	III (%)
G1	100 (n = 52)	-	-
G2	27.4 (n = 14)	56.8 (n = 29)	15.6 (n = 8)
G3	-	81 (n = 103)	19 (n = 24)

Friedman and Kruskal–Wallis test. G1—women undergoing conservative mastectomy alone; G2—women undergoing chemotherapy alone; G3—women undergoing conservative surgery and chemotherapy.

With regards to the clinical stages of the disease, stage II predominated reaching 57.4% (n = 132) of the assessed patients. Stage I had 28.7% (n = 66) and stage III had 13.9% (n = 32) (Table 1).

Considering the studied groups, the highest percentage of retinol deficiency was in G3 reaching 21.3% (n = 27), and of β-carotene in G1 reaching 38.5% (20). The highest percentage of the mineral zinc was also found in G1 and reached 30.8% (n = 16) (Table 2).

Table 2. Percentage of antioxidant micronutrients deficiency according to groups that received treatments prior to radiation therapy and according to breast cancer staging.

Variables	Retinol (%)	β-Carotene (%)	Zinc (%)
G1	15.5 (n = 8)	38.5 (n = 20)	30.8 (n = 16)
G2	11.8 (n = 6)	7.8 (n = 4)	37.3 (n = 19)
G3	21.3 (n = 27)	10.2 (n = 13)	17.3 (n = 22)
G1			
Stage I	15.5 (n = 8)	38.5 (n = 20)	30.8 (n = 16)
Stage II	-	-	-
Stage III	-	-	-
G2			
Stage I	0	0	0
Stage II	10.3 (n = 3)	13.8 (n = 4)	37.9 (n = 11)
Stage III	37.5 (n = 3)	-	100 (n = 8)
G3			
Stage I	-	-	-
Stage II	17.5 (n = 18)	12.6 (n = 13)	42.7 (n = 44)
Stage III	37.0 (n = 9)	-	58.3 (n = 14)

Friedman and Kruskal–Wallis test. G1—women undergoing conservative mastectomy alone; G2—women undergoing chemotherapy alone; G3—women undergoing conservative surgery and chemotherapy.

When assessing the serum concentrations of antioxidants in the studied groups, significant differences were only observed in retinol ($p < 0.01$) (Table 3).

Table 3. Serum concentrations of antioxidant micronutrients according to groups that received treatments prior to radiation therapy and according to breast cancer staging.

Variables	Retinol (μmol/L)	β-Carotene (μg/L)	Zinc (mcg/L)
G1	1.56 ± 0.073	171.11 ± 180.2	671.8 ± 170.2
G2	1.87 ± 0.072	203.6 ± 101.5	750.4 ± 249.8
G3	1.46 ± 0.050	227.1 ± 157.8	752.2 ± 193.6
p-value	<0.01	0.083	0.045
G1			
Stage I	1.57 ± 0.74	171.1 ± 180.2	671.6
Stage II	-	-	-
Stage III	-	-	-
G2			
Stage I	2.15 ± 0.42	245.3 ± 29.0	728.6 ± 14.1
Stage II	1.99 ± 0.78	196.7 ± 128.2	840.10 ± 278.8
Stage III	1.02 ± 0.18	156.0 ± 0.1	460.4 ± 54.7
p-value	<0.01	0.11	<0.01
G3			
Stage I	-	-	-
Stage II	1.56 ± 0.50	247.1 ± 166.3	823.7 ± 133.6
Stage III	1.04 ± 0.23	141.1 ± 64.5	500.9 ± 172.3
p-value	<0.01	<0.01	<0.01

Friedman and Kruskal–Wallis test. G1—women undergoing conservative mastectomy alone; G2—women undergoing chemotherapy alone; G3—women undergoing conservative surgery and chemotherapy.

After assessing serum concentrations, it was observed that these antioxidants decreased as stages of breast cancer increased (Table 3).

When the comparison among the means of serum concentrations of retinol was performed according to the stages of the disease in the studied groups, it was observed that in G2 the differences were significant between stage I and III, and between stage II and III (both with $p < 0.01$ values). β-carotene showed statistical difference only when stage I was compared to stage III ($p < 0.01$).

Zinc showed a behavior similar to retinol with statistical differences when stage I was compared to stage III and stage II to III (both with $p < 0.01$ values).

In G3, when the means of the micronutrients assessed in stage II were compared to stage III, it was observed that all showed statistically significant difference with $p < 0.01$ values.

With regard to comparison between the groups, it was observed that serum concentrations of retinol were significantly different between G1 and G2 ($p = 0.03$). However, the same did not occur with β-carotene ($p = 0.26$) and zinc ($p = 0.06$).

When assessing G1 and G3, no statistical difference was found in retinol and β-carotene ($p = 0.29$ and 0.07, respectively). However, statistical difference was found in zinc ($p = 0.01$).

When comparing G2 to G3, retinol was the only antioxidant nutrient that showed statistical difference ($p < 0.01$).

When analyzing the correlations between the assessed micronutrients, there was a positive correlation between retinol and β-carotene ($p < 0.01$ r = 0.358), between retinol and zinc ($p < 0.01$ r = 0.233), and between β-carotene and zinc ($p = 0.03$ r = 0.261).

4. Discussion

The results of the current study show that the more advanced stage of breast cancer, the smaller were the means of serum concentrations of retinol and β-carotene. Thus, our results corroborate the results of Matos et al. [16], who found a significant reduction in serum concentrations of vitamin A as breast cancer staging progressed. However, the percentage of β-carotene deficiency was different in G2 and G3, as no deficiency of this antioxidant in stage III was found in G3. This fact can be explained by an increase in the oxidative stress caused by the disease itself and made worse by the treatments received, which led to low-efficiency of β-carotene bioconversion to retinol [17], thus, causing an increase in retinol deficiency, as noted in our findings.

A similar behavior was observed in serum concentrations of zinc compared to retinol and β-carotene, i.e., the more advanced the stage of the disease, the greater the percentage of deficiency of this antioxidant nutrient. This finding corroborates the results of Kumar R. et al. (2017) [18], who found a significant decrease in serum concentrations of zinc as breast cancer staging progressed.

In our study, the highest prevalence of the disease was found in stage II, followed by stage I and III, with percentage values very close, corroborating the Instituto Nacional de Câncer(INCA) [National Institute of Cancer] national data (2012) [19] and the investigation carried out by Borges et al. (2013) [20], who found prevalence of stage II at the time of diagnosis. However, Soares et al. (2012) [21] reported a greater prevalence in stage III and IV at the time of diagnosis. It is noteworthy that the clinical stage of the disease is an important instrument for prognostic evaluation and that survival rates are related to the early detection of this disease [3].

The treatment of breast cancer is related to the clinical staging of the disease and depends on this classification. The procedures used are able to increase the production of free radicals and, consequently, to deplete antioxidants by the increase in oxidative stress [22]. In our study, among the treatments involved, the women who had only undergone surgery (G1) showed a more prominent reduction in serum concentrations of β-carotene and zinc. When assessing retinol, a reduction of serum concentrations in women who had undergone surgery and chemotherapy (G3) was observed, followed by the women who had only undergone surgery (G1), and no significant difference was observed between the groups. The trauma caused by surgery is associated with the increase in oxidative stress and excessive release of reactive oxygen species and reduction of antioxidant defenses [23]. Such findings demonstrate that the surgery alone, or in combination, had a negative impact similar to the one caused by the assessed antioxidants.

It is noteworthy that the women who had undergone surgery will still be exposed to radiation therapy, which may further increase the imbalance in the oxidant-antioxidant system, which is able to cause acute damage in the medium and long term, and may even result in secondary cancers [24]. In addition, free radicals can exacerbate the pre-existing comorbidities of cancer [25] and generate toxic effects such as cardiotoxicity, pulmonary, and renal toxicity [6].

In this context, retinol stands out for its antioxidant, proapoptotic, and anti-proliferative activity [25], and, as it reduces growth and cell division, it favors tumor cells death [26]. In addition, its adjuvant role in radiation therapy has been reported, making it more effective in the fight against the disease progression and in the reduction of side effects [27].

Carotenoids have antioxidant activity since they neutralize peroxyl radicals, in addition to singlet oxygen, thus reducing the oxidation of DNA and lipids. The mechanisms of action that contribute to their anticancer effects include antioxidant activity, inhibition of proliferation, effects on the immune system, and inhibition of the endogenous formation of carcinogens [28,29]. On the other hand, zinc has an important antioxidant action, has functions in metabolism and interacts with malignant cells, particularly with relation to apoptosis [30].

Although studies addressing these micronutrients in isolation have shown promising results in cancer therapy [25,26,29,30], studies have not yet considered the synergistic relationship between retinol, β-carotene, and zinc which, in addition to being potent antioxidants and closely linked to the immune system, have an important synergy.

Zinc is required for hepatic synthesis and secretion of retinol binding protein (RBP) and, in situations of deficiency, RBP synthesis may be impaired, resulting in secondary vitamin A deficiency [12]. According to Doldo et al. (2015) [25], in breast tumors a low regulation of RBP occurs, jeopardizing the transportation and the proapoptotic and anti-proliferative activity of retinol, thus, favoring tumor progression.

The low concentrations of zinc, often observed in patients with breast cancer who have undergone treatment protocols of this disease, generate an increase in oxidative stress [31–33], and may further worsen serum retinol deficiency as they cause a reduction in the liver mobilization of this vitamin [12]. Studies have reported that low concentrations of serum retinol are predictors of poor prognosis in patients with head and neck cancer [34] and hepatocellular carcinoma [35,36].

The synergy between the assessed micronutrients was observed in our study through the results that showed a positive correlation between retinol and β-carotene, between retinol and zinc, and between β-carotene and zinc. That is, as zinc deficiency occurred, the same occurred with respect to retinol, thus affecting serum concentrations of β-carotene. The better the status of retinol, the smaller will be the requirement of β-carotene to maintain its serum concentrations since this is the most powerful precursor of retinol [37]. This fact allows β-carotene to be more available in its antioxidant function, an action considered important in cancer control [29]. The results found in our study are in agreement with this finding, as the group with the lowest percentage of retinol deficiency (G2) also showed the lowest concentrations of β-carotene. However, we consider as a limitation of our study the impossibility of assessing other antioxidant micronutrients that could present synergy with the nutrients assessed in this study.

The findings presented here are important because, in addition to the role that these nutrients play in breast cancer treatment, they show that their joint use can promote the effectiveness of treatment by inhibiting the repair of the damage caused by irradiation in cancer cells, enhancing the expected damage caused by irradiation [26].

5. Conclusions

Our study showed a significant reduction in serum concentrations of retinol, β-carotene, and zinc, according to the increase in breast cancer staging. Considering the treatments prior to radiotherapy, patients undergoing surgery alone and chemotherapy associated with surgery had higher percentages of micronutrient deficiency, except for zinc in the group that only underwentchemotherapy.There was a positive correlation between deficiencies of zinc, retinol, and β-carotene, showing that the synergy between these micronutrients should be considered.

We recommend the follow-up of the nutritional status of the nutrients discussed in this study in conjunction with the different modalities of breast cancer treatments in order to maximize the benefits of treatment and minimize adverse effects to normal cells.

Author Contributions: A.R. conceived and designed the experiments; C.R., C.N. and A.P. performed the experiments; A.C., S.L.V. and C.F. analyzed the data; C.R., S.L. and A.R. wrote the paper.

References

1. Bray, F.; Ferlay, J.; Soerjomataram, I.; Siegel, R.L.; Torre, L.A.; Jemal, A. Global Cancer Statistics 2018: GLOBOCAN Estimates of Incidence and Mortality Worldwide for 36 Cancers in 185 Countries. *CA Cancer J. Clin.* **2018**, *68*, 394–424. [CrossRef] [PubMed]
2. National Institute of Cancer (INCA)a. Estimate 2016. Incidence of Cancer in Brazil. Available online: http://www.inca.gov.br/conteudo_view.asp?ID=101 (accessed on 17 October 2016).
3. National Institute of Cancer (INCA)b Ministry of Health Staging. Available online: http://www.inca.gov.br/conteudo_view.asp?ID=54 (accessed on 22 September 2016).
4. Cintra, J.R.D.; Guerra, M.R.; Bustamante-Teixeira, M.T. Specified survival of patients with non-metastatic breast cancer undergoing adjuvant chemotherapy. *Rev. Assoc. Med. Bras. Med.* **2008**, *54*, 339–346.
5. Fallowfield, L. Participation of patients in decisions about treatment for cancer. *BMJ* **2001**, *323*, 323–1144. [CrossRef]
6. National Cancer Institute (INCA)c -Ministry of Health-Treatment. Available online: http://www2.inca.gov.br/wps/wcm/connect/tiposdecancer/site/home/mama (accessed on 25 July 2016).
7. Moss, R.W. Do antioxidants interfere with radiation therapy for cancer? *Integr. Cancer Ther.* **2007**, *6*, 281–292. [CrossRef]
8. Lawenda, B.D.; Kelly, K.M.; Ladas, E.J.; Sagar, S.M.; Vickers, A.; Blumberg, J.B. Should supplemental antioxidant administration be avoided during chemotherapy and radiation therapy? *J. Natl. Cancer Inst.* **2008**, *100*, 773–783. [CrossRef]
9. Nechuta, S.; Lu, W.; Chen, Z.; Zheng, Y.; Gu, K.; Cai, H.; Zheng, W.; Shu, X. Vitamin supplement use during breast cancer treatment and survival: A prospective cohort study. *Cancer Epidemiol. Biomark. Prev.* **2011**, *20*, 261–271. [CrossRef]
10. Bouriez, D.; Giraud, J.; Gronnier, C.; Varon, C. Efficiency of All-Trans Retinoic Acid on Gastric Cancer: A Narrative Literature Review. *Int. J. Mol. Sci.* **2018**, *19*, 3388. [CrossRef]
11. John, E.; Laskow, T.C.; Buchser, W.J.; Pitt, B.R.; Basse, P.H.; Butterfield, L.H.; Kalinski, P.; Lotze, M.T. Zinc in innate and adaptive tumor immunity. *J. Transl. Med.* **2010**, *8*, 118. [CrossRef]
12. Ramalho, A.; Saunders, C.; Souza, G.; Thiapó, A.P.; Silva, L. Micronutrients in Pregnancy and Lactation. *Rev. Bras. Saude Mater. Infant.* **2007**, *7*, 237–244.
13. World Health Organization. *Indicators for Assessing Vitamin A Deficiency and Their Application in Monitoring and Evaluating Intervention Programmes*; World Health Organization: Geneva, Switzerland, 1996.
14. Hotz, C.; Peerson, J.M.; Brown, K.H. Suggested lower cutoffs of serum zinc concentrations for assessing zinc status: Reanalysis of the second National Health and Nutrition Examination Survey data (1976–1980). *Am. J. Clinnutr.* **2003**, *78*, 756–764. [CrossRef]
15. Ministry of Health; Secretariat of Health Care; National Cancer Institute. *TNM: Classification of Malignant Tumours*, 6th ed.; INCA: Rio de Janeiro, Brazil, 2004; p. 254.
16. Matos, A.; Nogueira, C.; Franca, C.; Carvalho, A.; Vieira, S.L.; Penna, A.; Ramalho, A. The relationship between serum vitamin A and breast cancer staging before and after radiotherapy. *Nutricion Hosp.* **2014**, *29*, 139–163.
17. Monroy, C.K.; Esparza, R.J.; Genaro, G.T.A.; Valencia, M.E.; Mendez, E.R.O.; Tortoledo, O.O.; Pacheco Moreno, B.; Astiazaran Garcia, H. Impacto del tratamento antineoplásicoenel estado nutricional em pacientes com cáncer de mama. *Nutricion Hosp.* **2014**, *30*, 876–882.
18. Kumar, R.; Razab, S.; Prabhu, K.; Ray, S. Serum butyrylcholinesterase and zinc in breast cancer. *J. Can. Res. Ther.* **2017**, *13*, 367–370.
19. National Cancer Institute. *Information on Cancer Hospital Records as a Transformation Strategy: Profile of the José Alencar Gomes da Silva National Cancer Institute in 25 years/José Alencar Gomes da Silva National Cancer Institute*; INCA: Rio de Janeiro, Brazil, 2012; p. 100.

20. Borges, G.S.; Rebelo, R.J.; Maman, S.A.K.; Zabel, M.C.J.; Almeida, A.M.; Custodio, G.S.; Anjos, P.T.; Senna, B.R.; Hasse, J.; Zimath, T.; et al. Epidemiological profile of patients with breast cancer treated at amastology out patient clinic in the Vale do Itajaí region. *Rev. Bras. Oncol. Clín.* **2013**, *9*, 88–92.
21. Soares, P.B.M.; Quirino Filho, S.; Souza, W.P.; Gonccalves, R.C.R.; Martelli, D.R.B.; Silveira, M.F.; Martelli, J.H. Characteristics of women with breast cancer assisted in referral services in the North of Minas Gerais. *Rev. Bras Epidemiol.* **2012**, *15*, 295–604.
22. Santos, H.; Cruz, W. The antioxidant vitamin nutritional therapy and the chemotherapy treatment in oncology. *Rev. Bras. De Cancerol.* **2001**, *47*, 303–308.
23. Szychta, P.; Zadrozny, M.; Lewinski, A.; Karbownik-Lewinska, M. Increased oxidative damage to membrane lipids following surgery for breast cancer. *Neuro Endocrinol. Lett.* **2014**, *7*, 602–607.
24. Koh, E.-S.; Tran, T.H.; Heydarian, M.; Sachs, R.K.; Tsang, R.W.; Brenner, D.J.; Pintilie, M.; Xu, T.; Chung, J.; Paul, N.; et al. A comparison of mantle versus involved-field radiotherapy for Hodgkin's lymphoma: Reduction in normal tissue dose and second cancer risk. *Radiat. Oncol.* **2007**, *2*, 1–13. [CrossRef]
25. Doldo, E.; Costanza, G.; Agostinelli, S.; Tarquini, C.; Ferlosio, A.; Arcuri, G.; Passeri, D.; Scioli, M.G.; Orlandi, A. Vitamin A, Cancer Treatment and Prevention: The New Role of Cellular Retinol Binding Proteins. *Biomed. Res. Int.* **2015**, *10*, 1–14. [CrossRef]
26. Prasad, K. Free Radicals: The Pros and Cons of Antioxidants. American Society for Nutritional Sciences. *J. Nutr.* **2004**, *134*, 3182–3183. [CrossRef]
27. Chen, M.; Hsu, S.; Lin, H. Ying Yang Tsung. Retinoic acid and cancer treatment. *BioMed.* **2014**, *4*, 1–6. [CrossRef] [PubMed]
28. Kobayashi, T.; Iijima, K.; Mitamura, T.; Toriizuka, K.; Cyong, J.C.; Nagasawa, H. Effects of lycopene, a carotenoid, on intrathymic T cell differentiation and peripheral CD4/CD8 ratio in a high mammary tumor strain of SHN retired mice. *Anticancer Drugs* **1996**, *7*, 195–203. [CrossRef] [PubMed]
29. Fiedor, J.; Burda, K. Potential role of carotenoids as antioxidants in human health and disease. *Nutrients* **2017**, *27*, 466. [CrossRef] [PubMed]
30. Dhawan, D.K.; Chadha, V.D. Zinc: A promising agent in dietary chemoprevention of cancer. *Indian J. Med. Res.* **2010**, *132*, 676–682. [PubMed]
31. Figueiredo Ribeiro, S.M.; Braga, C.B.M.; Peria, F.M.D.; Fernanda, A.; Martinez, E.Z.; Feres, O.; Da Rocha, J.J.R.; Da Cunha, S.F.D.C. Effect of Zinc Supplementation on Antioxidant Defenses and Oxidative Stress Markers in Patients Undergoing Chemotherapy for Colorectal Cancer: A Placebo-Controlled, Prospective Randomized Trial. *Biol Trace Elem Res.* **2015**, *5*, 1–9.
32. Takatani-Nakase, T.; Matsui, C.; Maeda, S.; Kawahara, S.; Takahashi, K. High Glucose Level Promotes Migration Behavior of Breast Cancer Cells through Zinc and Its Transporters. *PLoS ONE* **2014**, *9*, e90136. [CrossRef]
33. Veras, C.M.T.; Sousa, M.S.B.; Silva, B.B.; Cozzolino, S.M.F.; Pires, L.V.; Pimentel, J.A.C.; Nogueira, N.N.; Marreiro, N. Analysis of plasma and erythrocyte zinc levels in premenopausal women with breast cancer. *Nutr. Hosp.* **2011**, *26*, 293–297.
34. Hana, K.; Petra, H.; Jiri, P.; Pavel, V.; Michaela, Z.; Bohuslav, M.; Lenka, K.K.; Marketa, K.; Milosav, P.; Damgrar, S.; et al. Prognostic significance of serum retinol, serum alpha-tocopherol, and urinary neopterin in patients with head and neck carcinoma treated with external beam radiation. *Int. J. Vitam. Nutr. Res.* **2012**, *87*, 77–84.
35. Peres, W.A.F.; Chaves, G.V.; Gonccalves, J.C.S.; Ramalho, A.; Coelho, H.S.M. Vitamin A deficiency in patients with hepatitis C virus-related chronic liver disease. *Br. J. Nutr.* **2011**, *106*, 1724–1731. [CrossRef]
36. Arantes, F.P.; Villaça Chaves, G.; Saraiva Gonçalves, J.C.; Ramalho, A.; Moraes Coelho, H.S. Assessment of the relative dose response teste as indicators of hepatic vitamin A stores in various stages of chronic liver disease. *Nutr. Clin. Pract.* **2012**, *28*, 95–100. [CrossRef]
37. Rodriguez-Amaya, D.B.; Kiemura, M.; Farfan-Amaya, J. Brazilian Sources of Carotenoids. In *Brazilian Table of Carotenoid Composition in Foods*; Ministry of the Environment: Brasília, Brazil, 2008; p. 100.

2

Low-Dose and Long-Term Olaparib Treatment Sensitizes MDA-MB-231 and SUM1315 Triple-Negative Breast Cancers Spheroids to Fractioned Radiotherapy

Clémence Dubois [1,2], Fanny Martin [3,†], Chervin Hassel [4,†], Florian Magnier [5,†], Pierre Daumar [2,†], Corinne Aubel [6,†], Sylvie Guerder [4], Emmanuelle Mounetou [2,†], Frédérique Penault-Lorca [1,†] and Mahchid Bamdad [2,*]

1 Université Clermont Auvergne, INSERM, U1240, Imagerie Moléculaire et Stratégies Théranostiques, F-63000 Clermont Ferrand, France; clemence.dubois@uca.fr (C.D.); frederique.penault-llorca@clermont.unicancer.fr (F.P.-L.)
2 Université Clermont Auvergne, Institut Universitaire de Technologie, INSERM, U1240, Imagerie Moléculaire et Stratégies Théranostiques, F-63000 Clermont Ferrand, France; pierre.daumar@uca.fr (P.D.); emmanuelle.mounetou@inserm.fr (E.M.)
3 Département de Radiothérapie, Centre Jean Perrin, F-63000 Clermont Ferrand, France; fanny.martin@centre-saint-jean.fr
4 Centre Hospitalier Universitaire Purpan, Centre de Physiopathologie de Toulouse Purpan, INSERM, UMR 1043/CNRS UMR 5282, Antigen Presenting Cells and CD4 T cell responses, F-31024 Toulouse, France; chervin.hassel@gmail.com (C.H.); sylvie.guerder@inserm.fr (S.G.)
5 Service de Physique Médicale, Centre Jean Perrin, F-63000 Clermont Ferrand, France; Florian.magnier@centre-saint-jean.fr
6 Université Clermont Auvergne, Faculté de Médecine, INSERM, U1240, Imagerie Moléculaire et Stratégies Théranostiques, F-63000 Clermont Ferrand, France; corinne.aubel@uca.fr
* Correspondence: mahchid.bamdad@uca.fr
† These authors contributed equally to this work.

Abstract: The Triple-Negative Breast Cancer subtype (TNBC) is particularly aggressive and heterogeneous. Thus, Poly-ADP-Ribose Polymerase inhibitors were developed to improve the prognosis of patients and treatment protocols are still being evaluated. In this context, we modelized the efficacy of Olaparib (i.e., 5 and 50 μM), combined with fractioned irradiation (i.e., 5 × 2 Gy) on two aggressive TNBC cell lines MDA-MB-231 (BRCAness) and SUM1315 (BRCA1-mutated). In 2D cell culture and for both models, the clonogenicity drop was 95-fold higher after 5 μM Olaparib and 10 Gy irradiation than Olaparib treatment alone and was only 2-fold higher after 50 μM and 10 Gy. Similar responses were obtained on TNBC tumor-like spheroid models after 10 days of co-treatment. Indeed, the ratio of metabolic activity decrease was of 1.2 for SUM1315 and 3.3 for MDA-MB-231 after 5 μM and 10 Gy and of only 0.9 (both models) after 50 μM and 10 Gy. MDA-MB-231, exhibiting a strong proliferation profile and an overexpression of AURKA, was more sensitive to the co-treatment than SUM1315 cell line, with a stem-cell like phenotype. These results suggest that, with the studied models, the potentiation of Olaparib treatment could be reached with low-dose and long-term exposure combined with fractioned irradiation.

Keywords: Triple-Negative Breast Cancer; SUM1315; MDA-MB-231; PARPi Olaparib; fractioned radiotherapy; co-treatment; the three-dimensional cell culture; spheroid; transcriptomic analysis

1. Introduction

Breast cancer is a complex disease presenting various phenotypes with distinct prognosis and sensitivity to drugs [1]. Among the multiple classifications, the Triple-Negative breast cancers (TNBC) are characterized by the absence of estrogen and progesterone receptor expression, the absence of Human-Epidermal-Receptor Type 2 (HER2) overexpression, a high proliferation, and by the expression of the cytokeratins 5 and 6 [2]. Furthermore, approximately 10–15% of TNBC tumours carry hereditary mutations in the BReast CAncer early onset 1 and 2 genes (BRCA1/2 genes), which are responsible for hereditary predisposed cancers developments [3–5]. Given this aggressive phenotype, a great proportion of TNBC tumours recur within 3 years after conventional anticancer treatments such as surgery, chemotherapy or radiotherapy. Indeed, these TNBC tumours temporarily benefit from neo-adjuvant or adjuvant therapies, but then a rapid metastatic relapse occurs in almost 60% of the patients [6]. As a result, many efforts have been made to improve the prognosis of patients. Indeed, the treatment protocols have been optimized and targeted therapeutic agents exploiting the specificities of TNBC tumours developed, such as Poly-ADP-Ribose-Polymerase 1 inhibitors (PARPi such as Olaparib/Lynparza®, AstraZeneca) [2,7].

PARPi constitute a class of targeted therapeutics acting on DNA repair systems using the synthetic lethality concept. These open up new prospects for improving the treatment of TNBC aggressive subtype [8]. Since February 2019, the Lynparza® (Olaparib) was adopted by the Committee for Medicinal Products for Human Use (CHMP from European Medicines Agency) for the treatment of adult patients with germline BRCA1/2-mutations, who have HER2-negative locally advanced or metastatic breast cancer. In addition to being used as monotherapy treatment agents, PARPi may also be used in combination with chemotherapy or radiotherapy [8]. These combination methods exhibit a strong rationale due to the inhibition of DNA homologous recombination repair system induced by PARPi and the generation of DNA single and double-strand breaks induced by irradiation and are still being studied in the preclinical setting [9,10].

The pipeline of drug development is composed of several preclinical and clinical phases. The preclinical setting is divided into in vitro and in vivo experiments which goals are the determination of drug efficacy and toxicity. Recently, the three-dimensional cell culture (3D) has been integrated into these preclinical processes after the monolayer in vitro cell culture experiments. The 3D cell culture (spheroid) appears to be an adapted tool for the evaluation of drug efficacy for drug development and optimization in Oncology. Indeed, these 3D models mimic more precisely the tumour microenvironment by the formation of genetical, biochemical and phenotypical gradients, resembling intratumoral gradients and microenvironment [11–13].

In recent years, in order to optimize the treatment of these aggressive breast cancers, our research group has focused its works on the modeling of the balance between cytotoxicity/resistance of TNBC cell lines, in response to PARPi [14,15]. In this context, these works aimed to determine the effectiveness of a concomitant treatment combining increasing concentrations of Olaparib (PARPi) and fractioned irradiation (5×2 Gy) on two TNBC models i.e., MDA-MB-231 (wild-type BRCA1 gene, loss of heterozigoty) [16] and SUM1315 (BRCA1-mutated) [16] cultured in monolayer and 3D cell culture conditions. We first determined the efficacy of this co-treatment by the analysis of (i) DNA double strand breaks induction, (ii) cell survival decrease and (iii) clonogenic survival decrease, in 2D cell cultures. These tests allowed us to further validate this combination on tumor-like models (3D cell cultures), treated at long-term with specific efficient Olaparib concentrations, and daily irradiated (5×2 Gy). Finally, an in silico transcriptomic approach highlighted the different cell-line patterns leading to a promising perspective for the treatment of aggressive/metastatic breast cancer tumours.

2. Materials and Methods

2.1. Cell Lines and Culture

SUM1315 cell line (Asterand®, MO2) was cultured in Ham's F12 medium supplemented with 5% decomplemented fetal calf serum, 10 mM HEPES buffer, 20 µg/mL gentamycin, 10 ng/mL EGF and 4 µg/mL insulin. MDA-MB-231 cell line (HTB-26™, ATCC®) was cultured in RPMI medium 1640 supplemented with 10% decomplemented fetal calf serum and 20 µg/mL of gentamycin. Both cell lines were maintained at 37 °C under 5% CO_2 in a humidified incubator. The absence of mycoplasma contamination was checked before every experiment by the mycoplasmacheck test (GATC Biotech, Konstanz, Germany).

According to the experiments, cells were either seeded in Ibitreat microscopy chambers (Foci H2AX assay), six-well flat bottom microplates (clonogenic survival test) or 96-well flat-bottom microplates (cell survival test) at a concentration of 5000 cells/cm^2 and let in the incubator for 24 h before treatments.

Spheroid Formation

For spheroid formation and treatments, the liquid overlay technique (LOT) was performed in Ultra-Low-Attachment round-bottom microplates according to our previous works [13].

2.2. Olaparib Treatment

Olaparib (Carbosynth®) was solubilized in Dimethylsulfoxide (DMSO) at a concentration of 100 mM. For all experiments, the solubilized Olaparib was diluted in the culture medium at increasing concentrations with a final and constant DMSO concentration of 0.1%. Parallely, DMSO 0.1% controls without Olaparib were also performed. For Olaparib treatments and co-treatment (Olaparib/irradiation), Olaparib was added once, three hours before the first radiotherapy session. The treatment lasted for 24 h, 72 h or 120 h in 2D experiments, and for 6, 8 or 10 days in 3D experiments. The absence of DMSO 0.1% toxicity was systematically checked prior to results analysis.

Irradiation

The cells were irradiated at a daily dose of 2 Gy for one to five days, on a linear electron accelerator with a 6 MegaVolts X-ray beam used for routine treatment in clinic (Truebeam®, Varian Medical Systems, Palo Alto located in Centre Jean Perrin, Clermont-Ferrand, France). The dose rate applied to the accelerator was 400 Monitor Units per minute (MU/min), which corresponds to the dose rate conventionally used in radiotherapy. For this, the cells were placed 3 cm deep inside a 13 cm thick PolyMethyl MethAcrylate (PMMA) phantom in order to obtain a homogeneous distribution of dose and respect the charged particle equilibrium conditions. A computed tomography (CT) scanner examination of this phantom was performed with each device containing the irradiated cells. The dose was prescribed in the middle of the volume containing the cells and the calculation was performed with the Anisotropic Analytical Algorithm (AAA). The irradiated plates remained in the incubator outside of radiotherapy treatment session. The non-irradiated culture plates with or without Olaparib were maintained in the same experimental conditions.

2.3. Experiments in Monolayer Cell Culture

2.3.1. DNA DSBs Induction: Gamma H2AX Immunofluorescent Markings

Cells were treated with 5 and 50 µM Olaparib for 3 h and then were irradiated with a single X-ray dose of 2 Gy. After one hour, cells were fixed in 4% paraformaldehyde, permeabilized in ethanol, incubated with a saturation solution and then with the primary antibody (1/250, Anti-phospho-histone H2AX, Ser 139 clone JBW301) or the isotype control (1/1000, isotype IgG1a mouse). Cells were then incubated with the anti-mouse secondary antibody (1/800, Alexa Fluor 488 gloat anti-mouse) and with Hoechst 33258 for nuclear counterstaining. Finally, cells were dried, mounted and observed with Cytation™3MV plate reader (Biotek, Winooski, VT, USA). The number of γH2AX foci was calculated on >10 cellular fields for each condition with ImageJ® software, representing at least more than hundred cells. The results were represented as the mean number of γH2AX foci per nucleus with their standard deviation (s.d.).

2.3.2. SulfoRhodamine B Survival Test

Cells were treated with increasing concentrations of Olaparib (0.1 to 100 μM) for 24 h, 72 h or 120 h, corresponding to concomitant doses of radiotherapy of 2, 6 and 10 Gy, respectively. After each treatment endpoint, cells were fixed with a trichloroacetic acid (TCA) solution for 1 h, washed in water, dried and incubated with a SRB solution in 1% (v/v) acetic acid for 15 min. Again, cells were washed with 1% acetic acid, dried and a 10 mM Tris-base buffer solution was finally added to the wells for 30 min. The absorbance of SRB dye dissolved in each well was determined at 540 nm with Cytation3MV plate reader (Biotek, Winooski, VT, USA). Cell survival was calculated for each treatment condition by the comparison of 24 h, 72 h and 120 h aged untreated control wells with the following formula:

$$\text{Cell survival (\%)} = (OD_{540\ \text{nm treated wells}}/OD_{540\ \text{nm no X-Ray/no Olaparib = control}}) \times 100. \tag{1}$$

The results are presented as mean viability of $n > 45$ wells ± their standard deviation (s.d.).

2.3.3. Clonogenic Survival Test

The clonogenic potential of cells following a treatment with irradiation alone or combined with Olaparib (0.5, 5 and 50 μM) was evaluated after cumulative X-ray doses of 2, 6 or 10 Gy, corresponding to concomitant Olaparib exposures of 24 h, 72 h of 120 h. After each treatment endpoint, cells were recovered by trypsinisation, enumerated and re-seeded into new plates at an adapted concentration. The number of colonies formed was determined after nine doubling times (objective 10×). The Plating Efficiency (PE) corresponding to the cell repopulation factor after each treatment condition was calculated as follows:

$$\text{PE} = \text{Number of colonies formed/Number of seeded cells at } T_0. \tag{2}$$

Then, the survival fraction after each X-ray dose was calculated compared to the corresponding untreated control of each dose (= No X-ray and No Olaparib treatment) with the following formula:

$$\text{Survival fraction (\%)} = \text{PE treated condition}^{\text{(X-ray dose} \pm \text{Olaparib)}} / \text{PE control}^{\text{(no X-ray/no Olaparib)}} \text{ of each corresponding X-ray dose.} \tag{3}$$

The values of the clonogenic survival were expressed as mean survival ± their standard deviation (s.d.) of $n = 5$ replicates.

2.4. Experiments in 3D Cell Culture

2.4.1. Spheroid Treatment

Spheroids aged of 3 days were treated with 5 and 50 μM of Olaparib for 6, 8 and 10 days, corresponding to concomitant X-ray doses of 2 Gy (1 session), 6 Gy (three successive daily sessions) and 10 Gy (five successive daily sessions), respectively.

2.4.2. Spheroid Growth Monitoring

The size of spheroids after each treatment endpoint (6, 8 and 10 days) was monitored with the Cytation™3MV microplate reader (Biotek, Winooski, VT, USA) using the cellular analysis algorithm of the Gen 5 software (version 03, Biotek, Winooski, VT, USA). Results were expressed as the mean spheroid size of each treatment condition ($n > 45$) with their standard deviation (s.d.).

2.4.3. Spheroid Metabolic Activity Assessment With the Resazurin Test

Spheroids from every treatment condition were transferred in a new microplate containing 60 µM resazurin in PBS. The Fluorescence Intensity (FI) corresponding to the amount of resorufin formed after 17 h incubation was quantified in each well with Cytation3^{MV} plate reader (Biotek, Winooski, VT, USA). This allowed the determination of the percentage of spheroid metabolic activity as controls calculated as follows:

$$\text{Metabolic activity (\%)} = \text{FI treated spheroid}^{\,(\text{X-ray} \pm \text{Olaparib or Olaparib} \pm \text{X-ray})} / \text{FI control spheroid}^{\,(\text{no Olaparib/no X-ray})}. \tag{4}$$

The results were presented as mean spheroid metabolic activity of each treatment condition ($n > 16$ spheroids) ± their standard deviation (s.d.).

2.4.4. Spheroid Viability and Mortality Fluorescent Profile (Live/Dead)

Spheroids of each treatment condition were harvested, rinsed twice in PBS and incubated with 4 µM ethidium-homodimer (Etdh-1, red fluorescence, dead cells) and 2 µM Calcein-AM (green fluorescence, viable cells) for 45 min. The fluorescence of each fluorophore was then imaged with Cytation3MV plate reader (Biotek, Winooski, VT, USA). For the image analysis, same exposure time, LED intensity and gain were programmed for all image acquisitions.

2.5. Transcriptomic Analysis of TNBC Cell Lines

All available MDA-MB-231 and SUM1315 transcriptomic data from different studies were collected from the NCBI public dataset GEO DataSet. Accession number, sample and sequencing information are indicated in the Table 1 below:

Table 1. Accession number, sample and sequencing information from the NCBI public GEO DataSet.

Name	Accession N	Library Type	Sequencing	End Type	Reference
MDAMB231_A	GSE73526	TruSeq Stranded mRNA	Illumina HiSeq 2000	paired-end	[17]
MDAMB231_B	GSE48213	TruSeq RNA Sample Preparation Kit	Illumina Genome Analyzer IIx	paired-end	[18]
MDAMB231_C	GSE83132	TruSeq RNA Sample Prep Kit v2	Illumina HiSeq 2000	paired-end	[19]
MDAMB231_D	GSE83132	TruSeq RNA Sample Prep Kit v2	Illumina HiSeq 2000	paired-end	[19]
MDAMB231_E	GSE83132	TruSeq RNA Sample Prep Kit v2	Illumina HiSeq 2000	paired-end	[19]
SUM1315_B	GSE48213	TruSeq RNA Sample Preparation Kit	Illumina Genome Analyzer IIx	paired-end	[18]
SUM1315_A	GSE73526	TruSeq Stranded mRNA	Illumina HiSeq 2000	Illumina HiSeq 2000	[17]

Fastq files were analyzed on Genotoul Bio-informatic cluster. Input reads for each sample were aligned to the Human (GRCh38) reference genome using TopHat [20]. Two-dimensional principal component analysis (PCA) of all data was performed to assess quality samples. It depicted that the first principal component represents 63% of variance and separated the two cell lines. The R package Deseq2 was used to analyze the statistically significant Differential Expressed Genes (DEG) between MDA-MB-231 and SUM1315 cell lines. An adjusted p value of <0.1 was the cutoff to select specifically DEG between the two cell lines. This DEGs list was subject as query to Ingenuity Pathway Analysis (IPA, QIAGEN Inc., Hilden, Germany). IPA permits to infer functional and cellular processes that are modified between these two cell lines using the Ingenuity Knowledge Base. Two statistical indexes (p-value and z-score) are determined for each prediction. The p-value is calculated by a Fisher exact test and permits to identify significantly enriched pathways. The IPA z-score is the statistical measure of the match between altered genes and the inferred biological function. z-score let to predict the direction of change of a function. Indeed, a cellular function activity is increased when z-score is >2 and decreased when z-score <−2.

2.6. Statistical Analysis

All the data set was statistically compared with a Student's two-sided test, where significative values are indicated in the graphs as: * $p < 0.05$, ** $p < 0.01$, *** $p < 0.001$, **** $p < 0.0001$ and ***** $p < 0.00001$. The level of interaction between all treatment conditions was determined with a multivariate ANOVA analysis (mixed model), performed with the SEM software (developed by F.K., Centre Jean Perrin, Clermont-Fd, France).

3. Results

3.1. Olaparib and Radiotherapy Induce DNA Double Strand Breaks in TNBC Cell Lines

For MDA-MB-231 cell line (Figure 1A), after a 4 h treatment with Olaparib alone, the number of gH2AX foci per nuclei doubled in presence of 5 μM (8 ± 0.7 than 0.1% DMSO controls 4 ± 0.4, $p = 10^{-7}$) and tripled after 50 μM (13 ± 1.1, $p = 10^{-12}$). After 2 Gy irradiation alone, the number of foci increased up to 19 ± 1.1 ($p = 10^{-26}$). In presence of the co-treatment, this parameter kept increasing significantly than irradiation alone or Olaparib treatment alone with 23 ± 1.3 and 32 ± 1.6 foci per nuclei (for 5 μM/2 Gy and 50 μM/2 Gy, respectively) (Figure 1A). Parallely, same results were obtained for SUM1315 cell line (Figure 1B), with a 3.2-fold increase after 50 μM Olaparib treatment (15 ± 1.9 than 0.1% DMSO controls 5 ± 0.5, $p = 10^{-7}$), and a 1.8-fold increase after irradiation and Olaparib treatment (31 ± 2.9 for 50 μM than irradiated controls 17 ± 1.1, $p = 10^{-5}$)(Figure 1B). These results suggest a cumulative effect of the co-treatment in terms of DNA DSBs induction after 4 h of treatment, probably related to both the irradiation and the Olaparib treatment impact. We then modelized the impact of the co-treatment on 2D cell survival after one to five days of Olaparib exposure and 2 to 10 Gy cumulative X-ray doses.

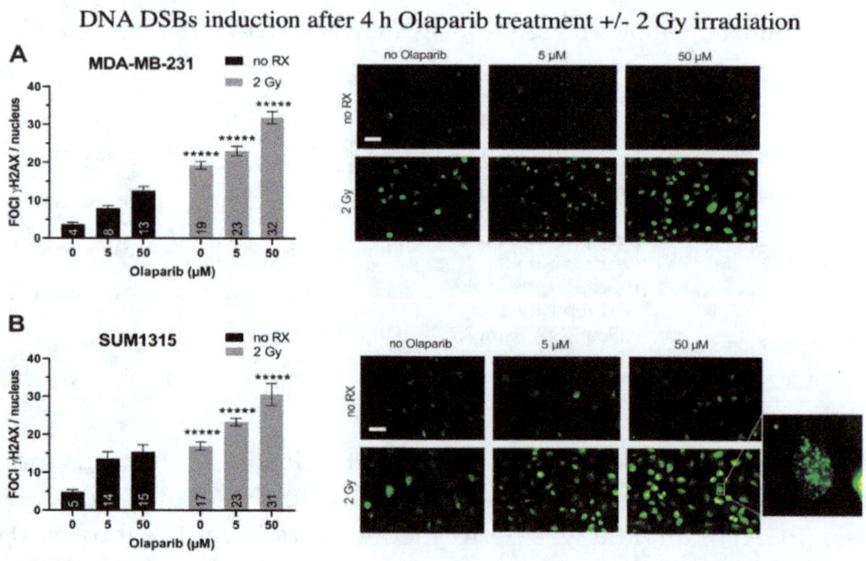

Figure 1. DNA Double Strand Breaks (DSBs) induction in MDA-MB-231 (**A**) and SUM1315 (**B**) cell lines cultured in monolayer after a treatment with 0.1% DMSO (control cells), 5 and 50 μM Olaparib for 4 h alone (no irradiation "no RX") or combined with 2 Gy of irradiation (4 h and 2 Gy). The number of foci gammaH2AX per cell in >10 fields per condition was determined with ImageJ software. Results are represented as mean number of foci gammaH2AX per nuclei with their standard deviation. A student *t*-test was performed for statistical comparison of all treatment conditions, where ns = non-significant and ***** $p < 0.00001$. Magnification = 40×, scale bar = 50 μm.

3.2. *The Cytotoxicity of Radiotherapy Is Optimized by Olaparib and is Potentiated in Presence of Low Doses of Olaparib*

Impact on TNBC Cell Survival in 2D Cell Culture

The cell survival of both MDA-MB-231 and SUM1315 cell lines was analyzed by an SRB survival test, either after treatment with 0.1–100 μM Olaparib concentrations for 24, 72, or 120 h, or combined with 2, 6 or 10 Gy cumulative irradiation doses. The 2 Gy radiation was prescribed daily. All data are presented in Figure S1. In order to determine the impact of each analyzed parameter on cell survival variance, i.e., (i) the type of cell line (MDA-MB-231, SUM1315), (ii) the Olaparib concentration (0.1–100 μM), (iii) the Olaparib time of exposure (24–120 h) and (iv) the irradiation dose (2–10 Gy), the overall cell survival results from both cell line models were compiled and processed in a multivariate ANOVA analysis (Table 2 and Figure 2).

Table 2. Multivariate ANOVA results obtained from the SRB monolayer cell survival dataset.

Experimental Parameters	Probability of Variance Influence	% of Variance Explanation
Type of cell line (MDA-MB-231; SUM1315)	<0.0000001	8%
Dose Olaparib (0; 0.1; 1; 5; 10; 25; 50; 75; 100 μM)	<0.0000001	14%
Olaparib exposure (24 h; 72 h; 120 h)	<0.0000001	40%
Irradiation dose (0; 2; 6; 10 Gy)	<0.0000001	38%

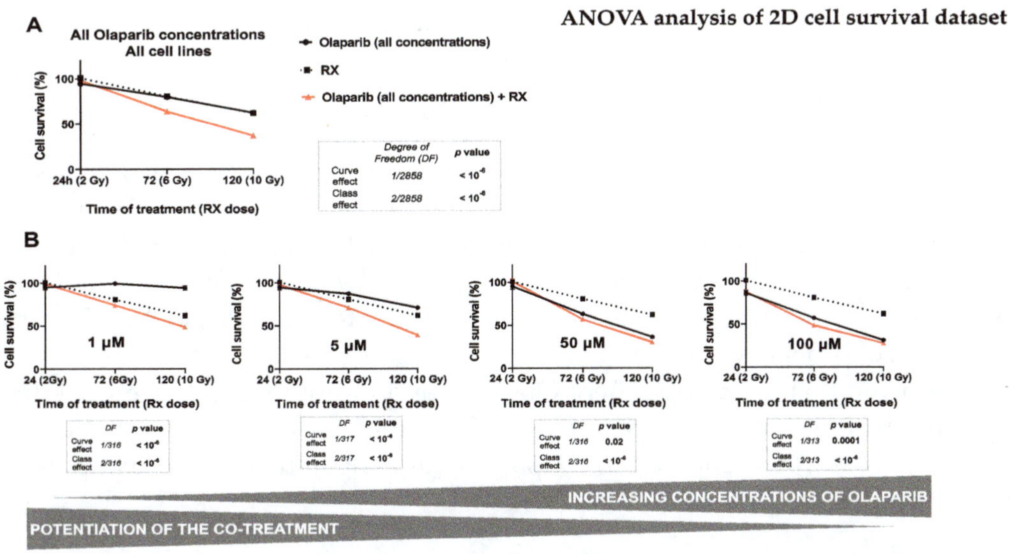

Figure 2. ANOVA analysis of monolayer cell culture sensitivity (SRB survival test) after the co-treatment: The graph (**A**) describes the decrease in the cell survival of both cell lines (MDA-MB-231 and SUM1315) by the time, according to (i) the Olaparib treatment alone (all concentrations), (ii) the treatment with fractioned irradiation alone or (iii) the co-treatment with Olaparib (all concentrations) and fractioned irradiation. The second set of graphs (**B**) describes the decrease of cell survival of both cell lines by the time according to (i) the Olaparib treatment alone after each concentration of 1 μM, 5 μM, 50 μM or 100 μM and (ii) the co-treatment Olaparib (same concentrations) with fractioned irradiation. For **A** and **B**, the curve effect (= significant decrease in cell survival by the time for a same condition) and the class effect (= significant difference in cell survival for a same incubation time between each condition) were determined by the ANOVA analysis, associated with their degree of freedom (= number of data of each analysis).

Firstly, the results presented in Table 2 showed a significant influence of all studied parameters on the variation of cell survival with a probability inferior to 10^{-6} for every parameter. Indeed, in our experimental conditions, the cell survival variance was impacted (i) at 40% by the time of Olaparib exposure, (ii) at 39% by the radiotherapy dose, (iii) at 14% by the Olaparib concentration, and at 9% by the type of cell line. These results suggest clearly that both the duration of Olaparib exposure and the dose of radiotherapy play a major role in the decrease of survival of these TNBC cell lines. Secondly, the multivariate ANOVA analysis allowed to determine the impact of each Olaparib dose with or without irradiation on cell survival (Figure 2).

The impact of all experimental parameters (type of cell line, dose of Olaparib, Olaparib time of exposure and dose of radiotherapy) on cell survival variance was analyzed in a multivariate ANOVA analysis, performed with the SEM software (Centre Jean Perrin, Clermont-Ferrand, France). The probability of variance influence in the analysis and the percentage of variance explanation were described for each experimental parameter. All parameters explained the survival variance (probabilities inferior to 10^{-6}) and the strongest parameters influencing this variation were the time of Olaparib exposure (40%) and the radiotherapy dose (38%).

For this, the impact of radiotherapy dose and the time of Olaparib exposure were studied on all the data of cell survival whatever the type of cell line, after a treatment with Olaparib alone (all concentrations), radiotherapy alone and Olaparib (all concentrations) combined with irradiation (Figure 2A). The results showed the same impact on cell survival after 24 h, 72 h and 120 h of exposure to Olaparib alone, with 95 ± 1%, 80 ± 1% and 62 ± 2% or after radiotherapy alone, with 2 Gy at 100 ± 2%, 6 Gy at 81 ± 3% and 10 Gy at 62 ± 3%, respectively. In contrast, the combination of Olaparib and radiotherapy caused a significant cell survival decrease from 6 Gy and 72 h exposure with 64 ± 1%, which kept decreasing after 10 Gy and 120 h exposure with 37 ± 1%. These results showed clearly that Olaparib combined with radiotherapy induced a significant decrease in cell survival compared to radiotherapy alone, or Olaparib alone, and this, independently of the Olaparib concentration or the type of cell line (curve effect and class effects inferior to 10^{-6}).

Then, the impact of several Olaparib tested concentration was represented in Figure 2B. This analysis showed a strong decrease in survival for cells treated with 1 to 5 μM Olaparib for 120 h and 10 Gy compared to 120 h Olaparib treatment alone. Indeed, cell survival was of 48 ± 2% vs. 94 ± 3% for 1 μM and of 39 ± 2% vs. 71 ± 2% for 5 μM, respectively. More, the curve effect probabilities for each dose were systematically inferior to 10^{-6}. In contrast, with higher Olaparib concentrations of 50 and 100 μM, cell survival remained relatively similar at 120 h between a treatment with Olaparib alone or combined with 10 Gy radiotherapy, with 36 ± 2 vs. 30 ± 2% for 50 μM and 31 ± 2% vs. 27 ± 2 for 100 μM, with curve effect probabilities of 0.02 and 0.0001, respectively.

These results showed that the co-treatment Olaparib and radiotherapy was more efficient than a treatment with Olaparib alone, or radiotherapy alone. Thus, this analysis showed that the beneficial of the co-treatment (Olaparib + RX) compared to Olaparib treatment alone was more important with low Olaparib concentrations.

3.3. Impact on TNBC Cell Clonogenic Potential of Repopulation

The clonogenic survival of cells treated with Olaparib alone (concentrations of 0.5, 5 or 50 μM for 24, 72 and 120 h) or concomitantly with radiotherapy (2, 6 and 10 Gy, respectively) was determined for both MDA-MB-231 (Figure 3A) and SUM1315 (Figure 3B) cell lines cultured in monolayer.

For MDA-MB-231 cell line, the 0.1% DMSO controls after 24 h, 72 h and 120 h incubation presented same clonogenic survivals as the controls with 89 ± 19%, 90 ± 6% and 92 ± 40%, respectively ($p > 0.05$ for all conditions) (Figure 3Aa,b). For MDA-MB-231 cell line treated with Olaparib 0.5 to 50 μM, the clonogenic survival decreased firstly during 72 h (22 ± 2% for 0.5 μM and 0.5 ± 0.1% for 50 μM, $p= 10^{-6}$ et $p = 10^{-6}$, respectively) and then increased again after 120 h treatment with 100 ± 3% and 1 ± 0.1% ($p = 0.05$ and $p = 0.007$, respectively) (Figure 3Aa). These results suggest that after a longtime exposure to Olaparib (120 h), the clonogenic capacity of MDA-MB-231 cell line may be restarted. Then, the radiotherapy alone induced strong clonogenic decrease with 10 ± 2% after 6 Gy to 3 ± 1% after 10 Gy, respectively ($p = 0.0006$) (Figure 3Ab). These results showed that fractioned irradiation induced a clear potential clonogenic decrease very effective at 10 Gy. More, after a co-treatment Olaparib/irradiation, this effect was amplified by the time (for 0.5 μM Olaparib, with 6 ± 2% after 6 Gy to 1 ± 0.8% after 10 Gy, $p = 0.01$) and according to Olaparib concentration with 1 ± 0.8% after 0.5 μM and 6 Gy and 0.2 ±

0.01% after 50 µM and 6 Gy ($p = 0.03$ and $p = 0.003$ compared to Rx alone, respectively) (Figure 3Ab). In contrast, the clonogenic repopulation remained the lowest and similar between 5 and 50 µM Olaparib treatment combined with 10 Gy (0.3 ± 0.2% and 0.2 ± 0.01%, respectively, $p = 0.09$).

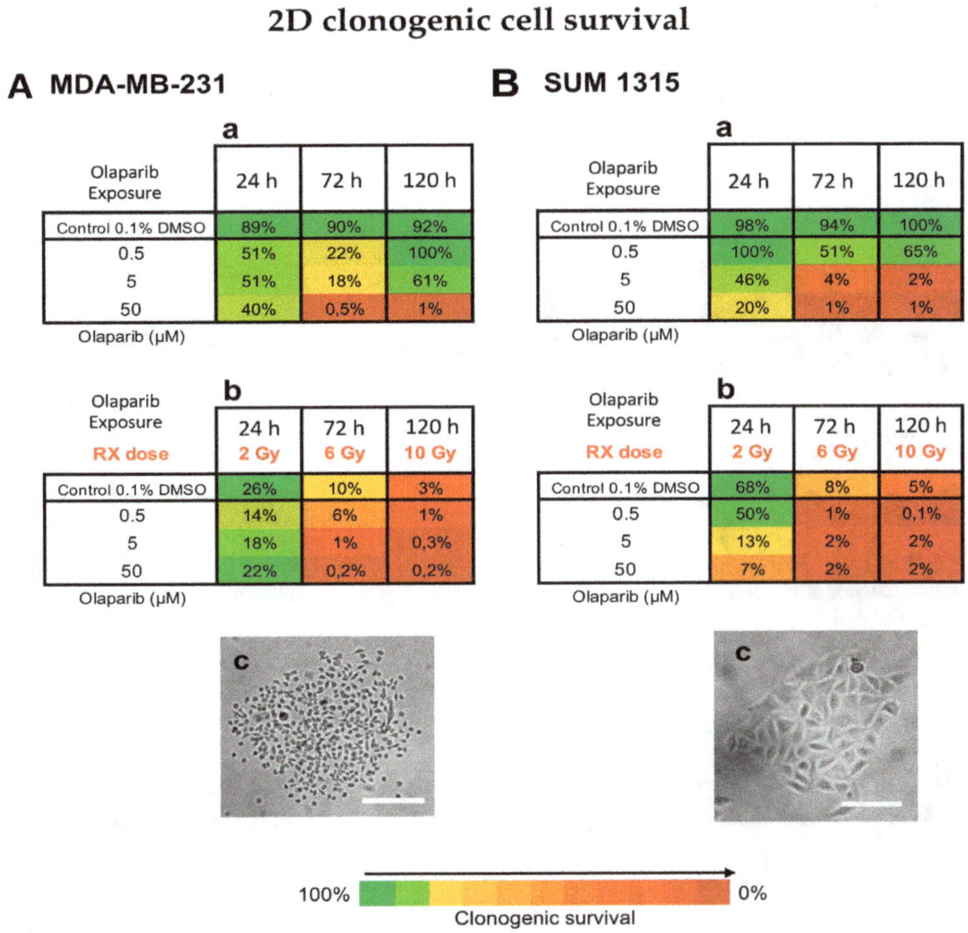

Figure 3. Clonogenic cell survival of MDA-MB-231 (**A**) and SUM1315 (**B**) cell lines cultured in monolayer, after a treatment with 0.5, 5 and 50 µM Olaparib alone for 24 h, 72 h, or 120 h (**a**), or combined with fractioned irradiation of 2, 6 or 10 Gy ("Rx dose") (**b**). For each treatment condition, the percentage of the clonogenic survival was determined by the ratio of the survival fraction of treated cells on the survival fraction of 0.1% DMSO control cells. Results are represented on a Heatmap. Standard errors are <10% for every treatment condition ($n > 3$). (**c**) Photographs of clonogenic populations of MDA-MB-231 and SUM1315, Magnification = 40×, scale bar = 50 µm.

For SUM1315 cell line, the 0.1% DMSO controls after 24 h, 72 h and 120 h incubation presented same clonogenic survivals as the controls with 98 ± 8%, 94 ± 2% and 100 ± 18%, respectively ($p > 0.05$ for all conditions) (Figure 3Ba). For this cell line after Olaparib treatment alone, the clonogenic repopulation capacity decreased in a time and dose-dependent manner, with 65 ± 1% for 0.5 µM to 1 ± 0.1% for 50 µM after 120h ($p = 10^{-5}$) (Figure 3Ba). Similarly, after irradiation, the clonogenic potential decreased strongly with 8 ± 2% after 6 Gy and 5 ± 1% after 10 Gy, compared to 2 Gy with 68 ± 14% ($p = 0.03$ and $p = 0.03$, respectively) (Figure 3Bb). More, after a co-treatment Olaparib/irradiation, this effect was intensified with 0.5 µM Olaparib and 10 Gy (0.1 ± 0.01%). Again, no difference in clonogenic survival of 5 and 50 µM treated cells was detected after 10 Gy ($p = 0.75$) (Figure 3Bb).

For both cell lines, the co-treatment with low dose of Olaparib (0.5 to 5 µM) and fractioned irradiation (10 Gy) induced very low clonogenic potential inferior to 1% indicating a nearly eradicated repopulation potential of these cell lines.

Impact on Tumor-Like Models

Thanks to preliminary 2D experiments, the long-term cell toxicity of Olaparib was highlighted as well as the interest of using low Olaparib doses (0.5–5 µM) compared to high doses (50–100 µM). Thus, for the tumor-like experiments, the spheroids were treated at long-term (6–10 days) with Olaparib alone (5 µM—low dose and 50 µM—high dose) and without/with fractioned irradiation (2, 6 and 10 Gy). For this, (i) the spheroid growth inhibition, (ii) the spheroid viability/mortality profiles and (iii) the spheroid metabolic activity were analyzed (Figures 4 and 5).

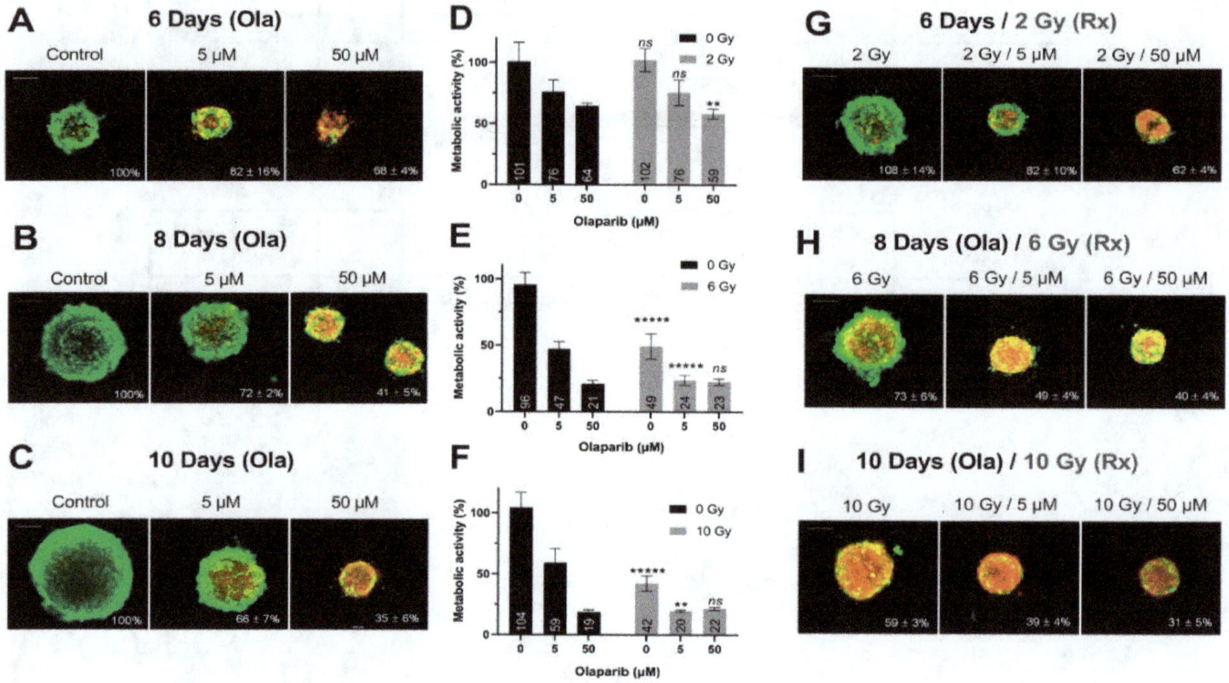

Figure 4. MDA-MB-231 spheroids live/dead profile (**A–C,G–I**) and metabolic activity (**D–F**) after a treatment with Olaparib ("Ola", 5 and 5 µM) for 6, 8 and 10 days with or without fractioned irradiation ("Rx"). (**A–C,G–I**) Spheroid viability/mortality profile and spheroid normalized size after a treatment with Olaparib and/or fractioned irradiation for 6 days (**A**,**G**), 8 days (**B**,**H**) and 10 days (**C**,**I**): Images were taken with Cytation3MV where green markings correspond to calcein-AM penetration (viable cells) and red markings correspond to ethidium homodimer-1 cell penetration (dead cells). The percentage of spheroid size was normalized by the size of spheroid controls. Scale bar = 200 µm. (**D–F**) MDA-MB-231 cell metabolic activity in spheroids with resazurin test after 6 (**D**), 8 (**E**) and 10 days of treatment (**F**). Corrected fluorescence intensity of resorufin (ex/em λ576/λ584 nm) was measured after 15 h incubation with 60 µM resazurin. The fluorescence intensity of treated spheroids ($n > 15$) was normalized by the fluorescence intensity of each associated 0.1% DMSO control spheroids. Results are expressed as mean metabolic activity (%) of each treatment conditions with their standard errors. A student t-test was performed for the statistical comparison of all treatment conditions and the p-value is represented in the graphs as ns = non-significant, ** $p < 0.01$ and ***** $p < 0.00001$.

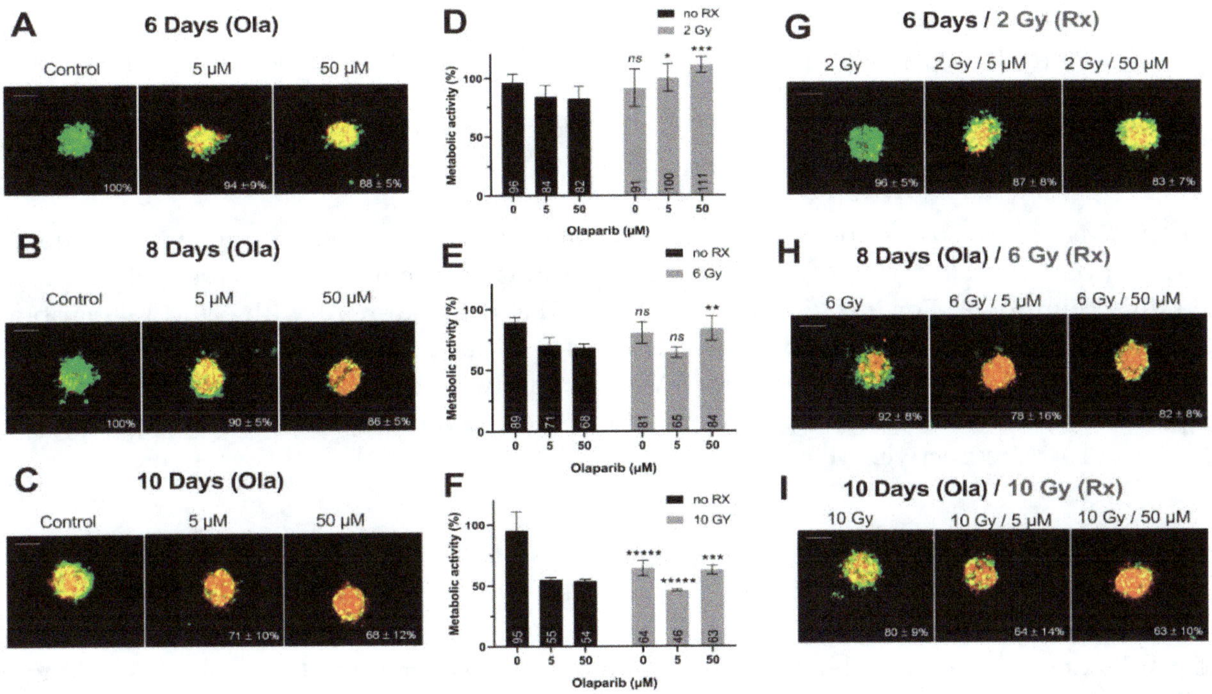

Figure 5. SUM1315 spheroids live/dead profile (**A–C,G–I**) and metabolic activity (**D–F**) after a treatment with Olaparib ("Ola", 5 and 5 μM) for 6, 8 and 10 days with or without fractioned irradiation ("Rx"). (**A–C,G–I**) Spheroid viability/mortality profile and spheroid normalized size after a treatment with Olaparib and/or fractioned irradiation for 6 days (**A**,**G**), 8 days (**B**,**H**) and 10 days (**C**,**I**): Images were taken with Cytation3MV where green markings correspond to calcein-AM penetration (viable cells) and red markings correspond to ethidium homodimer-1 cell penetration (dead cells). The percentage of spheroid size was normalized by the size of spheroid controls. Scale bar = 200 μm. (**D–F**) SUM1315 cell metabolic activity in spheroids with resazurin test after 6 (**D**), 8 (**E**) and 10 days of treatment (**F**). Corrected fluorescence intensity of resorufin (ex/em λ576/λ584 nm) was measured after 15 h incubation with 60 μM resazurin. The fluorescence intensity of treated spheroids ($n > 15$) was normalized by the fluorescence intensity of each associated 0.1% DMSO control spheroids. Results are expressed as mean metabolic activity (%) of each treatment conditions with their standard errors. A student t-test was performed for the statistical comparison of all treatment conditions and the p value is represented in the graphs as ns = non-significant, * $p < 0.05$, ** $p < 0.01$, *** $p < 0.001$ and ***** $p < 0.00001$.

Firstly, for all treatment conditions, no difference in spheroid size and metabolic activity was detected between 0.1% DMSO-treated spheroid controls and control spheroids (Figure S2). Secondly, the impact of all treatment strategies (Olaparib alone, radiotherapy or the co-treatment) was firstly analyzed according to the treatment duration (6, 8 or 10 days treatment), and then according to Olaparib concentrations (5 or 50 μM).

1. Impact of treatment duration

For MDA-MB-231 spheroids treated with 5 μM Olaparib alone, a significant decrease of spheroid size (82 ± 16% vs. 66 ± 7%, $p = 10^{-5}$) (Figure 4A–C) and metabolic activity (76 ± 10% vs. 59 ± 12%, $p = 0.04$) (Figure 4D–F) was detected from 6 to 10 days treatment duration, respectively. Similar results were highlighted after 50 μM Olaparib treatment alone (68 ± 4% vs. 35 ± 6% for spheroid size and 64 ± 2 vs. 19 ± 2% for metabolic activity, after 6 and 10 days, respectively, $p = 10^{-30}$ and $p = 10^{-12}$)

(Figure 4A–F). In addition, after irradiation alone, spheroid size and metabolic activity decreased significantly from 108 ± 14% to 59 ± 3% ($p = 10^{-18}$) and 102 ± 10% to 43 ± 6% ($p = 10^{-10}$) after 6 and 10 days, respectively (Figure 4D–I). Same results were also obtained for 5 and 50 μM co-treated spheroids (with 50 μM, spheroid size of 62 ± 4% vs. 31 ± 5%, $p = 10^{-33}$ and metabolic activity of 59 ± 4% vs. 21 ± 1%, $p = 10^{-7}$, after 6 and 10 days of co-treatment, respectively)(Figure 4D–I).

For SUM1315 spheroids, the comparison of spheroid size and metabolic activity, whatever the Olaparib concentration (5 or 50 μM) with or without irradiation, showed a similar significant decrease by the time (Figure 5). For instance, after 6 and 10 days of treatment with 5 μM Olaparib alone, spheroid size and metabolic activity decreased from 94 ± 9% to 71 ± 10% ($p = 10^{-12}$) and from 84 ± 10% to 55 ± 2% ($p = 0.0008$), respectively (Figure 5A–F). Similarly, with 5 μM Olaparib and irradiation, the same parameters decreased significantly from 87 ± 8% to 64 ± 14% ($p = 10^{-10}$) and from 100 ± 12% to 46 ± 1% ($p = 10^{-5}$), respectively (Figure 5D–I).

In addition, for both cell lines, the time-dependant decrease in terms of spheroid growth and metabolic activity was supported by an increase in the number of dead cells (red/yellow markings) within the spheroids, whatever the treatment condition (Figure 4A–C,G–I and Figure 5A–C,G–I). All these results demonstrated for both models, the importance of treating the spheroids at long-term, with Olaparib alone or combined with radiotherapy, in order to increase the tumor growth inhibition and the cell mortality.

2. Impact of Olaparib concentrations

The same spheroid parameters were compared for both models, according to the high/low Olaparib concentrations and without/with irradiation. For MDA-MD-231 model after 10 days, a significant decrease in spheroid size and metabolic activity was detected, from 66 ± 7% (5 μM Olaparib) to 39 ± 4% (5 μM and 10 Gy, $p = 10^{-23}$) and from 59 ± 12% (5 μM Olaparib) to 20 ± 1% (5 μM and 10 Gy, $p = 0.01$), respectively (Figure 4C,F,I). Similarly, SUM1315 spheroids size evolved from 71 ± 10% to 64 ± 14% ($p = 0.04$) and metabolic activity from 55 ± 2% to 46 ± 1% ($p = 10^{-7}$) after the same treatment condition, respectively (Figure 5C,F,I). More, for both models, the increase in Olaparib concentration (50 μM) and 10 Gy irradiation led to low additional toxicity on spheroid size (31 ± 5%, $p = 10^{-10}$ for MDA-MB-231 and 63 ± 10% for SUM1315, $p = 0.77$) and even induced an increase in spheroid metabolic activity (21 ± 1% for MDA-MB-231 and 63 ± 4%, for SUM1315, both superior to low dose Olaparib 5 μM, $p = 0.01$ and $p = 10^{-5}$)(Figure 4C,F,I and Figure 5C,F,I).

Finally, the sensitivity of each spheroid model was analyzed by the time after irradiation and 5 or 50 μM Olaparib treatment by the ANOVA analysis (Figure 6). It confirmed the efficacy of a long-term and low dose Olaparib treatment (5 μM) compared to a high dose (50 μM) (20 ± 1% and 46 ± 1% of metabolic activity for MDA-MB-231 and SUM1315 spheroids after 5 μM and 10 Gy compared to 22 ± 1% and 63 ± 3%, respectively, class effect $<10^{-6}$). Additionnaly, whatever the treatment condition, MDA-MB-231 spheroids seemed to be more sensitive to the treatment than SUM1315 spheroids (Figure 6). All these results with tumor-like models demonstrated the potentiation of irradiation combined with Olaparib treatment and confirmed the interest of administrating a long-term co-treatment with low-dose of Olaparib.

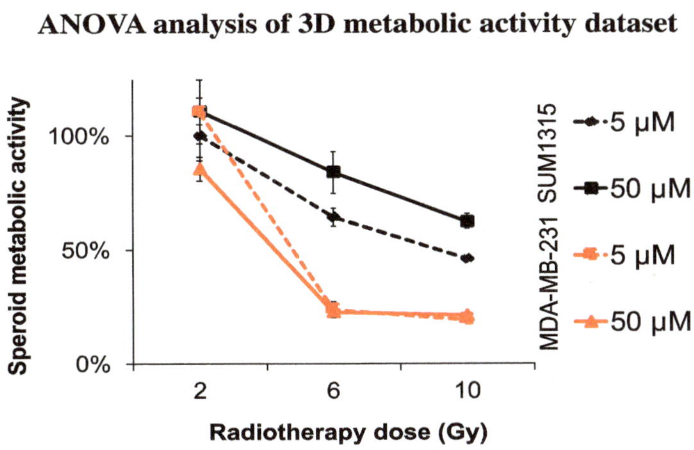

	DF	p value
Curve effect	2/116	**10^{-6}**
Class effect	3/116	**10^{-6}**

Figure 6. ANOVA analysis of spheroids sensitivity to the co-treatment with Olaparib and 2 to 10 Gy of fractioned irradiation: The decrease in spheroid metabolic activity is potentialized with 5 µM Olaparib and heterogenous between the two MDA-MB-231 and SUM1315 cell lines. The curve effect indicates a significant decrease in cell survival by the time for a same condition and the class effect indicates a significant difference in cell survival for a same incubation (DF = Degree of Freedom).

3.4. The Difference in SUM1315 and MDA-MB-231 TNBC Cell Lines Sensitivity in 2D and 3D Is Explained by a Strong Genomic Heterogeneity

In our experiments, the sensitivity was heterogeneous between the two cell lines as depicted in the ANOVA analysis. In both 2D and 3D cell cultures, MDA-MB-231 cell line was more sensitive to the co-treatment 5 µM Olaparib/irradiation than SUM1315 cell line. Thereby, in order to explain this difference, a in silico transcriptomic comparison was carried out from GEOdatasets (Figure 6). The transcriptome of both cell lines was analyzed using a classical bioinformatics pipeline including TOPHAT and DESeq2 package. First, this analysis underlined 3870 significant differentially expressed genes (DEGs) between the two cell lines (Figure 7A). Among these DEGs, 1704 (44%) were overexpressed in MDA-MB-231 cell line whereas 2166 (56%) were overexpressed in SUM1315 cell line.

Then, we focused on those DEGs involved in the DNA reparation pathways that play a major role in Olaparib and radiotherapy efficacy [21] (Figure 7B). Among all key selected genes, CHEK1 (log fold change LFG of 2.3, $p < 0.01$), AURKA (LFG = 2.1, $p < 0.01$), LIG1 (LFG = 1.7, $p < 0.01$), RAD51 (LFG = 1.5, $p < 0.01$) and EXO1 (LFG = 2.2, $p < 0.01$) were significantly overexpressed in MDA-MB-231 against SUM1315. Conversely, DNAPK (LFG = 1.88, $p < 0.01$), XLF (LFG = 2.82, $p < 0.01$), MRN (LFG = 5.5, $p < 0.01$), PMS2 (LFG = 2.1, $p < 0.01$) and PARP3 (LFG = 1.3, $p < 0.01$) were overexpressed in SUM1315 cell line compared to MDA-MB-231 cell line (Figure 7B). In contrast, concerning the principal targets of the PARP inhibitor Olaparib that are PARP1, and PARP2, no significant difference in gene expression was detected (Figure 7B).

Then, for a further insight into the differential phenotypes between the two cell lines, we next used the powerful Ingenuity Pathway Analysis (IPA) software to infer the functional phenotype of each cell line from their differential transcriptomic patterns (Figure 7C). First, for both cell lines, the cell survival pathway was highly activated (z-score > 7). In contrast, an important number of cellular functions were differentially activated between these two cell lines. Indeed, for MDA-MB-231 cell line, the proliferation, migration and invasion capacities were highly activated (z-score > 3 for cellular functions), as already reported in previous studies [13]. Conversely, SUM1315 cell line did not exhibit the same cellular pattern of proliferation and migration as MDA-MB-231 but presented a particular phenotype highly associated with neuron development and morphogenesis characteristics (z-score > 2.5). These results demonstrated the stem-cell like phenotype of SUM1315 cell line, suggesting a specific neuronal engagement profile.

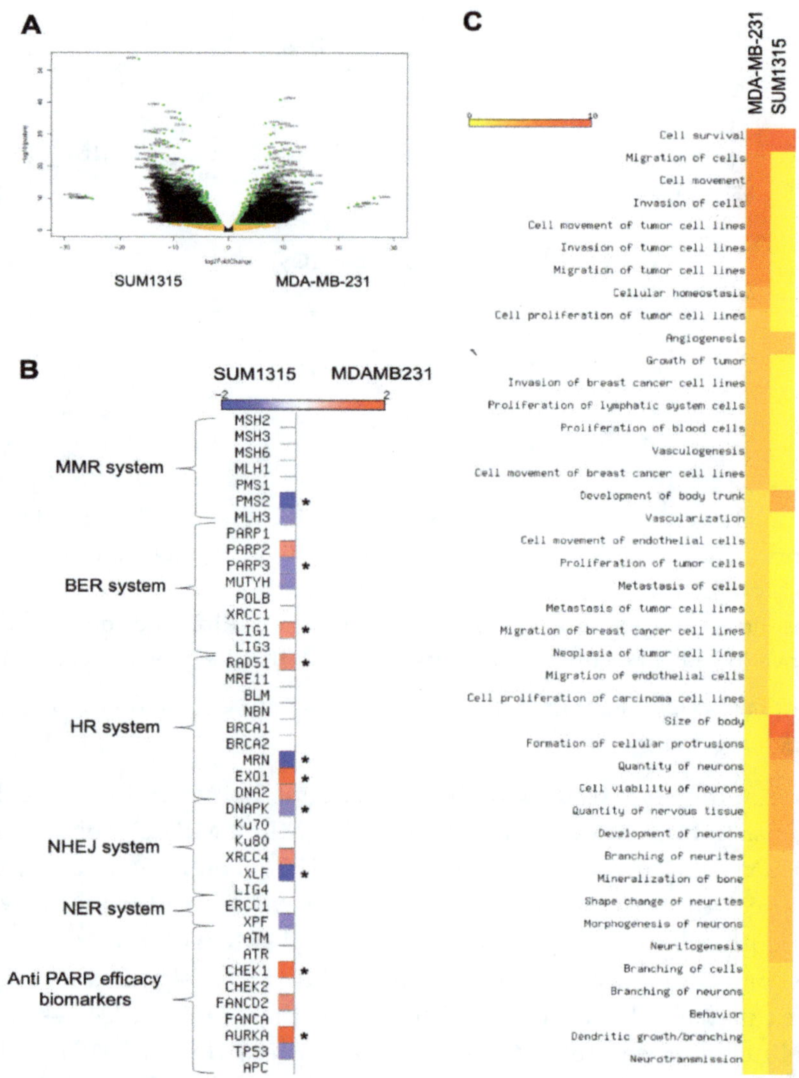

Figure 7. Transcriptomic analysis of MDA-MB-231 and SUM1315 cell lines: Determination of cell difference in sensitivity by a Differential Expressed Gene analysis (**A,B**) and a functional phenotype analysis (**C**). (**A**) Volcanoplot of the Differential Expressed Genes between MDA-MB-231 and SUM1315 cell lines. The y-axis corresponds to the mean expression value of log 10 (p-value), and the x-axis displays the log 2 fold change value. Each point represents a gene. The green dots represent the significant up/down expressed genes (adjusted p value < 0.05, log 10 >1) whereas the orange dots represent the non-significant differentially significant genes. Genes symbol are indicated. (**B**) Expression levels of keys genes involved in DNA reparation mechanisms (mismatch repair system "MMR", base excision repair system "BER", homologous recombination system "HR", non homologous end-joining repair system "NHEJ", nucleotide excision repair system "NER"). The heatmap shows the expression level of key genes involved in different DNA reparation pathways. These last are indicated beside the heatmap. Asterisk marks designated genes which are significantly differential expressed genes between the two cell lines: MDA-MB-231 and SUM1315, * $p < 0.01$. (**C**) Determination of MDA-MB-231 and SUM1315 cell lines functional phenotype by an Ingenuity Pathway (IPA) analysis. The heatmap shows the cellular functions that were inferred to be associated with enriched DGE clusters between MDA-MB-231 and SUM1315 cell lines.

4. Discussion

The Triple-Negative breast cancers (TNBC) are very aggressive and have a poor prognostic. TNBC cancer cells exhibit several DNA repair pathway deficiencies, such as deleterious mutations on the BRCA1/2 genes or assimilated "BRCAness" phenotypes. Thus, for this tumour subtype, the use of PARP inhibitors (PARPi), exploiting the concept of synthetic lethality, seem to be very promising [22–27].

In addition, the inhibition of PARPi has been described to increase the radio-sensitivity of tumour cells exhibiting a BRCAness phenotype [9,28–31]. Thus, PARPi could be administered in combination with chemotherapy targeting DNA or radiotherapy [10,29]. Indeed, PARPi induce an increase in the rate of unrepaired DNA single-strand breaks in proliferating cells, leading to the more frequent appearance of lethal DNA double-stranded breaks. Similarly, the cytotoxicity of irradiation is mainly related to the rate of DNA double-strand breaks, due to the accumulation of lethal lesions and sub lethal lesions [10]. In this context, our study aimed to model the effectiveness of a co-treatment anti-PARP (Olaparib) and fractioned irradiation, using two TNBC cell line models with metastatic origin i.e., MDA-MB-231 (highly proliferative, BRCA1-wild with BRCAness profile) and SUM1315 (low proliferative with stem-cell like phenotype, BRCA1-mutated), in 2D and 3D cell culture conditions.

Firstly, the DNA double-strand breaks induction further to the co-treatment Olaparib 4 h and 2 Gy irradiation was determined on both models by the analysis of focigammaH2AX increase. Indeed, these proteins are the first recruited in the process of DSBs reparation by the HR system and are usually used to determine the cell sensitivity to DNA damaging agents or radiations [28,32,33]. For both studied models treated with 5 and 50 μM Olaparib alone, the number of DNA double strand breaks per nuclei increased in an Olaparib-dose-dependent-manner with 2.1- to 2.3-fold higher levels than 0.1% DMSO controls, respectively. Similarly, the number of foci per nuclei was increased by 2.4 to 3.5-fold in the presence of 5 and 50 μM Olaparib and radiotherapy, as compared to the irradiated controls. These results suggest a cumulative induction of DNA double-strand breaks further to the co-treatment, probably related to (i) the irradiation and (ii) the accumulation of unrepaired single-strand breaks by the inhibition of the BER repair system, thus degenerating into DSBs.

Secondly, the cellular response further to the co-treatment Olaparib/fractioned irradiation was studied on both cell models cultured in 2D by cell survival and cell clonogenic repopulation tests. These experiments highlighted the low-dose efficacy of Olaparib combined with high dose of irradiation, in terms of (i) cell survival decrease and (ii) cell clonogenic repopulation capacity, compared to high dose Olaparib alone or high dose of irradiation alone. Indeed, the use of low-dose Olaparib potentialized the irradiation in terms of clonogenic repopulation decrease with a ratio "Olaparib/Olaparib + 10 Gy" of 100- to 650-fold after 0.5 μM, of 0.8- to 188-fold after 5 μM, compared to only 0.4- to 4-fold after 50 μM Olaparib (for SUM1315 and MDA-MB-231 cell lines, respectively). In the same way, other in vitro studies also showed a strong cytotoxic effect of the treatment combining hypofractioned irradiation (0 to 6 Gy) and 10 μM of PARPi Olaparib, on cholangiocarcinoma, a very malignant and radioresistant tumor model [34].

Our experiments in 2D cell culture conditions allowed us to choose the Olaparib concentrations (5 and 50 μM) for the treatment on more-predictive tumor-like models. More, the spheroid models allow long-term cultures up to 14 days [13]. Thus, a longer exposure time (up to 10 days) was designated in order to mimic the potential treatment strategy in vivo. For the proliferative MDA-MB-231 spheroid model, a cytostatic and cytotoxic effect of the co-treatment was detected, with a higher efficacy of the low-dose Olaparib compared to the high dose (50 μM). Indeed, the ratio of metabolic activity decrease "Ola/Ola + 10 Gy" was of 3.3-fold for 5 μM compared to 0.9 with 50 μM. Similarly, for the non-proliferative SUM1315 spheroid model, the co-treatment showed a cytotoxic activity, with always a higher efficacy of low-dose Olaparib (5 μM). The spheroid metabolic activity decreased was of 1.2-fold with 5 μM "Ola/Ola + 10 Gy" against 0.9-fold with 50 μM. These results suggest that the potentiation of the co-treatment could be reached with low-dose Olaparib and long-term exposure. More, the interest of using these tumor-like models resides also in their long-term preservation, mimicking the treatment strategies in vivo.

In the same way, the combination PARPi/radiotherapy has been studied for the treatment of various types of cancers in preclinical studies and has demonstrated improved efficacy compared to PARPi treatments alone or radiotherapy alone. Indeed, in vivo studies evaluated the impact of Olaparib combined with fractioned radiotherapy sessions (5 x 2 Gy) on bronchial cancer xenografts, leading to delayed tumor growths [30]. An in vivo study on prostate cancer showed significant growth delay and clonogenic kill after hypofractioned or fractioned radiotherapy coupled to Olaparib [28]. Other studies showed similar results on breast cancer xenografts (MCF-7 cell line), where veliparib (another PARP inhibitor) was associated with 6 Gy of hypofractioned X-ray session [35].

Furthermore, the cell ANOVA survival analysis in both 2D and 3D cell culture conditions highlighted the heterogeneous sensitivity between the two cell line models. MDA-MB-231 cell line was more sensitive to the co-treatment than SUM1315. Thereby, a in silico transcriptomic comparison was carried out. These analyses highlighted in MDA-MB-231 the overexpression of AURKA, a gene exhibiting cell cycle regulation function and known as a biomarker of PARPi sensitivity [36–39]. Therefore, this specific overexpression of AURKA could partially explain the increased sensitivity to the co-treatment of MDA-MB-231 model compared to SUM1315 model. Thus, these results suggest that AURKA overexpression might be a potential biomarker of the co-treatment efficacy. Secondly, according to the differential transcriptomic patterns between both models, MDA-MB-231 cell line exhibited strong proliferation, migration and invasion functions, already reported in previous studies [13]. In contrast, SUM1315 cell line expressed a stem-cell like phenotype, with a specific neuronal engagement profile. This general pattern could partially explain the resistant property of SUM1315 cell line, as undifferentiated stem cells exhibit slowed proliferation rates and develop specific resistance mechanisms [40]. Otherwise, the neuronal differentiation pattern in SUM1315 cell line might be explained by its metastatic tumoral origin [41]. Indeed, Triple-Negative breast tumors frequently develop metastases in brain, compared to other types that invade preferentially bones or lungs [4].

5. Conclusions

All these preclinical modeling experiments using the more-predictive and high throughput tumor-like models suggest the perspective of a low dose and long-term Olaparib administration alongside fractioned irradiation for resistant metastatic breast cancers. Other studies on Triple-Negative Breast Cancer cases have to be performed to assess whether AURKA overexpression/amplification could predict the "PARPi and irradiation" sensitivity regardless of the proliferation/stem-cell like status and the BRCA-status. These hypothesis are also to be corroborated on other tumor-like spheroid models that are PARPi candidates.

Author Contributions: Conceptualization, C.D., F.M., C.H., F.M., P.D., C.A., S.G., E.M., F.P.-L. and M.B.; Data curation, C.H. and S.G.; Formal analysis, C.D., F.M., C.H. and M.B.; Funding acquisition, E.M., F.P.-L. and M.B.; Investigation, C.D., F.M., C.H. and F.M.; Methodology, C.D., F.M., C.H., F.M. and M.B.; Project administration, C.D. and M.B.; Resources, C.D., C.H., F.M., S.G., E.M., F.P.-L. and M.B.; Software, C.H., F.M. and S.G.; Supervision, C.D., F.M., F.M., E.M., F.P.-L. and M.B.; Validation, C.D., F.M., C.H. and M.B.; Visualization, C.D.; Writing—original draft, C.D., F.M., C.H., F.M., E.M., F.P.-L. and M.B.; Writing—review & editing, C.D., F.M., C.H., F.M., P.D., C.A., S.G., E.M., F.P.-L. and M.B. All authors have read and agreed to the published version of the manuscript.

Acknowledgments: Our thanks to Michel Lapeyre, for kindly giving us the access to the radiotherapy department and the irradiators. Our thanks to Fabrice Kwiatkowski and Denise Donnarieix from the "Centre Jean Perrin" for their help in the ANOVA analysis and the irradiation methodology, respectively. We are grateful to the Genotoul bioinformatics platform Toulouse Midi-Pyrenees (Bioinfo Genotoul) for providing help and/or computing and/or storage resources.

References

1. Horton, J.K.; Jagsi, R.; Woodward, W.A.; Ho, A. Breast Cancer Biology: Clinical Implications for Breast Radiation Therapy. *Int. J. Radiat. Oncol. Biol. Phys.* **2018**, *100*, 23–37. [CrossRef] [PubMed]
2. Penault-Llorca, F.; Viale, G. Pathological and molecular diagnosis of triple-negative breast cancer: A clinical perspective. *Ann. Oncol. Off. J. Eur. Soc. Med. Oncol.* **2012**, *23* (Suppl. 6), vi19–vi22. [CrossRef] [PubMed]
3. Kobayashi, S. Basal-like subtype of breast cancer: A review of its unique characteristics and their clinical significance. *Breast Cancer Tokyo Jpn.* **2008**, *15*, 153–158. [CrossRef] [PubMed]
4. Rakha, E.A.; Elsheikh, S.E.; Aleskandarany, M.A.; Habashi, H.O.; Green, A.R.; Powe, D.G.; El-Sayed, M.E.; Benhasouna, A.; Brunet, J.-S.; Akslen, L.A.; et al. Triple-negative breast cancer: Distinguishing between basal and nonbasal subtypes. *Clin. Cancer Res. Off. J. Am. Assoc. Cancer Res.* **2009**, *15*, 2302–2310. [CrossRef] [PubMed]
5. De Ruijter, T.C.; Veeck, J.; de Hoon, J.P.J.; van Engeland, M.; Tjan-Heijnen, V.C. Characteristics of triple-negative breast cancer. *J. Cancer Res. Clin. Oncol.* **2011**, *137*, 183–192. [CrossRef] [PubMed]
6. Foulkes, W.D.; Smith, I.E.; Reis-Filho, J.S. Triple-negative breast cancer. *N. Engl. J. Med.* **2010**, *363*, 1938–1948. [CrossRef]
7. Marmé, F.; Schneeweiss, A. Targeted Therapies in Triple-Negative Breast Cancer. *Breast Care Basel Switz.* **2015**, *10*, 159–166. [CrossRef]
8. Duma, N.; Gast, K.C.; Choong, G.M.; Leon-Ferre, R.A.; O'Sullivan, C.C. Where Do We Stand on the Integration of PARP Inhibitors for the Treatment of Breast Cancer? *Curr. Oncol. Rep.* **2018**, *20*, 63. [CrossRef]
9. Pernin, V.; Mégnin-Chanet, F.; Pennaneach, V.; Fourquet, A.; Kirova, Y.; Hall, J. PARP inhibitors and radiotherapy: Rational and prospects for a clinical use. *Cancer Radiother. J. Soc. Fr. Radiother. Oncol.* **2014**, *18*, 790–798, quiz 799–802.
10. Chalmers, A.J.; Lakshman, M.; Chan, N.; Bristow, R.G. Poly (ADP-ribose) polymerase inhibition as a model for synthetic lethality in developing radiation oncology targets. *Semin. Radiat. Oncol.* **2010**, *20*, 274–281. [CrossRef]
11. Costa, E.C.; Moreira, A.F.; de Melo-Diogo, D.; Gaspar, V.M.; Carvalho, M.P.; Correia, I.J. 3D tumor spheroids: An overview on the tools and techniques used for their analysis. *Biotechnol. Adv.* **2016**, *34*, 1427–1441. [CrossRef] [PubMed]
12. Fang, Y.; Eglen, R.M. Three-Dimensional Cell Cultures in Drug Discovery and Development. *SLAS Discov. Adv. Life Sci. RD* **2017**, *22*, 456–472.
13. Dubois, C.; Dufour, R.; Daumar, P.; Aubel, C.; Szczepaniak, C.; Blavignac, C.; Mounetou, E.; Penault-Llorca, F.; Bamdad, M. Development and cytotoxic response of two proliferative MDA-MB-231 and non-proliferative SUM1315 three-dimensional cell culture models of triple-negative basal-like breast cancer cell lines. *Oncotarget* **2017**, *8*, 95316–95331. [PubMed]
14. Daumar, P.; Dufour, R.; Dubois, C.; Penault-Llorca, F.; Bamdad, M.; Mounetou, E. Development and validation of a high-performance liquid chromatography method for the quantitation of intracellular PARP inhibitor Olaparib in cancer cells. *J. Pharm. Biomed. Anal.* **2018**, *152*, 74–80. [CrossRef] [PubMed]
15. Dufour, R.; Daumar, P.; Mounetou, E.; Aubel, C.; Kwiatkowski, F.; Abrial, C.; Vatoux, C.; Penault-Llorca, F.; Bamdad, M. BCRP and P-gp relay overexpression in triple negative basal-like breast cancer cell line: A prospective role in resistance to Olaparib. *Sci. Rep.* **2015**, *5*, 12670. [CrossRef] [PubMed]
16. Elstrodt, F.; Hollestelle, A.; Nagel, J.H.A.; Gorin, M.; Wasielewski, M.; van den Ouweland, A.; Merajver, S.D.; Ethier, S.P.; Schutte, M. BRCA1 mutation analysis of 41 human breast cancer cell lines reveals three new deleterious mutants. *Cancer Res.* **2006**, *66*, 41–45. [CrossRef]
17. Marcotte, R.; Sayad, A.; Brown, K.R.; Sanchez-Garcia, F.; Reimand, J.; Haider, M.; Virtanen, C.; Bradner, J.E.; Bader, G.D.; Mills, G.B.; et al. Functional Genomic Landscape of Human Breast Cancer Drivers, Vulnerabilities, and Resistance. *Cell* **2016**, *164*, 293–309. [CrossRef]
18. Daemen, A.; Griffith, O.L.; Heiser, L.M.; Wang, N.J.; Enache, O.M.; Sanborn, Z.; Pepin, F.; Durinck, S.; Korkola, J.E.; Griffith, M.; et al. Modeling precision treatment of breast cancer. *Genome Biol.* **2013**, *14*, R110. [CrossRef]

19. Boire, A.; Zou, Y.; Shieh, J.; Macalinao, D.G.; Pentsova, E.; Massagué, J. Complement Component 3 Adapts the Cerebrospinal Fluid for Leptomeningeal Metastasis. *Cell* **2017**, *168*, 1101–1113. [CrossRef]
20. Trapnell, C.; Pachter, L.; Salzberg, S.L. TopHat: Discovering splice junctions with RNA-Seq. *Bioinform. Oxf. Engl.* **2009**, *25*, 1105–1111. [CrossRef]
21. Ollier, M.; Radosevic-Robin, N.; Kwiatkowski, F.; Ponelle, F.; Viala, S.; Privat, M.; Uhrhammer, N.; Bernard-Gallon, D.; Penault-Llorca, F.; Bignon, Y.-J.; et al. DNA repair genes implicated in triple negative familial non-BRCA1/2 breast cancer predisposition. *Am. J. Cancer Res.* **2015**, *5*, 2113–2126. [PubMed]
22. Dhillon, K.K.; Bajrami, I.; Taniguchi, T.; Lord, C.J. Synthetic lethality: The road to novel therapies for breast cancer. *Endocr. Relat. Cancer* **2016**, *23*, T39–T55. [CrossRef] [PubMed]
23. Fang, B. Development of synthetic lethality anticancer therapeutics. *J. Med. Chem.* **2014**, *57*, 7859–7873. [CrossRef] [PubMed]
24. Fang, L.; Barekati, Z.; Zhang, B.; Liu, Z.; Zhong, X. Targeted therapy in breast cancer: What's new? *Swiss Med. Wkly.* **2011**, *141*, w13231. [CrossRef] [PubMed]
25. Farmer, H.; McCabe, N.; Lord, C.J.; Tutt, A.N.J.; Johnson, D.A.; Richardson, T.B.; Santarosa, M.; Dillon, K.J.; Hickson, I.; Knights, C.; et al. Targeting the DNA repair defect in BRCA mutant cells as a therapeutic strategy. *Nature* **2005**, *434*, 917–921. [CrossRef]
26. Lord, C.J.; Ashworth, A. PARP inhibitors: Synthetic lethality in the clinic. *Science* **2017**, *355*, 1152–1158. [CrossRef]
27. O'Neil, N.J.; Bailey, M.L.; Hieter, P. Synthetic lethality and cancer. *Nat. Rev. Genet.* **2017**, *18*, 613–623. [CrossRef]
28. Gani, C.; Coackley, C.; Kumareswaran, R.; Schütze, C.; Krause, M.; Zafarana, G.; Bristow, R.G. In vivo studies of the PARP inhibitor, AZD-2281, in combination with fractionated radiotherapy: An exploration of the therapeutic ratio. *Radiother. Oncol. J. Eur. Soc. Ther. Radiol. Oncol.* **2015**, *116*, 486–494. [CrossRef]
29. Kötter, A.; Cornils, K.; Borgmann, K.; Dahm-Daphi, J.; Petersen, C.; Dikomey, E.; Mansour, W.Y. Inhibition of PARP1-dependent end-joining contributes to Olaparib-mediated radiosensitization in tumor cells. *Mol. Oncol.* **2014**, *8*, 1616–1625. [CrossRef]
30. Senra, J.M.; Telfer, B.A.; Cherry, K.E.; McCrudden, C.M.; Hirst, D.G.; O'Connor, M.J.; Wedge, S.R.; Stratford, I.J. Inhibition of PARP-1 by olaparib (AZD2281) increases the radiosensitivity of a lung tumor xenograft. *Mol. Cancer Ther.* **2011**, *10*, 1949–1958. [CrossRef]
31. Verhagen, C.V.M.; de Haan, R.; Hageman, F.; Oostendorp, T.P.D.; Carli, A.L.E.; O'Connor, M.J.; Jonkers, J.; Verheij, M.; van den Brekel, M.W.; Vens, C. Extent of radiosensitization by the PARP inhibitor olaparib depends on its dose, the radiation dose and the integrity of the homologous recombination pathway of tumor cells. *Radiother. Oncol. J. Eur. Soc. Ther. Radiol. Oncol.* **2015**, *116*, 358–365. [CrossRef] [PubMed]
32. Mah, L.-J.; El-Osta, A.; Karagiannis, T.C. gammaH2AX: A sensitive molecular marker of DNA damage and repair. *Leukemia* **2010**, *24*, 679–686. [CrossRef] [PubMed]
33. Olive, P.L.; Banáth, J.P. Phosphorylation of histone H2AX as a measure of radiosensitivity. *Int. J. Radiat. Oncol. Biol. Phys.* **2004**, *58*, 331–335. [CrossRef] [PubMed]
34. Mao, Y.; Huang, X.; Shuang, Z.; Lin, G.; Wang, J.; Duan, F.; Chen, J.; Li, S. PARP inhibitor olaparib sensitizes cholangiocarcinoma cells to radiation. *Cancer Med.* **2018**, *7*, 1285–1296. [CrossRef]
35. Efimova, E.V.; Mauceri, H.J.; Golden, D.W.; Labay, E.; Bindokas, V.P.; Darga, T.E.; Chakraborty, C.; Barreto-Andrade, J.C.; Crawley, C.; Sutton, H.G.; et al. Poly (ADP-ribose) polymerase inhibitor induces accelerated senescence in irradiated breast cancer cells and tumors. *Cancer Res.* **2010**, *70*, 6277–6282. [CrossRef]
36. Ihnen, M.; zu Eulenburg, C.; Kolarova, T.; Qi, J.W.; Manivong, K.; Chalukya, M.; Dering, J.; Anderson, L.; Ginther, C.; Meuter, A.; et al. Therapeutic potential of the poly (ADP-ribose) polymerase inhibitor rucaparib for the treatment of sporadic human ovarian cancer. *Mol. Cancer Ther.* **2013**, *12*, 1002–1015. [CrossRef]
37. Ohmoto, A.; Yachida, S. Current status of poly (ADP-ribose) polymerase inhibitors and future directions. *Onco Targets Ther.* **2017**, *10*, 5195–5208. [CrossRef]
38. Telli, M.L.; Stover, D.G.; Loi, S.; Aparicio, S.; Carey, L.A.; Domchek, S.M.; Newman, L.; Sledge, G.W.; Winer, E.P. Homologous recombination deficiency and host anti-tumor immunity in triple-negative breast cancer. *Breast Cancer Res. Treat.* **2018**, *171*, 21–31. [CrossRef]
39. Wang, X.; Shi, Y.; Huang, D.; Guan, X. Emerging therapeutic modalities of PARP inhibitors in breast cancer. *Cancer Treat. Rev.* **2018**, *68*, 62–68. [CrossRef]

40. Fillmore, C.M.; Kuperwasser, C. Human breast cancer cell lines contain stem-like cells that self-renew, give rise to phenotypically diverse progeny and survive chemotherapy. *Breast Cancer Res. BCR* **2008**, *10*, R25. [CrossRef]

41. Barnabas, N.; Cohen, D. Phenotypic and Molecular Characterization of MCF10DCIS and SUM Breast Cancer Cell Lines. *Int. J. Breast Cancer* **2013**, *2013*, 872743. [CrossRef] [PubMed]

3

The Composition of Surgical Wound Fluids from Breast Cancer Patients is Affected by Intraoperative Radiotherapy Treatment and Depends on the Molecular Subtype of Breast Cancer

Katarzyna Kulcenty [1,2,*], Igor Piotrowski [1,2,†], Joanna Patrycja Wróblewska [3,†], Janusz Wasiewicz [4] and Wiktoria Maria Suchorska [1,2]

1 Radiobiology Lab, Department of Medical Physics, Greater Poland Cancer, 61-866 Poznań, Poland; igor.piotrowski@wco.pl (I.P.); wiktoria.suchorska@wco.pl (W.M.S.)

2 Department of Electroradiology, Poznan University of Medical Sciences, ul. Garbary 15, 61-866 Poznan, Poland

3 Department of Pathology, Poznan University of Medical Sciences and Greater Poland Cancer Center, ul. Garbary 15, 61-866 Poznan, Poland; joanna.wroblewska@wco.pl

4 Department of Breast Cancer Surgery, Greater Poland Cancer Centre, ul. Garbary 15, 61-866 Poznań, Poland; janusz.wasiewicz@wco.pl

* Correspondence: katarzyna.kulcenty@wco.pl

† These authors contribute equally.

Abstract: Invasive oncological procedures affect the remaining tumor cells by increasing their survival, proliferation, and migration through the induction of wound healing response. The phenomena of local relapse after breast-conserving surgery (BCS) has resulted in a series of research and clinical trials with the aim of assessing whether localized intraoperative radiotherapy (IORT), may be beneficial in inhibiting local recurrences. Therefore, it is essential to assess the impact of intraoperative radiotherapy in modulating the immunological response and wound healing process. Thus, we decided to perform a quantitative analysis of the composition of surgical wound fluids (SWF) in two groups of breast cancer (BC) patients: those treated with BCS followed by IORT, and those who underwent BCS alone. We found that several cytokines, which are believed to have anti-tumor properties, were highly expressed in the luminal A breast cancer subtype in the IORT treatment group. Interestingly, we also found significant differences between IORT patients with tumors of different molecular subtypes. Based on these findings, we hypothesized that IORT treatment might be beneficial in changing the tumor bed microenvironment, making it less favorable for tumor recurrence due to decreased concentration of tumor-facilitating cytokines, especially in the luminal A subtype of BC.

Keywords: surgery-induced inflammation; cytokines; breast cancer; breast-conserving surgery, intraoperative radiation therapy

---

1. Introduction

Breast cancer (BC) is the most common cancer in women. After lung cancer, it is the second most common cause of cancer-related death. Conservative breast cancer surgery followed by radiation therapy is currently the standard treatment for this type of cancer. Local recurrence is, however, of major concern after conservative breast cancer (BCS) treatment. Numerous studies have demonstrated that approximately 90% of post-surgical local recurrences occur in the same quadrant as the primary cancer. It has been shown that local recurrence originates from residual cancer cells which are present in the interstitial peritumoral tissue, peritumoral vascular spaces, or in resection margins positive for residual cancer cells. It has also been shown that peritumoral lymphatic invasion is a predictor of both local and distant metastases [1]. Breast cancer surgery of the primary tumor is required to reduce the potential of cancer cells to mutate and metastasize. However, the clinical and experimental data suggest that surgery itself may be responsible for local relapse and metastasis [2]. It has been demonstrated that invasive procedures (both surgery and biopsy) affect the remaining tumor cells, increasing their survival, proliferation, and migration [3,4]. One of the concepts explaining this phenomenon is the induction of a wound healing response. In normal tissue, such a response is necessary for tissue repair. However, induction of adaptive and innate immune response in tumor tissue stimulates cell survival, angiogenesis, and extravasation of circulating tumor cells. It has become evident that some types of immune response, or immune cells, can promote tumor progression more than others [3]. For example, tumor-resident macrophages (M2 polarized macrophages) secret vascular endothelial growth factor (VEGF) and epidermal growth factor (EGF), which induce angiogenesis and the recruitment of neutrophils contribute to tumor progression and metastasis [5,6]. Using an in vitro model, Krall et al. proved that the systemic consequences of surgery could promote the regrowth of tumor cells even at distal anatomical sites. They found out that surgery-induced tumor regrowth was associated with both local and systemic inflammatory responses characterized by the release of cytokines and the mobilization of myeloid cells into the circulation of wounded mice [7]. Several studies revealed that surgical wound fluids (SWF) derived from the surgical sites act as a stimulant factor for tumor progression. Although SWF is rich in biological factors, the expression of these factors and how they interact with tumor cells, has not been entirely explained. Agresti et al. and Wang et al. analyzed the composition of SWF from breast cancer patients in detail [8,9]. They found that the composition of SWF differs between patients depending on the treatment (quadrantectomy or mastectomy), type (invasive or in situ) and the molecular subtype of breast cancer (BC) (luminal or triple-negative). Moreover, they also found that SWF stimulated proliferation of breast cancer cells of the intrinsic subtypes in vitro. This effect was more pronounced in triple negative breast cancer (TNBC) cells than in luminal cell lines. Tagliabue et al. confirmed that higher proliferation of human epidermal growth factor receptor 2 (HER2) positive breast cancer cells occurs after stimulation with SWF [4]. Moreover, it has been demonstrated that surgery-induced inflammation promotes the stem-like phenotype and tumor-initiating abilities of breast cancer cells via STAT3 signaling [10].

The phenomenon of local relapse initiated a series of research and clinical trials aimed at assessing whether localized intraoperative radiotherapy could be as effective in inhibiting local recurrence as standard postoperative whole breast radiotherapy but better tolerated by patients in terms of shortening the therapy course. Intraoperative radiation therapy (IORT) involves the direct irradiation of diseased tissue during surgery, within the tumor bed, with doses of either 10 Gy (dose used in the Greater Poland Cancer Center, from which SWFs for the presented experiments were collected) or 23 Gy. This approach reduces the potential risk of re-population of tumor cells during the process of wound healing [11]. The studies by Belletti and Tagliabue studies showed that SWF obtained from patients who had undergone surgical removal of the breast tumor could stimulate motility and invasiveness of tumor cells in vitro. They demonstrated that wound fluid could serve as an "attractant" for residual cancer cells in the tumor bed [4,12]. Moreover, we have previously reported that SWF from patients who underwent surgery alone (BCS, WF), and those who received IORT (IORT, RT-WF) affect the stem cell phenotype in breast cancer cell lines. We also revealed reduced stimulation of the cancer stem cell (CSC) phenotype, and migratory capabilities after incubation with SWF from IORT treated patients [13,14]. Moreover, it has been shown, that SWF from IORT patients decrease the proliferation of breast cancer cells comparing to SWF after BCS alone [12]. Previously, we demonstrated that luminal (MCF7) and basal (MDA-MB-468) cell lines transit from being more epithelial to more mesenchymal cells by stimulation with BCS and IORT, and that the mesenchymal features are more pronounced after stimulation with BCS alone [14]. Our previous experiments also proved that the biological effect of

SWF after IORT treatment depends on the radiation induced bystander effect (RIBE), which induces a radiobiological response in unirradiated cells [14,15]. Our results stay in compliance with the targeted intraoperative radiotherapy (TARGIT) clinical trial studies demonstrating that IORT significantly inhibits the stimulatory effects of SWF on tumor cells in vitro. This effect may be due to both cell death caused directly by ionizing radiation and to changes in the tumor microenvironment. Using proteomic analyses, Belletti et al. revealed, that TARGIT could have an antitumor effect, surpassing radiation-induced cancer cell kill through changes in the growth factors and cytokines present in the resection cavity [12].

Thereafter, it is important to assess the impact of intraoperative radiotherapy in modulating the immunological response and wound healing process. Thus, the main aim of this study was to perform an analysis of the SWF composition in two groups of breast cancer patients: those patients who underwent BCS followed by IORT treatment, and those who underwent BCS only. Clarification of the composition of SWF will allow a better understanding of the clinical observations obtained through the frequent utility of IORT treatment, which reduces the risk of local recurrence not only through direct cell killing, but also through modification of local microenvironment.

2. Results

Analysis of the Composition of SWF from BCS Patients and BCS Patients after IORT Treatment

The main aim of this study was to perform the quantitative analysis of the SWF composition in two groups of breast cancer patients: patients which undergo BCS followed by IORT treatment, and those who underwent BCS only. Thus, surgical wound fluids from 18 BCS and 20 IORT patients were collected 48 h after the surgery. Patients classified to IORT treatment are early breast cancer patients, usually with luminal A or luminal B molecular subtype. Thus, only patients with those classification were subjected to the study. The comparison without distinguishing molecular subtype diagnosis of BCS versus IORT SWF revealed 10 cytokines which differ significantly between analyzed groups. We found that the concentration of IL-7, IL-8, IL-13, MIF (macrophage migration inhibitory factor), and TNF-beta were significantly decreased in IORT SWF compared to BCS SWF (Figure 1A). On the other hand, IORT SWF is characterized by increased concentration of CTACK, G-CSF, HGF, IL-1 beta, and TNF-alpha (Figure 1B).

To dissect the composition of SWF according to BC molecular subtype, we divided the group of BCS and IORT SWF to luminal A and luminal B subtype (Figure 2).

We found that seven cytokines were significantly changed between BCS and IORT SWF, and they were characteristic only for luminal A subtype of BC: G-CSF, HGF, IL-1 beta, IL-12 (p40), MIP-1 alpha, SCGF, and TNF-alpha (Figure 3).

In luminal B subtype of BC, we found five cytokines which differ significantly between BCS and IORT group: IL-9, MIF, PDGF-BB, RANTES, and TNF-beta (Figure 4).

It is worth pointing out that concentration of HGF cytokine in SWF from luminal A subtype was also significantly decreased in IORT luminal A group in comparison with IORT luminal B group (Figure 3). Moreover, we found that the concentration of SCGF (Figure 3), IL-9, PDGF-BB, RANTES, and TNF-beta, differ significantly between luminal A and luminal B BCS group.

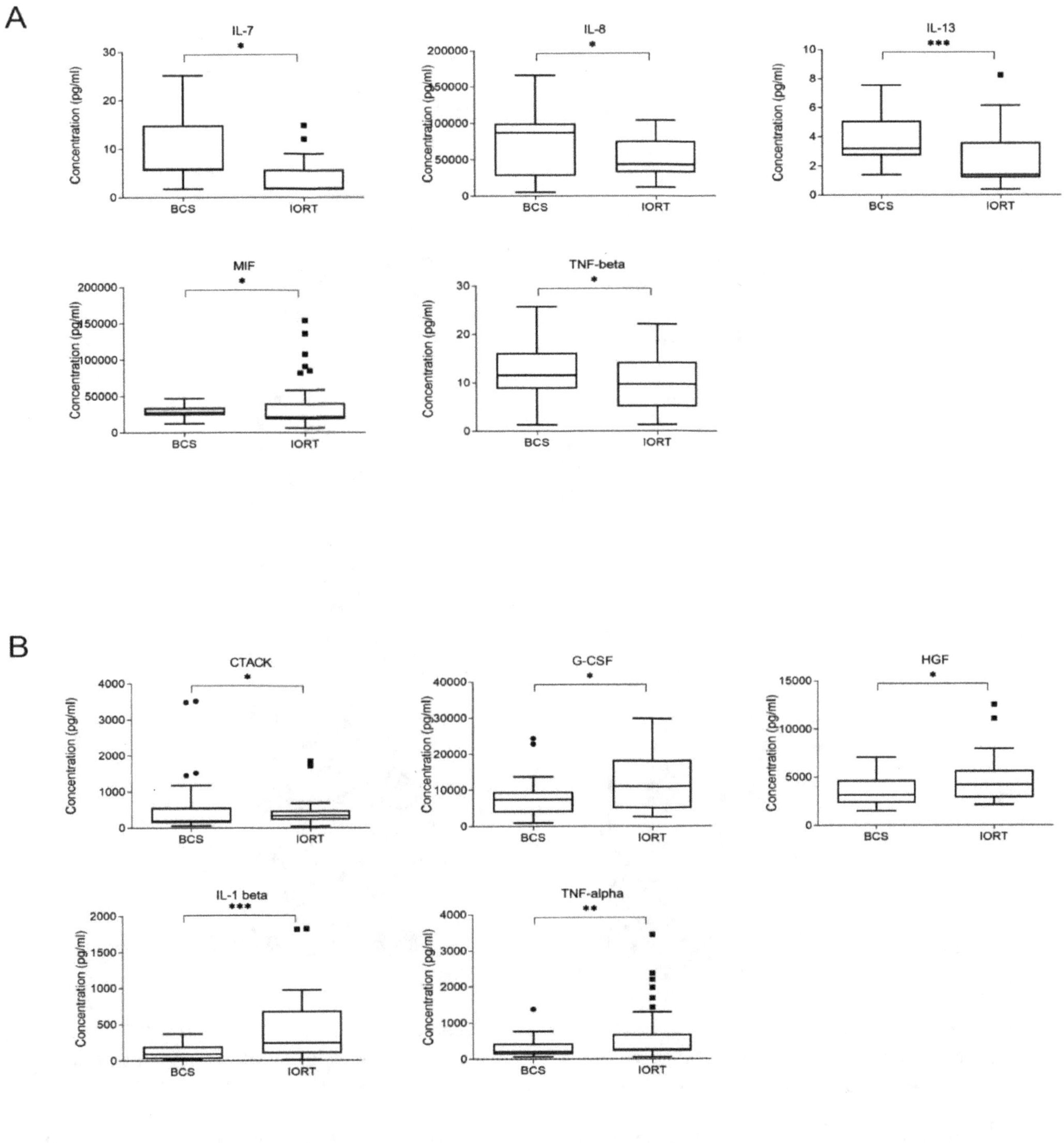

Figure 1. Box plots (median and whiskers) presenting concentration of cytokines (pg/ml) of surgical wound fluids (SWF) collected from patients after breast conserving surgery (BCS) and breast conserving surgery followed by intraoperative radiation therapy (IORT). (**A**) Cytokines with decreased concentrations in IORT group. (**B**) Cytokines with increased concentrations in IORT group. Whiskers were calculated using Tuckey method based on GraphPad Prism software. Outliners are shown as dots. * $p < 0.05$, ** $p < 0.01$, *** $p < 0.001$: based on Mann–Whitney test.

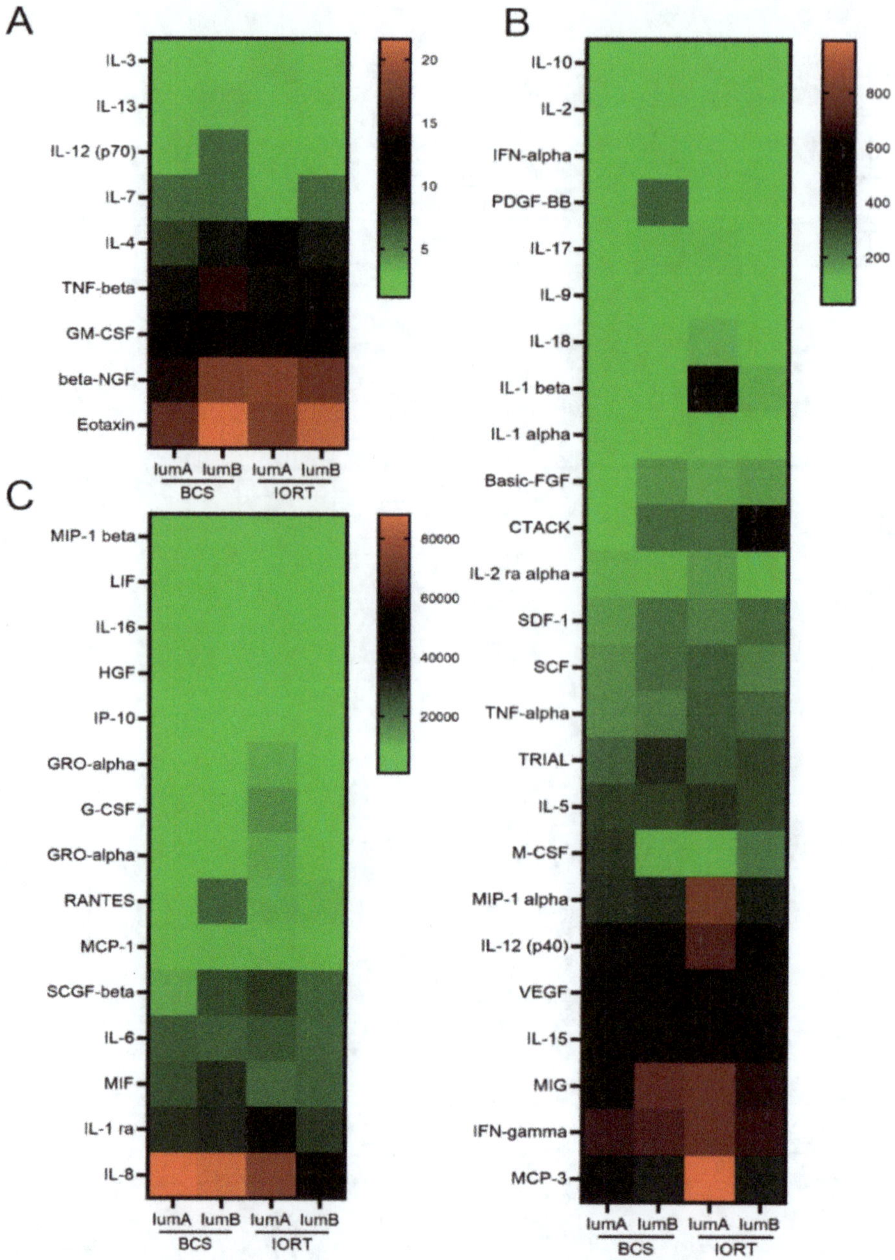

Figure 2. Heatmap representing concentration of all analyzed cytokines in BCS and IORT group distinguishing the molecular subtype of BC. To clarify the differences in cytokine concentrations, heatmap was divided into three: (**A**) 0–20 pg/ml, (**B**) 20–1000 pg/ml, (**C**) 1000–90000 pg/ml.

We found only three small molecules, which concentration differs significantly in both luminal A and luminal B subtypes of breast cancer: IL-13, MCP-1 (CCL2), and MCP-3 (CCL7). While the IL-13 concentration is significantly decreased in IORT group in both luminal A and luminal B subtype of BC, in the case of MCP-1, we observe an inverse correlation in the concentration difference between the molecular subtypes (Figure 5). In luminal A subtype, the concentration of MCP-1 is increased in the IORT group, while in luminal B subtype, its concentration is decreased in the IORT group. Moreover, a statistically significant change in MCP-1 concentration is also observed between two IORT groups (decrease in luminal B subtype). Similar differences between the IORT groups were also found in other monocytes chemotactic protein—MCP-3. Again, in IORT treated patients of luminal B subtype, the concentration of analyzed chemokine (MCP-3) in SWF is significantly decreased while comparing to luminal A subtype of BC.

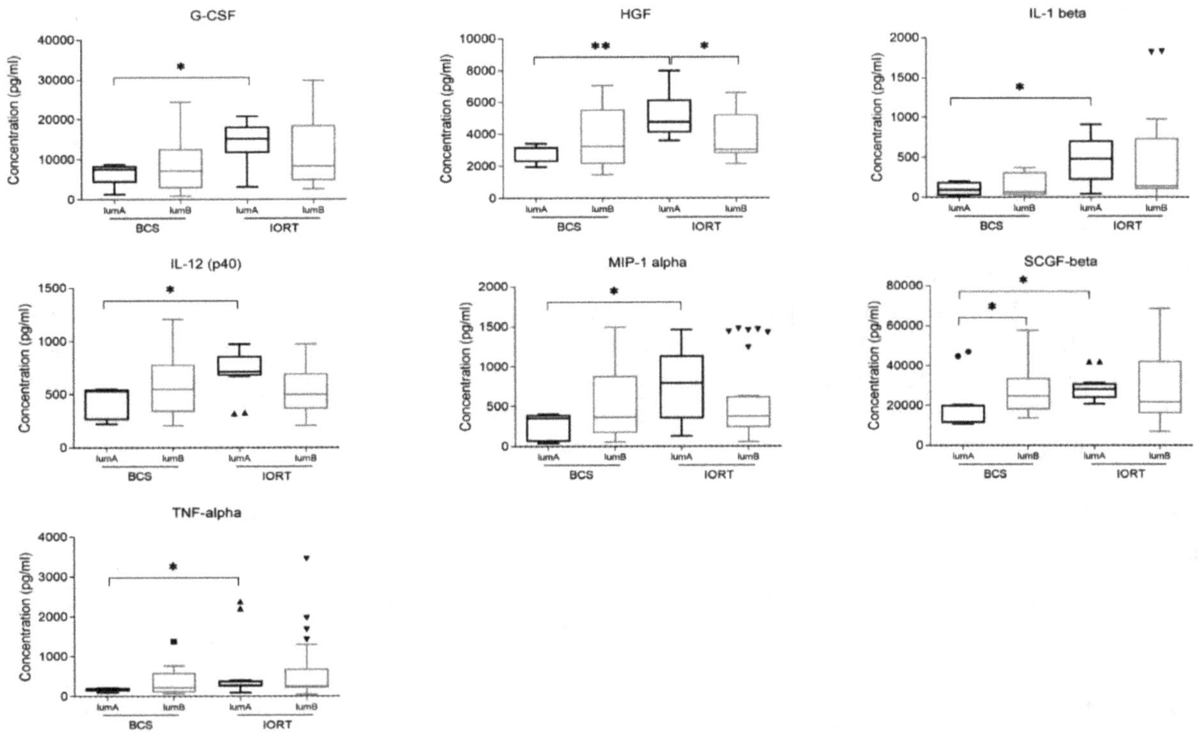

Figure 3. Box plots (median and whiskers) presenting concentration of cytokines (pg/ml) of surgical wound fluids (SWF) collected from patients after breast conserving surgery (BCS) and breast conserving surgery followed by IORT (IORT) in luminal A subtype of breast cancer. Whiskers were calculated using Tuckey method based on GraphPad Prism software. Outliners are shown as dots. * $p < 0.05$, ** $p < 0.01$, *** $p < 0.001$: based on Kruskal–Wallis test with Dunn's post hoc multiple comparison test.

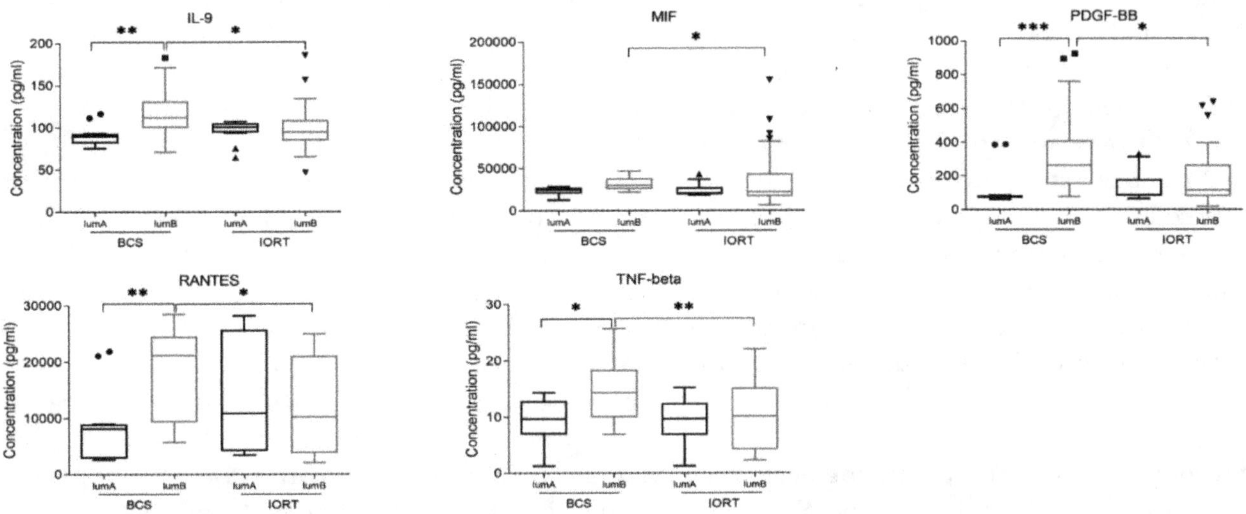

Figure 4. Box plots (median and whiskers) presenting concentration of cytokines (pg/ml) of surgical wound fluids (SWF) collected from patients after breast conserving surgery (BCS) and breast conserving surgery followed by IORT (IORT) in luminal B subtype of breast cancer. Whiskers were calculated using Tukey method based on GraphPad Prism software. Outliners are shown as dots. * $p < 0.05$, ** $p < 0.01$, *** $p < 0.001$: based on Kruskal–Wallis test with Dunn's post hoc multiple comparison test.

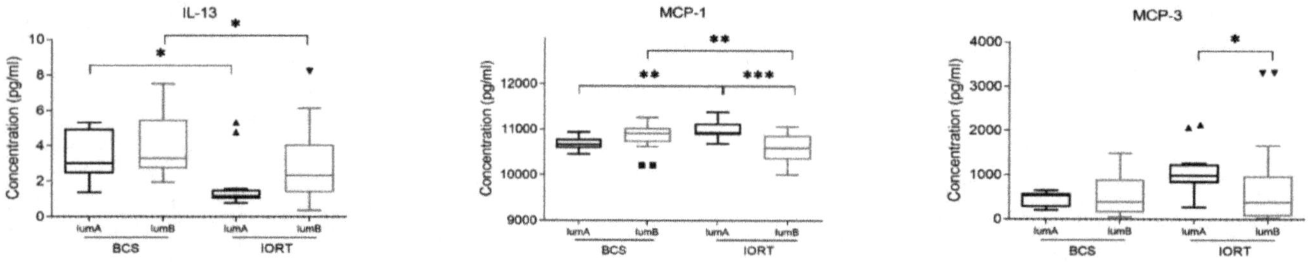

Figure 5. Box plots (median and whiskers) presenting concentration of cytokines (pg/ml) of surgical wound fluids (SWF) collected from patients after breast conserving surgery (BCS) and breast conserving surgery followed by IORT (IORT) in luminal A and luminal B subtype of breast cancer. Whiskers were calculated using Tukey method based on GraphPad Prism software. Outliners are shown as dots. * $p < 0.05$, ** $p < 0.01$, *** $p < 0.001$: based on Kruskal–Wallis test with Dunn's post hoc multiple comparison test.

3. Discussion

For many years it was believed, that the incidence of local recurrence and remote metastasis was much higher in patients who underwent breast-conserving surgery than those after radical mastectomy [1]. The 20-year follow up of randomized trial comparing BCS and radical mastectomy for patients with early breast cancer confirmed that BCS introduces a higher incidence of local recurrence ($p < 0.001$), although, there were no differences in the rates of contralateral-breast carcinomas, remote metastasis, or second primary cancers. Moreover, the long-term survival rate among those two groups was almost the same [16]. Thus, BCS followed by external beam radiation therapy (EBRT), delivered in fractionated doses in order to significantly reduce the risk of local recurrence [17], is now the treatment of choice for early breast cancer patients. Although the standard EBRT achieves good results, the duration of the treatment remains an obstacle. Due to breast cancer cell density (highest at up to 4 cm from the tumor edge), the probability of local recurrence is highest in the tumor bed. Therefore an additional single boost dose delivered directly to the tumor bed during the surgery, such as IORT, can significantly reduce local recurrence rates and the time of therapy comparing to standard EBRT [18,19]. This firstly is due to direct killing of residual cancer cells and also due to radiation-induced inflammation, which in turn can enhance the immunologic elimination of cancer cells. Moreover, recent studies of Meng et al. revealed that high single dose of irradiation is beneficial over fractionated irradiation due to lower activation of ATX-LPA-inflammatory cycle, which protects cancer cells from radiation induced cell death [20].

It has been suggested, that invasive procedures (such as surgery or biopsy) affect the remaining tumor cells by improving their survival and by stimulating proliferation and migration [3,4]. One of the concepts explaining this phenomenon is the induction of wound healing responses, which are responsible for tissue repair in normal tissues. However, the induction of adaptive and innate immune responses in tumor tissues stimulates cell survival and induces angiogenesis and the extravasation of circulating tumor cells. Studies of in vivo mouse models conducted by Krall et al. confirmed that the systemic inflammatory response induced after breast cancer surgery promotes the emergence of tumor cells. Moreover, the authors showed that perioperative anti-inflammatory treatment reduced the tumor regrowth, thus reducing early metastatic recurrence in breast cancer patients. This effect was associated with a release of cytokines and the mobilization of myeloid cells into the circulation of wounded mice [7]. Thus, it is believed that molecules present in SWF may affect residual cancer cells as well as modulating the immune response. It is important, therefore, to assess the impact of intraoperative radiotherapy in modulating the immunological response and wound healing processes. Thus, the main aim of this study was to carry out an analysis of the SWF composition in two groups of breast cancer patients: those patients who underwent BCS followed by IORT treatment, and those who underwent BCS alone.

To clarify the composition of SWF in BC patients, Wang et al. performed high-throughput screening of cytokines, chemokines and matrix metalloproteinases. In their analysis the authors focused on the time of SWF collection (1, 2, 3, and 4 days after the surgery), additional treatments such as neoadjuvant chemotherapy, TNM stage, and pathological type (carcinoma in situ, invasive breast cancer). They found that the highest concentration of cytokines was detected 1 day after the surgery and subsequently decreased day by day. They also found significant differences in levels of factors in SWF in relation to neoadjuvant chemotherapy, TNM stage, and the pathological type of BC [9]. In their in vitro studies, Wang et al. also confirmed the results of previous experiments [4,12], showing that SWF significantly stimulates proliferation of breast cancer cells. Similar experiments were also conducted by Agresti et al. who confirmed that the composition of SWF depends not only on the type of surgical procedure (quadrantectomy, mastectomy), but also on the aggressiveness of the tumor (in situ vs invasive), molecular subtype (luminal vs. triple-negative), the size of the tumor, staging (G2 or G3), and lymph node status (positive or negative for cancer cells). They suggested that the composition of surgical wound fluids collected from the tumor bed of breast cancer patients reflects the inflammatory nature and aggressiveness of the breast tumor [8]. The authors analyzed a panel of 34 cytokines, chemokines, and growth factors in the SWF of breast cancer patients and found, that the concentrations of IP-10, IL-6, G-CSF, osteoponin, MIP-1 alpha, MIP-1 beta, and MCP1-MCAF were higher in more aggressive tumors.

In this study, we have demonstrated that intraoperative radiation electron therapy treatment (10 Gy, 9 MeV, Mobetron) changes the composition of surgical wound fluids collected from breast cancer patients after breast-conserving therapy. We have also shown that the composition of SWF differs between two of the molecular subtypes of BC: luminal A and luminal B. In our study, we focused on quantitative analysis of individual SWF samples collected 48 h after BCS (Table 1).

Table 1. Role of immuno-modulatory molecules significantly changed in surgical wound fluids from BCS and IORT patients.

Molecule	Mechanism	Reference
CTACK	Regulates T cell recruitment under homeostatic and inflammatory conditions	[5]
G-CSF	Controls the maturation of neutrophils	[8]
HGF	Induces cancer cell migration and invasion, wound healing, angiogenesis	[21]
IL-1 beta	Inhibits the proliferation of some cancers, amplifies the function of dendritic cells, stimulates the proliferation and differentiation of CD4, CD8 and natural killer (NK) cells, increases antibody production by lymphocytes B, and finally increases the expression of adhesion molecules on vascular endothelium	[22]
IL-12	Induction of Th1 cells	[23,24]
IL-13	Induces the activation of M2 macrophages, polarizes M2a macrophages and induces migration and invasion of breast cancer cells	[25,26]
IL-7	Development of B cells and T cells, regulation of epithelial to mesenchymal transition (EMT) process in cancer	[27,28]
IL-8	Increased the formation of primary and secondary tumor spheres, as well as the cancer stem cell phenotype in BC	[29]
MCP-1	Increases monocyte mobilization and poor survival and is involved in monocyte polarization to M2-cells	[30]
MCP-3	Attracts monocytes, dendritic cells (DCs), and activated T lymphocytes, to invasion sites	[31]
MIF	Induces myeloid-derived suppressor cells in tumor microenvironment	[32]
PDGF-beta	Regulates metastasis and vascular remodeling in cancer	[33]

Table 1. *Cont.*

Molecule	Mechanism	Reference
RANTES	Promotes breast cancer progression, contributes to monocyte migration into tumor site, induces angiogenesis, promotes matrix metalloproteinase expression	[34]
SCGF-beta	Previously not reported in cancer	
TNF	Pleiotropic cytokine, stimulates survival, proliferation, migration, and angiogenesis; induces apoptosis and inhibits proliferation	[35–37]

The levels of cytokines in SWF from patients with benign breast lesions and breast cancer of different histopathological types and grades has already been investigated by Lyon et al. [38]. However, the difference between SWFs collected from cases of the luminal A, and luminal B molecular subtypes of BC have not been previously studied. An analysis comprising a comparison of the cytokines in SWF collected from IORT treated patients with those in the SWF of BCS patients has also never been performed. The approaches of the groups mentioned above differ significantly from ours, however. Firstly, the IORT patients in Belletti's study were treated in TARGIT trial, where 50 keV photon energy was used to deliver a dose of 20 Gy to the tumor bed. Secondly, a global analysis of cytokines was performed on pooled patient samples, and finally, patients were not grouped based on histopathological type or grading. Moreover, little of the presented data was based on quantitative analysis. In the studies conducted by Belletti et al., the authors named 10 cytokines to be increased by TARGIT and 20 to be decreased by TARGIT. Among these were cytokines which were also found to differ between groups in our studies. Cytokines which were found to be reduced after IORT treatment in both Belletti's work and ours include IL-7, MCP-1 (only in the luminal B subtype in our study), RANTES, PDGF-BB, and IL-8. Among the cytokines of increased concentration, only G-CSF was found in both studies. We found differences between several cytokines in the two studies: HGF and MIP-1 alpha were decreased in Belletti's studies, whereas we found a significant increase in their concentration in the IORT treated group compared to BCS only, and IL-13 which was increased in TARGIT patients but significantly decreased in our study. The discrepancies of those results may be caused by the different radiation doses used, different energy, and the selection of the study group. An essential feature of our work is the fact that the SWF samples were analyzed individually. Although sample pooling can be an attractive approach in proteomic analysis, it can also introduce errors and biases for broadly heterogenic samples. As we and others confirmed, the profile of cytokines differs significantly due to grading, histopathological type, molecular subtype, and lymph node status. Those features should be taken into consideration while performing proteomic analyses on patients' samples.

IL-8, the level of which was significantly decreased after IORT treatment, is a pro-inflammatory chemokine which plays an important role in tumor progression and metastasis in a variety of human cancers. It is also often associated with epithelial to mesenchymal transition and cancer stem cell features of breast cancer cells [39,40]. Studies of Charafe-Jauffret et al. on breast cancer cell lines [41] revealed that IL-8 treatment increased the formation of primary and secondary tumorospheres in a dose-dependent manner, as well as the cancer stem cell phenotype measured by aldehyde dehydrogenase (ALDH) activity. Moreover, IL-8 has also been implicated in the promotion of angiogenesis in endothelial cells, facilitating the development of cancer [29]. Epithelial to mesenchymal transition is associated with the increased invasive capacity of cancer cells and thus promotes tumor infiltration, growth, and metastasis. We have previously demonstrated that SWF stimulates the CSC phenotype and EMT program in breast cancer cell lines [14]. This effect was partially abolished when the cells were incubated in SWF collected from IORT treated patients. In this study, we showed a significant decrease of IL-8 after IORT treatment. Thus, our results agree with previously published papers, indicating that higher IL-8 concentrations correlate with EMT and CSC phenotype. Moreover, we have shown that intraoperative radiotherapy decreases the IL-8 concentration and thus EMT and CSC. The exact relationship between

IL-8-IORT-EMT/CSC needs further study, however. It is also important to point out that, in the work of Belletti et al., IL-8 concentration was also reduced in SWF from IORT treated patients.

IL-13 is another cytokine which we confirmed to be greatly reduced in SWF collected from patients after IORT treatment (Figures 1 and 5). IL-13 induces the activation of M2 macrophages. These cells are responsible for the promotion of inflammation, which induces angiogenesis and tissue remodeling [25]. M2 macrophages have also been implicated in tumor growth [42,43], and their presence has been correlated with a poor prognosis [44]. Recent data published by Little et al. showed that IL-4/IL-13 polarizes M2a macrophages and induces migration and invasion of breast cancer cells [26]. Based on those findings, we can assume that IORT treatment may be beneficial not only but direct tumor cell killing but also in changing the tumor bed microenvironment, making it less favorable for tumor recurrence due to decreased concentration of tumor-facilitating cytokines.

Haabeth et al. discovered that tumor-suppressive inflammation is regulated by a small number of cytokines, early in the immune response [22]. They pointed out that cancer-related inflammation processes cannot be seen as solely negative or positive. Based on their findings, as well as other data in the literature, they suggest that some of the well-known pro-inflammatory cytokines may either be cancer-suppressive or cancer-promoting [22,45]. In our study, we found increased concentrations of Il-12(p40), Il-1 beta and TNF-alpha in SWF from the luminal A subtype of BC in the group treated with IORT compared to BCS. IL-12 is known to stimulate Th1-dominant immunity, and thus has a strong anti-tumor activity [46]. It stimulates cytotoxic T lymphocytes and Th1 cells to produce IFN-γ, which inhibits the tumor cell cycle [45]. IL-12(p40) is the most important cytokine in the induction of Th1 cells. It has been suggested that activation of Th1 cells may be especially beneficial against cancer [23,24]. Th1 cells can induce the secretion of IL-1 beta and TNF-alpha by M1 macrophages and thus suppress the tumor. It has been proposed that IL-1 beta inhibits the proliferation of some cancers; amplifies the function of dendritic cells; stimulates the proliferation and differentiation of CD4, CD8, and NK cells; increases antibody production by lymphocytes B and finally increases the expression of adhesion molecules on vascular endothelium thus promoting the migration of leukocytes (reviewed in [22]).

The concentration of IL-1 beta is very high 24 h after surgery and decreases daily thereafter. It is one of the major cytokines present in SWF after surgery, especially in patients after neoadjuvant chemotherapy [9]. Agresti et al. also found a higher concentration of this cytokine in patients after radical mastectomy than in those after quadrantectomy [8].

TNF (tumor necrosis factor) has an important role in the tumor microenvironment. It is a pleiotropic cytokine which could be either pro- or anti-tumorigenic. On the one hand, it is connected to tumor promotion by stimulating survival, proliferation, migration, and angiogenesis in most cancer cells that are resistant to TNF-induced cytotoxicity [35,36,47]. However, TNF, by acting directly on cancer cells, can induce apoptosis and inhibit proliferation, processes that could be used for cancer therapy [37,48]. We have previously shown that SWF from patients treated by IORT significantly stimulates the apoptotic pathway in the luminal A subtype of breast cancer cells by activating the TNF-induced extrinsic apoptotic pathway [49].

In our study, we analyzed the composition of SWF not only dependent on the type of treatment (BCS or BCS followed by IORT), but also on two molecular subtypes—luminal A and luminal B—which have not been studied before in this context. The 10-year follow up of the clinical trial, "Intraoperative tumor bed boost with electrons in breast cancer", revealed that two analyzed parameters: metastasis-free survival and overall survival in the luminal B subtype of BC are significantly lower compared to the luminal A subtype [50]. Our small molecules analysis revealed that the concentration of HGF, SCF, MCP-1, and MCP-3 differed significantly between SWF samples from luminal A and luminal B subtype patients after BCS followed by IORT. The MCP-1 and MCP-3 concentrations correlate with TNM stage of breast cancer patients, as shown by Wang et al [9]. They found that MCP-1 concentration decreases with TNM staging, the higher the lymph node status, the lower the concentration, while MCP-3 increases with TNM staging (the highest in T2). While in our studies we did not see any changes in inflammatory chemokine MCP-1 (CCL2) concentrations between BCS and the IORT group

(Figure 1), more detailed analysis based on BC subtypes revealed significant differences. In the luminal A subtype, we observed a higher concentration of this chemokine in the IORT group than in the BCS group while in luminal B, the effect of IORT treatment was the opposite. As shown by Feng et al. [51], in breast cancer patients, high levels of MCP-1 correlates with increased monocyte mobilization and poor survival. Moreover, MCP-1 may also be involved in monocyte polarization to M2-cells [30]. A recent finding by Valeta-Magara et al. [39] showed that M2 macrophages are also associated with highly aggressive breast cancer—inflammatory breast cancer—which is characterized by a high percentage of cancer stem cells and increased mesenchymal features.

4. Materials and Methods

4.1. Surgical Wound Fluids Collection

Surgical wound fluids were collected as previously described [14]. Shortly, SWF were collected continuously for up to 48 h after BCS from BC patients. This time point was chosen as most of the drainages from patients after BCS in Greater Poland Cancer Center are usually collected at this time. Drainages are collected 24 h after BCS only if a high quantity of SWF is produced. Following tumor resection, one group of patients (denominated IORT group) underwent IORT boost (up to 10 Gy) to the tumor bed. For this procedure dedicated treatment accelerator Mobetron®from IntraOp®is used. This accelerator can produce a four treatment beams of electrons with energies 4,6,9, and 12 MeV and with dose rate about 1000 MU/min (usually 9 MeV is used). The therapeutic range is up to 4 cm tissue thickness. 10 Gy dose is delivered to the 90% isodose. The applicator (field size) is selected individually for each patient. Irradiated volume must contain tumor bed with resection margin (high-risk areas). The second group of patients did not receive IORT (BCS group). SWF were collected to drainage bottles, centrifuged for 25 min at 300 × g at 4 °C, sterile filtered and stored at −80 °C. The study was approved by the Bioethics Committee of Poznań University of Medical Sciences, study number 756/16.

4.2. Study Group

The study group was firstly divided into two groups based on the treatment scheme (BCS and IORT, see above). The BCS group consisted of 18 patients, and IORT—20 patients of both luminal A (ER receptor positive, PR receptor +/−, Her2−, Ki67 < 20) and luminal B subtype (ER receptor positive, PR receptor +/−, Her2−/+, Ki67 ≥ 20. We focused on these two molecular subtypes, as most of the IORT treated patients in Greater Poland Cancer Center are classified to those subtypes. None of the patients classified to the study underwent neoadjuvant therapy or had any incidence of earlier cancer. Each SWF sample was analyzed twice. For the analysis, we did not include SWF from ER−, PR−, HER+, and triple-negative subtypes of BC. Moreover, all patients were chosen based on histological subtype (all were classified as NST) and similar TNM status: T1, N0, or N1. In further statistical analysis, we classified patients from each treatment group to corresponding molecular subtype of BC: luminal A and luminal B. Histopathological and molecular classification of BC patients included in this study was done according to Fourth Edition of WHO Classification of Tumors of the Breast and current CAP/ASCO guidelines, respectively. Detailed patients' characteristics are shown in Table 2.

4.3. Analysis of SWF Composition

The composition of SWF was analyzed on the Bio-Plex 200 system (BioRad Laboratories, Hercules, CA, USA). We took used Bio-Plex Pro Human Cytokine 48-plex, to analyze cytokines, chemokines, and growth factors that may be involved in the inflammation process, initiation, and progression of cancer. The benefit of this system is the quantitative and qualitative analysis of 48 small molecules in one sample. The concentrations (pg/ml) of analyzed molecules are compared to the standard curve of serial dilutions of standard molecules. The analysis was performed according to the manufacturer's instructions. Each SWF sample was analyzed in technical duplicate.

Table 2. Patients' characteristics.

Feature	BCS Group (n = 18)	IORT Group (n = 20)
Age	61.6 ± 10.1	61.5 ± 12.2
Luminal subtype		
A	8	8
B	10	12
Her2 positive	3	5
Lymph node status		
N0	11	11
N1	7	9
T1 classification		
a	0	1
b	5	6
c	13	13

4.4. Statistical Analysis

Statistical analyses were performed using the GraphPad Prism software program, v.6 (GraphPad Software, Inc., La Jolla, CA, USA). As the data (pg/ml) did not follow Gaussian distribution, they were examined using Mann–Whitney test (comparing BCS versus IORT group) on the Kruskal–Wallis test. $p < 0.05$ was considered to indicate a statistically significant difference. The means of technical duplicates were visualized as box plots (median and whiskers) presenting concentration of cytokines (pg/ml). Whiskers were calculated using Tukey method based on GraphPad Prism software. Outliners are shown as dots. * $p < 0.05$, ** $p < 0.01$, *** $p < 0.001$: based on Mann–Whitney or Kruskal–Wallis test with Dunn's post hoc multiple comparison test. Heatmaps displaying median concentrations of analyzed cytokines were prepared in GraphPad Prism. The cut-offs were adjusted empirically to visualize changes (if present) both at the top and bottom of the heatmap.

5. Conclusions

In this study, we have conducted the quantitative analysis of SWF composition in BC patients treated with BCS only, and BCS followed by IORT. While choosing the study group, we also considered the molecular subtype of breast cancer: luminal A and luminal B. The performed analysis revealed changes based not only on the applied treatment but also on the molecular subtype of BC. We found many cytokines, which are believed to have anti-tumor properties, to be highly expressed in luminal A subtype of breast cancer in IORT treated group. What is interesting, we also found significant differences in the composition of SWF collected from IORT treated patients with tumors of different molecular subtypes.

Based on those findings we can assume that IORT treatment may be beneficial in changing tumor bed microenvironment in addition to direct killing of residual cancer cells. IORT makes tumor microenvironment less favorable for tumor recurrence due to decreased concentration of tumor-facilitating cytokines, especially in luminal A subtype of BC. By correlating the long-term results of IOERT as a boost in the breast cancer [19] and results presented in this study, we can speculate, that changes in tumor microenvironment due to different cytokine concentration may have an impact on metastasis-free survival of BC patients after IORT. In relation to this, we also confirmed the decreased concentration of cytokines connected to EMT and CSC in IORT treated patients, which confirms our previously published results of in vitro experiments showing lower EMT and CSC phenotype in BC cells treated with SWF from IORT [14].

Author Contributions: Conceptualization, K.K.; Formal analysis, K.K.; Funding acquisition, K.K. and W.M.S.; Investigation, K.K., J.P.W., and I.P.; Methodology, K.K. and I.P.; Project administration, K.K. and W.M.S.; Resources, J.P.W. and J.W.; Supervision, W.M.S.; Validation, K.K. and I.P.; Visualization, K.K., J.P.W., and J.W.; Writing—original draft, K.K.; Writing—review and editing, K.K., I.P., J.P.W., and W.M.S. All authors have read and agreed to the published version of the manuscript.

References

1. Veronesi, U.; Marubini, E.; Del Vecchio, M.; Manzari, A.; Andreola, S.; Greco, M.; Luini, A.; Merson, M.; Saccozzi, R.; Rilke, F.; et al. Local recurrences and distant metastases after conservative breast cancer treatments: Partly independent events. *J. Natl. Cancer Inst.* **1995**, *87*, 19–27. [CrossRef] [PubMed]
2. Al-Sahaf, O.; Wang, J.H.; Browne, T.J.; Cotter, T.G.; Redmond, H.P. Surgical injury enhances the expression of genes that mediate breast cancer metastasis to the lung. *Ann. Surg.* **2010**, *252*, 1037–1043. [CrossRef] [PubMed]
3. Alieva, M.; Margarido, A.S.; Wieles, T.; Abels, E.R.; Colak, B.; Boquetale, C.; Jan Noordmans, H.; Snijders, T.J.; Broekman, M.L.; van Rheenen, J. Preventing inflammation inhibits biopsy-mediated changes in tumor cell behavior. *Sci. Rep.* **2017**, *7*, 7529. [CrossRef] [PubMed]
4. Tagliabue, E.; Agresti, R.; Carcangiu, M.L.; Ghirelli, C.; Morelli, D.; Campiglio, M.; Martel, M.; Giovanazzi, R.; Greco, M.; Balsari, A.; et al. Role of HER2 in wound-induced breast carcinoma proliferation. *Lancet* **2003**, *362*, 527–533. [CrossRef]
5. Azab, B.; Bhatt, V.R.; Phookan, J.; Murukutla, S.; Kohn, N.; Terjanian, T.; Widmann, W.D. Usefulness of the neutrophil-to-lymphocyte ratio in predicting short- and long-term mortality in breast cancer patients. *Ann. Surg. Oncol.* **2012**, *19*, 217–224. [CrossRef]
6. Ruffell, B.; Affara, N.I.; Coussens, L.M. Differential macrophage programming in the tumor microenvironment. *Trends Immunol.* **2012**, *33*, 119–126. [CrossRef]
7. Krall, J.A.; Reinhardt, F.; Mercury, O.A.; Pattabiraman, D.R.; Brooks, M.W.; Dougan, M.; Lambert, A.W.; Bierie, B.; Ploegh, H.L.; Dougan, S.K.; et al. The systemic response to surgery triggers the outgrowth of distant immune-controlled tumors in mouse models of dormancy. *Sci. Transl. Med.* **2018**, *10*. [CrossRef]
8. Agresti, R.; Triulzi, T.; Sasso, M.; Ghirelli, C.; Aiello, P.; Rybinska, I.; Campiglio, M.; Sfondrini, L.; Tagliabue, E.; Bianchi, F. Wound Healing Fluid Reflects the Inflammatory Nature and Aggressiveness of Breast Tumors. *Cells* **2019**, *8*, 181. [CrossRef]
9. Wang, D.; Hu, K.; Gao, N.; Zhang, H.; Jiang, Y.; Liu, C.; Wang, S.; Zhao, Z. High throughput screening of cytokines, chemokines and matrix metalloproteinases in wound fluid induced by mammary surgery. *Oncotarget* **2015**, *6*, 29296–29310. [CrossRef]
10. Segatto, I.; Berton, S.; Sonego, M.; Massarut, S.; Perin, T.; Piccoli, E.; Colombatti, A.; Vecchione, A.; Baldassarre, G.; Belletti, B. Surgery-induced wound response promotes stem-like and tumor-initiating features of breast cancer cells, via STAT3 signaling. *Oncotarget* **2014**, *5*, 6267–6279. [CrossRef]
11. Vaidya, J.S.; Wenz, F.; Bulsara, M.; Tobias, J.S.; Joseph, D.J.; Keshtgar, M.; Flyger, H.L.; Massarut, S.; Alvarado, M.; Saunders, C.; et al. Risk-adapted targeted intraoperative radiotherapy versus whole-breast radiotherapy for breast cancer: 5-year results for local control and overall survival from the TARGIT-A randomised trial. *Lancet* **2014**, *383*, 603–613. [CrossRef]
12. Belletti, B.; Vaidya, J.S.; D'Andrea, S.; Entschladen, F.; Roncadin, M.; Lovat, F.; Berton, S.; Perin, T.; Candiani, E.; Reccanello, S.; et al. Targeted intraoperative radiotherapy impairs the stimulation of breast cancer cell proliferation and invasion caused by surgical wounding. *Clin. Cancer Res.* **2008**, *14*, 1325–1332. [CrossRef] [PubMed]
13. Zaleska, K.; Suchorska, W.M.; Przybyla, A.; Murawa, D. Effect of surgical wound fluids after intraoperative electron radiotherapy on the cancer stem cell phenotype in a panel of human breast cancer cell lines. *Oncol. Lett.* **2016**, *12*, 3707–3714. [CrossRef] [PubMed]
14. Kulcenty, K.; Piotrowski, I.; Zaleska, K.; Wichtowski, M.; Wroblewska, J.; Murawa, D.; Suchorska, W.M. Wound fluids collected postoperatively from patients with breast cancer induce epithelial to mesenchymal transition but intraoperative radiotherapy impairs this effect by activating the radiation-induced bystander effect. *Sci. Rep.* **2019**, *9*, 7891. [CrossRef]
15. Piotrowski, I.; Kulcenty, K.; Murawa, D.; Suchorska, W. Surgical wound fluids from patients treated with intraoperative radiotherapy induce radiobiological response in breast cancer cells. *Med. Oncol.* **2018**, *36*, 14. [CrossRef]

16. Veronesi, U.; Cascinelli, N.; Mariani, L.; Greco, M.; Saccozzi, R.; Luini, A.; Aguilar, M.; Marubini, E. Twenty-year follow-up of a randomized study comparing breast-conserving surgery with radical mastectomy for early breast cancer. *N. Engl. J. Med.* **2002**, *347*, 1227–1232. [CrossRef]
17. Veronesi, U.; Marubini, E.; Mariani, L.; Galimberti, V.; Luini, A.; Veronesi, P.; Salvadori, B.; Zucali, R. Radiotherapy after breast-conserving surgery in small breast carcinoma: Long-term results of a randomized trial. *Ann. Oncol.* **2001**, *12*, 997–1003. [CrossRef]
18. Piotrowski, I.; Kulcenty, K.; Wichtowski, M.; Murawa, D.; Suchorska, W. Intraoperative Radiotherapy of Breast Cancer and Its Biological Effects. *Breast Care* **2017**, *12*, 109–113. [CrossRef]
19. Kaiser, J.; Reitsamer, R.; Kopp, P.; Gaisberger, C.; Kopp, M.; Fischer, T.; Zehentmayr, F.; Sedlmayer, F.; Fastner, G. Intraoperative Electron Radiotherapy (IOERT) in the Treatment of Primary Breast Cancer. *Breast Care* **2018**, *13*, 162–167. [CrossRef]
20. Meng, G.; Wuest, M.; Tang, X.; Dufour, J.; Zhao, Y.; Curtis, J.M.; McMullen, T.P.W.; Murray, D.; Wuest, F.; Brindley, D.N. Repeated Fractions of X-Radiation to the Breast Fat Pads of Mice Augment Activation of the Autotaxin-Lysophosphatidate-Inflammatory Cycle. *Cancers* **2019**, *11*, 1816. [CrossRef]
21. Xiang, C.; Chen, J.; Fu, P. HGF/Met Signaling in Cancer Invasion: The Impact on Cytoskeleton Remodeling. *Cancers* **2017**, *9*, 44. [CrossRef]
22. Haabeth, O.A.; Bogen, B.; Corthay, A. A model for cancer-suppressive inflammation. *Oncoimmunology* **2012**, *1*, 1146–1155. [CrossRef] [PubMed]
23. Shankaran, V.; Ikeda, H.; Bruce, A.T.; White, J.M.; Swanson, P.E.; Old, L.J.; Schreiber, R.D. IFNgamma and lymphocytes prevent primary tumour development and shape tumour immunogenicity. *Nature* **2001**, *410*, 1107–1111. [CrossRef]
24. Haabeth, O.A.; Lorvik, K.B.; Hammarstrom, C.; Donaldson, I.M.; Haraldsen, G.; Bogen, B.; Corthay, A. Inflammation driven by tumour-specific Th1 cells protects against B-cell cancer. *Nat. Commun.* **2011**, *2*, 240. [CrossRef]
25. Murray, P.J.; Allen, J.E.; Biswas, S.K.; Fisher, E.A.; Gilroy, D.W.; Goerdt, S.; Gordon, S.; Hamilton, J.A.; Ivashkiv, L.B.; Lawrence, T.; et al. Macrophage activation and polarization: Nomenclature and experimental guidelines. *Immunity* **2014**, *41*, 14–20. [CrossRef] [PubMed]
26. Little, A.C.; Pathanjeli, P.; Wu, Z.; Bao, L.; Goo, L.E.; Yates, J.A.; Oliver, C.R.; Soellner, M.B.; Merajver, S.D. IL-4/IL-13 Stimulated Macrophages Enhance Breast Cancer Invasion Via Rho-GTPase Regulation of Synergistic VEGF/CCL-18 Signaling. *Front. Oncol.* **2019**, *9*, 456. [CrossRef]
27. Seol, M.A.; Kim, J.H.; Oh, K.; Kim, G.; Seo, M.W.; Shin, Y.K.; Sim, J.H.; Shin, H.M.; Seo, B.Y.; Lee, D.S.; et al. Interleukin-7 Contributes to the Invasiveness of Prostate Cancer Cells by Promoting Epithelial-Mesenchymal Transition. *Sci. Rep.* **2019**, *9*, 6917. [CrossRef] [PubMed]
28. Lin, J.; Zhu, Z.; Xiao, H.; Wakefield, M.R.; Ding, V.A.; Bai, Q.; Fang, Y. The role of IL-7 in Immunity and Cancer. *Anticancer Res.* **2017**, *37*, 963–967.
29. Vegran, F.; Boidot, R.; Michiels, C.; Sonveaux, P.; Feron, O. Lactate influx through the endothelial cell monocarboxylate transporter MCT1 supports an NF-kappaB/IL-8 pathway that drives tumor angiogenesis. *Cancer Res.* **2011**, *71*, 2550–2560. [CrossRef]
30. Roca, H.; Varsos, Z.S.; Sud, S.; Craig, M.J.; Ying, C.; Pienta, K.J. CCL2 and interleukin-6 promote survival of human CD11b+ peripheral blood mononuclear cells and induce M2-type macrophage polarization. *J. Biol. Chem.* **2009**, *284*, 34342–34354. [CrossRef]
31. Liu, Y.; Cai, Y.; Liu, L.; Wu, Y.; Xiong, X. Crucial biological functions of CCL7 in cancer. *Peer J.* **2018**, *6*, e4928. [CrossRef] [PubMed]
32. Simpson, K.D.; Templeton, D.J.; Cross, J.V. Macrophage migration inhibitory factor promotes tumor growth and metastasis by inducing myeloid-derived suppressor cells in the tumor microenvironment. *J. Immunol.* **2012**, *189*, 5533–5540. [CrossRef] [PubMed]
33. Hosaka, K.; Yang, Y.; Seki, T.; Nakamura, M.; Andersson, P.; Rouhi, P.; Yang, X.; Jensen, L.; Lim, S.; Feng, N.; et al. Tumour PDGF-BB expression levels determine dual effects of anti-PDGF drugs on vascular remodelling and metastasis. *Nat. Commun.* **2013**, *4*, 2129. [CrossRef] [PubMed]
34. Azenshtein, E.; Luboshits, G.; Shina, S.; Neumark, E.; Shahbazian, D.; Weil, M.; Wigler, N.; Keydar, I.; Ben-Baruch, A. The CC chemokine RANTES in breast carcinoma progression: Regulation of expression and potential mechanisms of promalignant activity. *Cancer Res.* **2002**, *62*, 1093–1102.

35. Arnott, C.H.; Scott, K.A.; Moore, R.J.; Hewer, A.; Phillips, D.H.; Parker, P.; Balkwill, F.R.; Owens, D.M. Tumour necrosis factor-alpha mediates tumour promotion via a PKC alpha- and AP-1-dependent pathway. *Oncogene* **2002**, *21*, 4728–4738. [CrossRef]
36. Kulbe, H.; Thompson, R.; Wilson, J.L.; Robinson, S.; Hagemann, T.; Fatah, R.; Gould, D.; Ayhan, A.; Balkwill, F. The inflammatory cytokine tumor necrosis factor-alpha generates an autocrine tumor-promoting network in epithelial ovarian cancer cells. *Cancer Res.* **2007**, *67*, 585–592. [CrossRef]
37. Wang, L.; Du, F.; Wang, X. TNF-alpha induces two distinct caspase-8 activation pathways. *Cell* **2008**, *133*, 693–703. [CrossRef]
38. Lyon, D.E.; McCain, N.L.; Walter, J.; Schubert, C. Cytokine comparisons between women with breast cancer and women with a negative breast biopsy. *Nurs. Res.* **2008**, *57*, 51–58. [CrossRef]
39. Valeta-Magara, A.; Gadi, A.; Volta, V.; Walters, B.; Arju, R.; Giashuddin, S.; Zhong, H.; Schneider, R.J. Inflammatory Breast Cancer Promotes Development of M2 Tumor-Associated Macrophages and Cancer Mesenchymal Cells through a Complex Chemokine Network. *Cancer Res.* **2019**, *79*, 3360–3371. [CrossRef]
40. Fernando, R.I.; Castillo, M.D.; Litzinger, M.; Hamilton, D.H.; Palena, C. IL-8 signaling plays a critical role in the epithelial-mesenchymal transition of human carcinoma cells. *Cancer Res.* **2011**, *71*, 5296–5306. [CrossRef]
41. Charafe-Jauffret, E.; Ginestier, C.; Iovino, F.; Wicinski, J.; Cervera, N.; Finetti, P.; Hur, M.H.; Diebel, M.E.; Monville, F.; Dutcher, J.; et al. Breast cancer cell lines contain functional cancer stem cells with metastatic capacity and a distinct molecular signature. *Cancer Res.* **2009**, *69*, 1302–1313. [CrossRef] [PubMed]
42. Mantovani, A.; Allavena, P.; Sica, A.; Balkwill, F. Cancer-related inflammation. *Nature* **2008**, *454*, 436–444. [CrossRef] [PubMed]
43. Pollard, J.W. Tumour-educated macrophages promote tumour progression and metastasis. *Nat. Rev. Cancer* **2004**, *4*, 71–78. [CrossRef] [PubMed]
44. Qian, B.Z.; Pollard, J.W. Macrophage diversity enhances tumor progression and metastasis. *Cell* **2010**, *141*, 39–51. [CrossRef]
45. Burkholder, B.; Huang, R.Y.; Burgess, R.; Luo, S.; Jones, V.S.; Zhang, W.; Lv, Z.Q.; Gao, C.Y.; Wang, B.L.; Zhang, Y.M.; et al. Tumor-induced perturbations of cytokines and immune cell networks. *Biochim. Biophys. Acta* **2014**, *1845*, 182–201. [CrossRef]
46. Nishimura, T.; Iwakabe, K.; Sekimoto, M.; Ohmi, Y.; Yahata, T.; Nakui, M.; Sato, T.; Habu, S.; Tashiro, H.; Sato, M.; et al. Distinct role of antigen-specific T helper type 1 (Th1) and Th2 cells in tumor eradication in vivo. *J. Exp. Med.* **1999**, *190*, 617–627. [CrossRef] [PubMed]
47. Ziprin, P.; Ridgway, P.F.; Pfistermuller, K.L.; Peck, D.H.; Darzi, A.W. ICAM-1 mediated tumor-mesothelial cell adhesion is modulated by IL-6 and TNF-alpha: A potential mechanism by which surgical trauma increases peritoneal metastases. *Cell Commun. Adhes.* **2003**, *10*, 141–154. [CrossRef]
48. Kim, Y.S.; Morgan, M.J.; Choksi, S.; Liu, Z.G. TNF-induced activation of the Nox1 NADPH oxidase and its role in the induction of necrotic cell death. *Mol. Cell* **2007**, *26*, 675–687. [CrossRef]
49. Kulcenty, K.I.; Piotrowski, I.; Zaleska, K.; Murawa, D.; Suchorska, W.M. Wound fluids collected from patients after IORT treatment activates extrinsic apoptotic pathway in MCF7 breast cancer cell line. *Ginekol. Pol.* **2018**, *89*, 175–182. [CrossRef]
50. Kaiser, J.; Kronberger, C.; Moder, A.; Kopp, P.; Wallner, M.; Reitsamer, R.; Fischer, T.; Fussl, C.; Zehentmayr, F.; Sedlmayer, F.; et al. Intraoperative Tumor Bed Boost With Electrons in Breast Cancer of Clinical Stages I Through III: Updated 10-Year Results. *Int. J. Radiat. Oncol. Biol. Phys.* **2018**, *102*, 92–101. [CrossRef]
51. Feng, A.L.; Zhu, J.K.; Sun, J.T.; Yang, M.X.; Neckenig, M.R.; Wang, X.W.; Shao, Q.Q.; Song, B.F.; Yang, Q.F.; Kong, B.H.; et al. CD16+ monocytes in breast cancer patients: Expanded by monocyte chemoattractant protein-1 and may be useful for early diagnosis. *Clin. Exp. Immunol.* **2011**, *164*, 57–65. [CrossRef] [PubMed]

4

APOBEC3B Gene Expression in Ductal Carcinoma In Situ and Synchronous Invasive Breast Cancer

Anieta M. Sieuwerts [1,2,†], Shusma C. Doebar [3,†], Vanja de Weerd [1], Esther I. Verhoef [3], Corine M. Beauford [1], Marie C. Agahozo [3], John W.M. Martens [1,2] and Carolien H.M. van Deurzen [3,*]

1 Department of Medical Oncology and Erasmus MC Cancer Institute, 3015 GD Rotterdam, The Netherlands
2 Cancer Genomics Netherlands, Erasmus MC Cancer Institute, 3015 GD Rotterdam, The Netherlands
3 Department of Pathology, Erasmus MC Cancer Institute, 3015 GD Rotterdam, The Netherlands
* Correspondence: c.h.m.vandeurzen@erasmusmc.nl
† These authors contributed equally to the manuscript.

Abstract: The underlying mechanism of the progression of ductal carcinoma in situ (DCIS), a non-obligate precursor of invasive breast cancer (IBC), has yet to be elucidated. In IBC, Apolipoprotein B mRNA Editing Enzyme, Catalytic Polypeptide-Like 3B (APOBEC3B) is upregulated in a substantial proportion of cases and is associated with higher mutational load and poor prognosis. However, APOBEC3B expression has never been studied in DCIS. We performed mRNA expression analysis of *APOBEC3B* in synchronous DCIS and IBC and surrounding normal cells. RNA was obtained from 53 patients. The tumors were categorized based on estrogen receptor (ER), progesterone receptor (PR), human epidermal growth factor receptor 2 (Her2) and phosphoinositide-3-kinase, catalytic, alpha polypeptide (PIK3CA) mutation status. *APOBEC3B* mRNA levels were measured by RT-qPCR. The expression levels of paired DCIS and adjacent IBC were compared, including subgroup analyses. The normal cells expressed the lowest levels of *APOBEC3B*. No differences in expression were found between DCIS and IBC. Subgroup analysis showed that *APOBEC3B* was the highest in the ER subgroups of DCIS and IBC. While there was no difference in *APOBEC3B* between wild-type versus mutated PIK3CA DCIS, *APOBEC3B* was higher in wild-type versus PIK3CA-mutated IBC. In summary, our data show that *APOBEC3B* is already upregulated in DCIS. This suggests that APOBEC3B could already play a role in early carcinogenesis. Since APOBEC3B is a gain-of-function mutagenic enzyme, patients could benefit from the therapeutic targeting of APOBEC3B in the early non-invasive stage of breast cancer.

Keywords: APOBEC3B; gene expression; breast cancer; ductal carcinoma in situ; infiltrating breast cancer; PIK3CA

---

1. Introduction

Ductal carcinoma in situ (DCIS) is a non-obligate precursor of invasive breast cancer (IBC) [1]. This is supported by previous studies that reported a high genomic concordance of synchronous DCIS and IBC [2–4]. However, despite molecular similarities, recent in-depth genetic studies also reported specific mutations that were either restricted to the in situ or the invasive component [3,5]. Increased insight in the molecular changes during DCIS progression has the potential to reveal novel, potentially targetable drivers of progression.

A major role of Apolipoprotein B mRNA Editing Enzyme, Catalytic Polypeptide-Like 3B (APOBEC3B) has been reported in breast cancer and several other cancers [6–9]. This enzyme is a member of the APOBEC family of deaminases and is involved in DNA cytosine deaminase activity, which has diverse biological functions, including activities in the innate immune system by restricting virus replication [10]. The upregulation of APOBEC3B is correlated with increased C-to-T transitions and increased mutational load, including known driver mutations in PIK3CA and tumor protein 53 (TP53) [10–12]. *APOBEC3B* mRNA is upregulated in a substantial proportion of IBC cases and an association with poor clinical outcome has been reported in Estrogen receptor (ER)-positive subtypes [13]. In addition, we recently reported higher mRNA levels of *APOBEC3B* in breast cancer metastasis as compared to the corresponding primary tumor, which implied that breast cancer progression is associated with the upregulation of APOBEC3B [14].

In this study we investigated *APOBEC3B* mRNA expression levels in synchronous DCIS and IBC and correlated the expression with PIK3CA mutation status in order to increase our understanding regarding the expression levels of this enzyme during progression from the in situ to the invasive stage. We believe this could improve breast cancer care in the future since APOBEC3B is a gain-of-function mutagenic enzyme, so patients could potentially be treated with small molecules at a very early, non-invasive stage.

2. Results

2.1. General Clinicopathological Data

In total, 53 patients were included. Table 1 provides an overview of the clinicopathological data of all patients. The overall median age was 53 years (range 28–102 years). The majority of DCIS and IBC samples were high grade (62.3 and 54.7%, respectively). There was no difference in grade between DCIS and adjacent IBC (Fisher Exact Probability Test $p = 0.92$). Based on immunohistochemical staining, IBCs were categorized into the following five breast cancer subtype categories: ER+/PR high/Her2− ($n = 13$), ER+/PR− or low/Her2− ($n = 12$), ER+/any PR/Her2+ ($n = 11$), ER−/PR−/Her2+ ($n = 8$), or ER−/PR−/Her2− ($n = 9$).

Table 1. Clinicopathological features of patients with ductal carcinoma in situ (DCIS) and adjacent invasive breast cancer (IBC) ($n = 53$).

Characteristic	n	(%)
Age at diagnosis	53	
years, median (range)	(28–102)	
Type of surgery		
Breast-conserving surgery	24	45.3
Mastectomy	29	54.7
Grade DCIS		
1	1	49.1
2	19	39.6
3	33	7.5
Grade IBC		
1	1	49.1
2	21	39.6
3	31	7.5
Tumor size		
≤2 cm	28	49.1
>2–5 cm	21	39.6
>5 cm	4	7.5
Missing	0	3.8
Subtypes based on immunohistochemistry		
ER+/PR high/Her2−	13	24.5
ER+/PR− or low/Her2−	12	22.6
ER+/any PR/Her2+	11	20.8
ER−/PR−/Her2+	8	15.1
ER−/PR−/Her2−	9	17.0

2.2. *APOBEC3B Expression in Synchronous Normal, DCIS and IBC Cells*

Both the Kruskal-Wallis Test and the Median Test indicated that there was a significant difference ($p < 0.001$) in APOBEC3B mRNA levels between the normal controls, DCIS and IBC. APOBEC3B mRNA was lower expressed in the normal mammary epithelial tissue adjacent DCIS and IBC (unpaired Mann-Whitney *U* Test and paired Wilcoxon Signed Ranks Test $p < 0.001$) (Figure 1). There was no statistically significant difference in APOBEC3B mRNA expression between DCIS and IBC (unpaired Mann–Whitney *U* Test $p = 0.065$ (Figure 1), Wilcoxon Signed Ranks Test $p = 0.082$). (Figure 2).

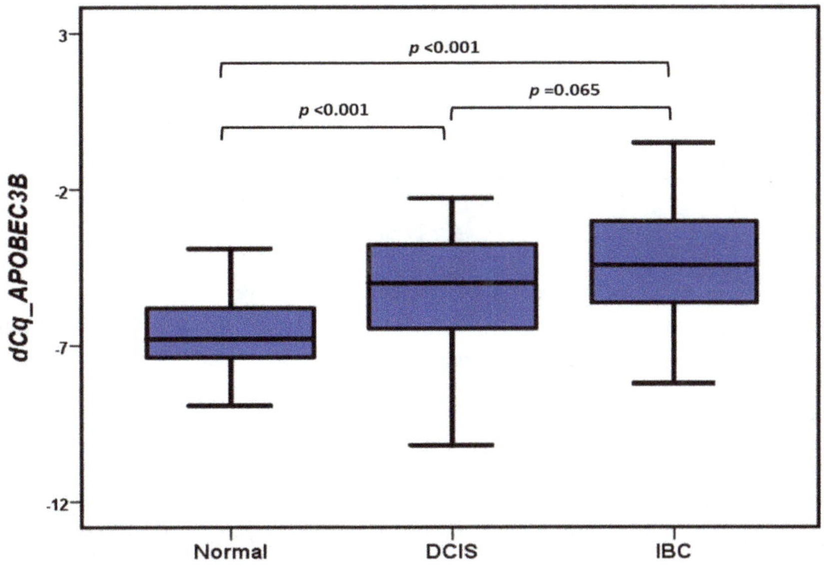

Figure 1. Boxplots of APOBEC3B mRNA expression levels in paired normal, DCIS and IBC ($n = 53$). Differences between normal, DCIS and IBC were analyzed by the Mann-Whitney *U* test.

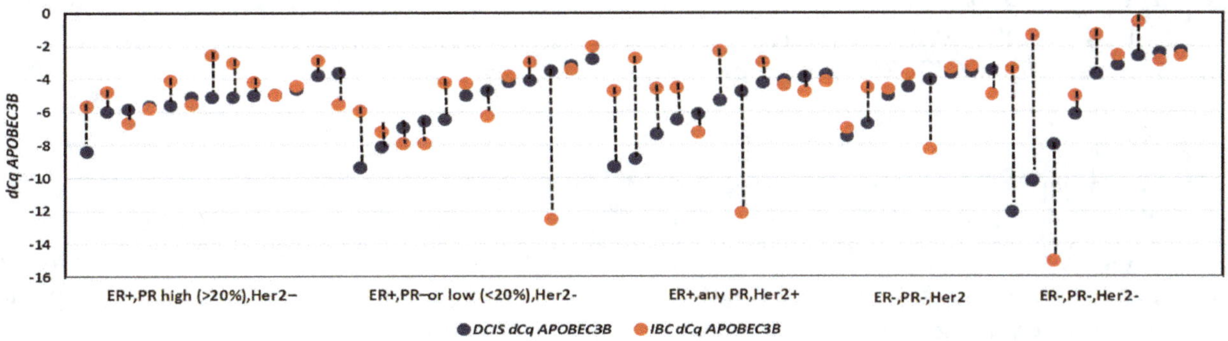

Figure 2. APOBEC3B expression levels in paired DCIS and IBC ($n = 53$). Wilcoxon Signed Ranks Test $p = 0.082$.

2.3. *APOBEC3B mRNA Subgroup Analysis*

Previous studies reported elevated *APOBEC3B* mRNA levels in breast cancers with otherwise aggressive characteristics, including high histological grade and lack of estrogen expression [7,13,15]. For both DCIS and IBC, there was no correlation between APOBEC3B expression levels and tumor diameter (Spearman Rank Correlation Test $p > 0.05$) or histological grade (Kruskal-Wallis Test $p > 0.05$). Our breast cancer subtype analysis showed that the expression of APOBEC3B was the highest in the ER− subgroup (Mann–Whitney *U* Test, $p = 0.037$) (Figure 3).

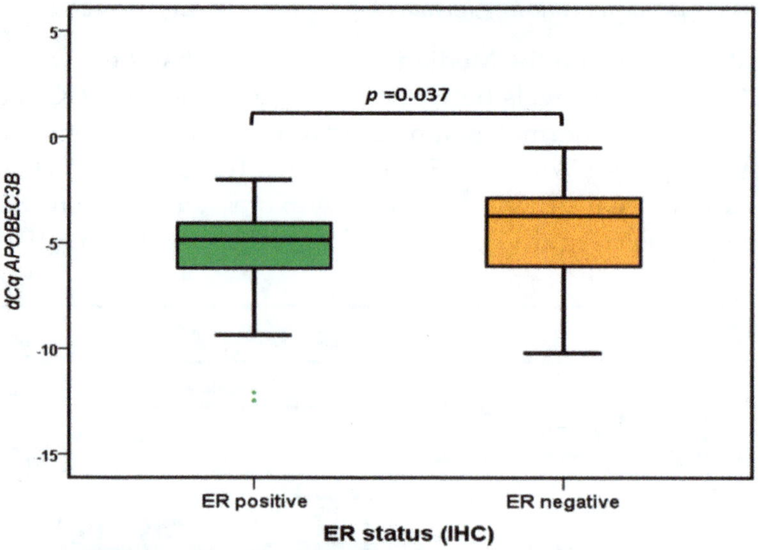

Figure 3. Boxplots of Apolipoprotein B mRNA Editing Enzyme, Catalytic Polypeptide-Like 3B (APOBEC3B) mRNA expression levels according to ER status. The difference between ER+ and ER− cases was analyzed by the Mann-Whitney *U* test.

2.4. APOBEC3B Expression in Epithelial Versus Inflammatory Cells

Based on the positive correlation between APOBEC3B and marker for epithelial content (EPCAM) mRNA levels (Spearman Rank Correlation test, $p = 0.005$ for DCIS, $p = 0.001$ for IBC), APOBEC3B mRNA was mostly expressed by epithelial cells. Of note, there was no significant difference in the levels of EPCAM mRNA between DCIS and synchronous IBC (Wilcoxon Signed Ranks Test, $p = 0.18$).

Since inflammatory cells also express APOBEC3B [16], we investigated whether the number of inflammatory cells could have biased our results by comparing Protein Tyrosine Phosphatase Receptor Type C (PTPRC, gene for the common leukocyte antigen CD45) mRNA levels from DCIS and IBC. There was no correlation between APOBEC3B and PTPRC mRNA levels (Spearman Rank Correlation test, $p = 0.18$ for DCIS and $p = 0.29$ for IBC). However, IBC expressed slightly higher levels of PTPRC when compared with DCIS (Wilcoxon Signed Ranks Test, $p = 0.023$).

2.5. APOBEC3B Expression and PIK3CA Mutation Status

In a recently published study [17], we detected a PIK3CA somatic hotspot mutation in 24.7% (18 out of 73) patients. For these 18 PIK3CA-positive patients, a significantly higher PIK3CA variant allele frequency (VAF) was detected in the DCIS component (45.8%) when compared with the synchronous IBC component (31.7%) ($p = 0.007$). For the $n = 14$ PIK3CA mutation-positive patients (26.4%) included in the current study, a significantly higher PIK3CA VAF was also detected in the DCIS component (52.3%) when compared with the synchronous IBC component (37.2%) ($p = 0.027$). The correlation of PIK3CA VAF with APOBEC3B showed a negative Spearman Rank correlation in IBC (rs = −0.33, $p = 0.001$, $n = 53$). For the DCIS cases, there was no such correlation (rs = 0.02, $p = 0.89$, $n = 53$). Analyzing these data irrespective of the degree of the PIK3CA VAF levels revealed that for the 53 patients analyzed in this study, APOBEC3B mRNA levels in IBC were significantly lower in the eight patients with exon 9 (G to A)-mutated PIK3CA when compared with the $n = 39$ wild-type PIK3CA cases (Mann-Whitney *U* test $p = 0.017$). No such difference was observed for the DCIS cases ($p = 0.28$) (Figure 4). Albeit not statistically significant, APOBEC3B mRNA levels were higher overall in the $n = 39$ PIK3CA wild-type IBC samples when compared with the PIK3CA wild-type DCIS samples (Mean ± SEM: −4.54 ± 0.36 for IBC versus −5.38 ± 0.35 for DCIS) and lower in the $n = 8$ G-to-A PIK3CA-mutated IBC samples when compared with G-to-A PIK3CA-mutated DCIS samples (Mean ± SEM: −6.52 ± 1.66 for IBC versus −6.14 ± 0.74 for DCIS). Although the majority of samples with a PIK3CA mutation were

ER+, there was no significant interaction effect between ER status and the absence or presence of the two types of tested PIK3CA mutations ($p = 0.46$ for DCIS and $p = 0.20$ for IBC).

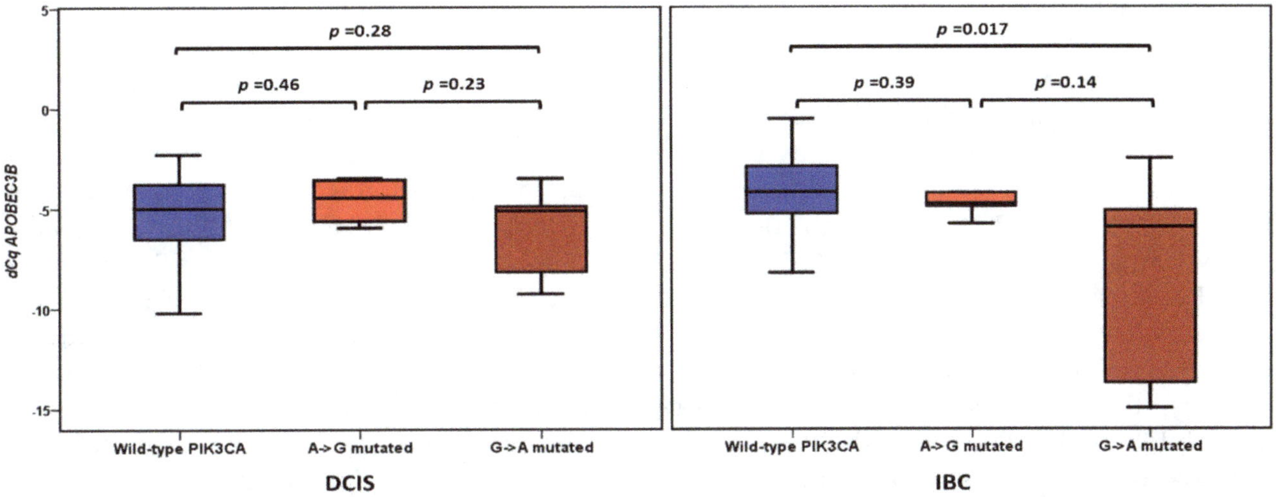

Figure 4. Boxplots of APOBEC3B mRNA expression levels according PIK3CA mutation status. The differences between wild-type (blue boxes) and mutated (red boxes) PIK3CA cases were analyzed by the Mann-Whitney *U* test.

3. Discussion

APOBEC3B has been identified as an important factor in the evolution of breast cancer [8]. In a recently published pan-tissue, pan-cancer analysis of RNA-seq data specific to the seven APOBEC3 genes in 8951 tumors, 786 cancer cell lines and 6119 normal tissues, *APOBEC3B* consistently demonstrated its association with proliferative cells and processes, in contrast to other APOBEC3s, especially *APOBEC3G* and *APOBEC3H*, which were revealed as more immune cell related [9]. Our current data showed that *APOBEC3B* mRNA is already upregulated in the in situ stage of breast cancer, which is in line with the high genomic resemblances between DCIS and IBC [18]. In a study we performed earlier, we observed higher mRNA levels of *APOBEC3B* in breast cancer metastasis as compared to the corresponding primary tumor [14], supporting our hypothesis that, already starting from DCIS, breast cancer progression is associated with deregulated expression of *APOBEC3B*.

Tumors with upregulated *APOBEC3B* demonstrate a higher mutational load, which could explain the aggressive behavior of these tumors [7,12]. Two hotspot G-to-A mutations in exon 9 of the—often mutated in breast cancer—PIK3CA gene (E542K and E545K) are thought to be generated by *APOBEC3B* induced C-to-T (G-to-A) transitions [11]. Whether *APOBEC3B* is still needed once the mutations are present needs further investigation. In the study of Kosumi et al., *APOBEC3B* expression in esophageal squamous cell carcinoma was significantly correlated with PIK3CA mutations in exon 9 [10]. However, no correlation was found between *APOBEC3B* expression and PIK3CA mutations status in a Japanese breast cancer cohort [15]. Although PIK3CA mutations are known to be more prevalent in ER+ cases [19], and thus might have been a confounder in our analysis, we found no significant difference in the distribution of wild-type and mutated PIK3CA in ER+ and ER− cases. In our cohort, *APOBEC3B* levels were decreased in specifically the G-to-A PIK3CA-mutated IBC samples when compared with wild-type PIK3CA IBC tumors. In the synchronous DCIS counterpart, however, there was no difference in *APOBEC3B* levels between mutated and PIK3CA wild-type tumors. This might suggest that, in contrast to DCIS, the invasive tumors no longer need *APOBEC3B* to proliferate and metastasize. Previous studies reported elevated *APOBEC3B* mRNA levels in breast cancers with otherwise aggressive characteristics, including high histological grade and lack of estrogen expression [7,13,15]. This is consistent with our subgroup analysis, which showed higher *APOBEC3B* levels in synchronous DCIS and IBC of ER− tumors as compared to ER+ tumors. However, in our study, no significant correlations were found between *APOBEC3B* levels and histological grade and/or tumor diameter. This could be due to the fact that the majority of our samples were high grade.

This is the first study evaluating *APOBEC3B* levels within DCIS and co-existing IBC, including different breast cancer subtypes. However, our study has several limitations, such as the relatively small size of our cohort and the analysis of a limited mRNA panel only, with the main focus on *APOBEC3B*. Since upregulated *APOBEC3B* is associated with higher mutational load, evaluation of the mutational status of additional markers besides PIK3CA will be interesting. Another limitation is that *APOBEC3B* is also expressed by inflammatory cells, which could have influenced our data because we performed manual microdissection, and thus contamination with inflammatory cells was not completely avoidable. Although IBC expressed slightly higher levels of *PTPRC* (the gene for leukocyte antigen CD45) than DCIS, there was no correlation between *APOBEC3B* and *PTPRC* mRNA levels. Based on this analysis, it seems unlikely that the number of inflammatory cells biased our data.

Increased insight in molecular mechanisms that contribute to DCIS progression will improve the development of a personalized treatment strategy for patients with DCIS. APOBEC3B could be a potential therapeutic target since it is non-essential, but it has an active enzymatic activity that may be inhibited [7]. Patients with DCIS could therefore benefit from such therapeutic molecules by inhibiting tumor evolution. Concept inhibitors have already been developed for the related enzyme APOBEC3G [20,21]. Additional clinical and pharmaceutical assays are necessary to develop and explore the potential benefit of APOBEC3B inhibitors.

4. Materials and Methods

4.1. Patient Materials

Fifty-three patients with synchronous DCIS and IBC were enrolled. We used coded leftover patient material in accordance with the Code of Conduct of the Federation of Medical Scientific Societies in the Netherlands (http://www.federa.org/codes-conduct). This article is approved by the Medical Ethics Committee of the Erasmus MC (approval number MEC 02.953). According to national guidelines, no informed consent was needed for this study.

Formalin-fixed-paraffin-embedded (FFPE) hematoxylin and eosin (H&E)-stained whole sections of excision specimens were collected and reviewed by two pathologists (Carolien H. M. van Deurzen and Shusma C. Doebar). Histopathological features included the grade of IBC [22], IBC diameter, ER, PR and Her2 status, and grade of DCIS [23]. Tumors were divided into subtypes based on immunohistochemistry (ER, PR and Her2), including the following 5 categories: ER+/PR high/Her2−; ER+/PR− or low/Her2−; ER+/any PR/Her2+; ER−/PR−/Her2+; ER−/PR−/Her2−. ER was considered positive when at least 10% of the tumor cells were positive, irrespective of intensity, according to national guidelines (https://richtlijnendatabase.nl). Low PR was defined as $\leq$ 20% [24]. Immunohistochemical HER2 expression was scored according to international guidelines [25]. Equivocal cases were evaluated by silver in situ hybridization.

4.2. RT-qPCR

RNA was extracted from tissue areas composed of at least 50% IBC or DCIS cells and analyzed by RT-qPCR as described before [14,17]. In brief, these cells were obtained by microdissection from FFPE tissue, which was performed with a sterile needle under a stereomicroscope. RNA was extracted from these cells using the Qiagen (Hamburg, Germany) AllPrep DNA/RNA FFPE Kit according the manufacturer's instructions. RNA concentrations were measured with a Nanodrop 2000 system. cDNA was generated from 50 ng/μL cDNA and was generated for 30 min at 48 °C with the RevertAid H minus kit (Thermo Fisher Scientific, Breda, The Netherlands) and gene-specific pre-amplified with Taqman PreAmp Master mix (Thermo Fisher Scientific) for 15 cycles, followed by Taqman probe based real-time PCR according to the manufacturer's instructions in a MX3000P Real-Time PCR System (Agilent, Amsterdam, The Netherlands). The following intron-spanning gene expression assays (all from Thermo

Fisher Scientific) were evaluated: *APOBEC3B*, assay ID: hs00358981_m1; *EPCAM*, hs00158980_m1, and *PTPRC*, hs00236304_m1. Messenger RNA levels were quantified relative to the average expression of 2 reference genes (*GUSB*, hs9999908_m1 and *HMBS*, hs00609297_m1) using the delta Cq (average Cq reference genes −Cq target gene) method. According GeNorm and NormFinder, the average of these two reference genes was the most stable expressed across our samples (M-value = 0.59, SD = 0.29). Also, when taking the different groups into account, the inter and intra variation was the lowest for the average of our 2 reference genes (SD = 0.19 for the NormFinder analysis across the control, DCIS and IBC groups and SD = 0.24 for the NormFinder analysis across the ER/PR/Her2 groups). Samples with an average reference gene expression of Cq > 25 were considered to be of insufficient RNA quality and excluded from further analysis, together with their paired samples. A serially diluted RNA pool of FFPE breast tumor samples was included in each experiment to evaluate the linear amplification and efficiencies for all genes included in the panel and absence of amplification in the absence of reverse transcriptase. All gene transcripts were equally efficient amplified (range 94–106%) and were negative in the absence of reverse transcriptase. A summary of the performance of our assays on these serially diluted samples is shown in Supplementary Table S1.

4.3. *PIK3CA Mutation Status*

PIK3CA mutation status and VAFs were measured as described before [17]. In brief, DNA was extracted from the same micro-dissected FFPE tissues used for RNA extraction using the Qiagen (Hamburg, Germany) AllPrep DNA/RNA FFPE Kit. The SNaPshot Multiplex System for SNP Genotyping (Thermo Fisher Scientific) was used to identify samples positive for PIK3CA hotspot mutations in exon 9 and exon 20. Next, we used digital PCR (dPCR) to validate the SNaPshot results and quantify the relative number of PIK3CA-mutated copies (of E542K, E545K in exon 9 and H1047R and H1047L in exon 20) in both the DCIS and IBC component of those patients with a PIK3CA mutation identified by SNaPshot analysis.

4.4. *Statistical Analyses*

GeNorm and NormFinder [26,27], present in GenEx qPCR data analysis software (version 6.1, MultiD, Götenborg, Sweden), were used to assess the stability of our reference genes. SPSS version 24 was used for the statistical analyses. Because our APOBEC3B mRNA data were not normally distributed (skewness −1.01 ± 0.33 and −1.75 ± 0.33, kurtosis 0.80 ± 0.64 and 3.60 ± 0.64 for DCIS and IBC, respectively), we only used non-parametric tests. The Wilcoxon Signed Ranks Test was used to compare levels in paired DCIS and IBC and unpaired analyses were performed using the Wilcoxon or Mann-Whitney *U* Test or the Fisher Exact Probability Test for contingency tabled data. Continuous variables were analyzed by the Spearman Rank Correlation test. *p*-values ≤ 0.05 were considered statistically significant.

5. Conclusions

In conclusion, our results indicate that *APOBEC3B* mRNA is similarly upregulated in DCIS and IBC, but declines in PIK3CA-mutated IBC, which suggests that APOBEC3B plays a role in the early stages of breast carcinogenesis. Since APOBEC3B is a gain-of-function mutagenic enzyme, it could be a candidate for therapeutic targeting in an early, non-invasive stage of breast cancer.

Author Contributions: Conceptualization, A.M.S., S.C.D. and C.H.M.v.D. Methodology, A.M.S., S.C.D., E.I.V., V.d.W., C.M.B., M.C.A. and C.H.M.v.D.; Formal analysis, A.M.S.; Validation, S.C.D., C.H.M.v.D. Writing—Original Draft Preparation, A.M.S. and S.C.D.; Writing—Review and Editing, A.M.S., S.C.D., J.M.W.M. and C.H.M.v.D.; Visualization, A.M.S.; Supervision, J.W.M.M. and C.H.M.v.D. All co-authors have read and approved of the manuscript and acknowledge their contributions.

Acknowledgments: A.M.S. was supported by Cancer Genomics Netherlands (CGC.nl) funded by the Netherlands Organization for Scientific Research (NWO).

References

1. Cowell, C.F.; Weigelt, B.; Sakr, R.A.; Ng, C.K.; Hicks, J.; King, T.A.; Reis-Filho, J.S. Progression from ductal carcinoma in situ to invasive breast cancer: Revisited. *Mol. Oncol.* **2013**, *7*, 859–869. [CrossRef] [PubMed]
2. Casasent, A.K.; Edgerton, M.; Navin, N.E. Genome evolution in ductal carcinoma in situ: Invasion of the clones. *J. Pathol.* **2017**, *241*, 208–218. [CrossRef] [PubMed]
3. Kim, S.Y.; Jung, S.H.; Kim, M.S.; Baek, I.P.; Lee, S.H.; Kim, T.M.; Chung, Y.J.; Lee, S.H. Genomic differences between pure ductal carcinoma in situ and synchronous ductal carcinoma in situ with invasive breast cancer. *Oncotarget* **2015**, *6*, 7597–7607. [CrossRef] [PubMed]
4. Casasent, A.K.; Schalck, A.; Gao, R.; Sei, E.; Long, A.; Pangburn, W.; Casasent, T.; Meric-Bernstam, F.; Edgerton, M.E.; Navin, N.E. Multiclonal Invasion in Breast Tumors Identified by Topographic Single Cell Sequencing. *Cell* **2018**, *172*, 205–217.e12. [CrossRef] [PubMed]
5. Hernandez, L.; Wilkerson, P.M.; Lambros, M.B.; Campion-Flora, A.; Rodrigues, D.N.; Gauthier, A.; Cabral, C.; Pawar, V.; Mackay, A.; A'Hern, R.; et al. Genomic and mutational profiling of ductal carcinomas in situ and matched adjacent invasive breast cancers reveals intra-tumour genetic heterogeneity and clonal selection. *J. Pathol.* **2012**, *227*, 42–52. [CrossRef] [PubMed]
6. Smith, H.C.; Bennett, R.P.; Kizilyer, A.; McDougall, W.M.; Prohaska, K.M. Functions and regulation of the APOBEC family of proteins. *Semin. Cell Dev. Biol.* **2012**, *23*, 258–268. [CrossRef] [PubMed]
7. Roberts, S.A.; Lawrence, M.S.; Klimczak, L.J.; Grimm, S.A.; Fargo, D.; Stojanov, P.; Kiezun, A.; Kryukov, G.V.; Carter, S.L.; Saksena, G.; et al. An APOBEC cytidine deaminase mutagenesis pattern is widespread in human cancers. *Nat. Genet.* **2013**, *45*, 970–976. [CrossRef]
8. Harris, R.S. Molecular mechanism and clinical impact of APOBEC3B-catalyzed mutagenesis in breast cancer. *Breast Cancer Res.* **2015**, *17*, 8. [CrossRef]
9. Ng, J.C.F.; Quist, J.; Grigoriadis, A.; Malim, M.H.; Fraternali, F. Pan-cancer transcriptomic analysis dissects immune and proliferative functions of APOBEC3 cytidine deaminases. *Nucleic Acids Res.* **2019**, *47*, 1178–1194. [CrossRef]
10. Kosumi, K.; Baba, Y.; Ishimoto, T.; Harada, K.; Nakamura, K.; Ohuchi, M.; Kiyozumi, Y.; Izumi, D.; Tokunaga, R.; Taki, K.; et al. APOBEC3B is an enzymatic source of molecular alterations in esophageal squamous cell carcinoma. *Med. Oncol.* **2016**, *33*, 26. [CrossRef]
11. Henderson, S.; Chakravarthy, A.; Su, X.; Boshoff, C.; Fenton, T.R. APOBEC-mediated cytosine deamination links PIK3CA helical domain mutations to human papillomavirus-driven tumor development. *Cell Rep.* **2014**, *7*, 1833–1841. [CrossRef] [PubMed]
12. Burns, M.B.; Lackey, L.; Carpenter, M.A.; Rathore, A.; Land, A.M.; Leonard, B.; Refsland, E.W.; Kotandeniya, D.; Tretyakova, N.; Nikas, J.B.; et al. APOBEC3B is an enzymatic source of mutation in breast cancer. *Nature* **2013**, *494*, 366–370. [CrossRef] [PubMed]
13. Sieuwerts, A.M.; Willis, S.; Burns, M.B.; Look, M.P.; Meijer-Van Gelder, M.E.; Schlicker, A.; Heideman, M.R.; Jacobs, H.; Wessels, L.; Leyland-Jones, B.; et al. Elevated APOBEC3B correlates with poor outcomes for estrogen-receptor-positive breast cancers. *Horm. Cancer* **2014**, *5*, 405–413. [CrossRef]
14. Sieuwerts, A.M.; Schrijver, W.A.; Dalm, S.U.; de Weerd, V.; Moelans, C.B.; Ter Hoeve, N.; van Diest, P.J.; Martens, J.W.; van Deurzen, C.H. Progressive APOBEC3B mRNA expression in distant breast cancer metastases. *PLoS ONE* **2017**, *12*, e0171343. [CrossRef] [PubMed]
15. Tsuboi, M.; Yamane, A.; Horiguchi, J.; Yokobori, T.; Kawabata-Iwakawa, R.; Yoshiyama, S.; Rokudai, S.; Odawara, H.; Tokiniwa, H.; Oyama, T.; et al. APOBEC3B high expression status is associated with aggressive phenotype in Japanese breast cancers. *Breast Cancer* **2016**, *23*, 780–788. [CrossRef] [PubMed]
16. Siriwardena, S.U.; Chen, K.; Bhagwat, A.S. Functions and Malfunctions of Mammalian DNA-Cytosine Deaminases. *Chem. Rev.* **2016**, *116*, 12688–12710. [CrossRef] [PubMed]

17. Agahozo, M.C.; Sieuwerts, A.M.; Doebar, S.C.; Verhoef, E.; Beaufort, C.M.; Ruigrok-Ritstier, K.; de Weerd, V.; Sleddens, H.; Dinjens, W.N.; Martens, J.; et al. PIK3CA mutations in ductal carcinoma in situ and adjacent invasive breast cancer. *Endocr. Relat. Cancer* **2019**, *26*, 471–482. [CrossRef] [PubMed]
18. Aubele, M.; Mattis, A.; Zitzelsberger, H.; Walch, A.; Kremer, M.; Welzl, G.; Hofler, H.; Werner, M. Extensive ductal carcinoma In situ with small foci of invasive ductal carcinoma: Evidence of genetic resemblance by CGH. *Int. J. Cancer* **2000**, *85*, 82–86. [CrossRef]
19. Pang, B.; Cheng, S.; Sun, S.P.; An, C.; Liu, Z.Y.; Feng, X.; Liu, G.J. Prognostic role of PIK3CA mutations and their association with hormone receptor expression in breast cancer: A meta-analysis. *Sci. Rep.* **2014**, *4*, 6255. [CrossRef]
20. Olson, M.E.; Harris, R.S.; Harki, D.A. APOBEC Enzymes as Targets for Virus and Cancer Therapy. *Cell Chem. Biol.* **2018**, *25*, 36–49. [CrossRef]
21. Li, M.; Shandilya, S.M.; Carpenter, M.A.; Rathore, A.; Brown, W.L.; Perkins, A.L.; Harki, D.A.; Solberg, J.; Hook, D.J.; Pandey, K.K.; et al. First-in-class small molecule inhibitors of the single-strand DNA cytosine deaminase APOBEC3G. *ACS Chem. Biol.* **2012**, *7*, 506–517. [CrossRef] [PubMed]
22. Elston, C.W.; Ellis, I.O. Pathological prognostic factors in breast cancer. I. The value of histological grade in breast cancer: Experience from a large study with long-term follow-up. *Histopathology* **1991**, *19*, 403–410. [CrossRef] [PubMed]
23. Consensus Conference Committee. Consensus Conference on the classification of ductal carcinoma in situ. Thomas Jefferson University in Philadelphia, Pennsylvania, USA, Nov 1. *Cancer* **1997**, *80*, 1798–1802. [CrossRef]
24. Prat, A.; Cheang, M.C.; Martín, M.; Parker, J.S.; Carrasco, E.; Caballero, R.; Tyldesley, S.; Gelmon, K.; Bernard, P.S.; Nielsen, T.O.; et al. Prognostic significance of progesterone receptor-positive tumor cells within immunohistochemically defined luminal A breast cancer. *J. Clin. Oncol.* **2013**, *31*, 203–209. [CrossRef] [PubMed]
25. Wolff, A.C.; Hammond, M.E.; Hicks, D.G.; Dowsett, M.; McShane, L.M.; Allison, K.H.; Allred, D.C.; Bartlett, J.M.; Bilous, M.; Fitzgibbons, P.; et al. Recommendations for human epidermal growth factor receptor 2 testing in breast cancer: American Society of Clinical Oncology/College of American Pathologists clinical practice guideline update. *J. Clin. Oncol.* **2013**, *31*, 3997–4013. [CrossRef] [PubMed]
26. Andersen, C.L.; Jensen, J.L.; Orntoft, T.F. Normalization of real-time quantitative reverse transcription-PCR data: A model-based variance estimation approach to identify genes suited for normalization, applied to bladder and colon cancer data sets. *Cancer Res.* **2004**, *64*, 5245–5250. [CrossRef] [PubMed]
27. Wang, Q.; Ishikawa, T.; Michiue, T.; Zhu, B.L.; Guan, D.W.; Maeda, H. Stability of endogenous reference genes in postmortem human brains for normalization of quantitative real-time PCR data: Comprehensive evaluation using geNorm, NormFinder, and BestKeeper. *Int. J. Legal Med.* **2012**, *126*, 943–952. [CrossRef] [PubMed]

5

Therapy Landscape in Patients with Metastatic HER2-Positive Breast Cancer: Data from the PRAEGNANT Real-World Breast Cancer Registry

Michael P. Lux [1,†], Naiba Nabieva [1,†], Andreas D. Hartkopf [2], Jens Huober [3], Bernhard Volz [1], Florin-Andrei Taran [2], Friedrich Overkamp [4], Hans-Christian Kolberg [5], Peyman Hadji [6], Hans Tesch [7], Lothar Häberle [1,8], Johannes Ettl [9], Diana Lüftner [10], Markus Wallwiener [11], Volkmar Müller [12], Matthias W. Beckmann [1], Erik Belleville [13], Pauline Wimberger [14], Carsten Hielscher [15], Matthias Geberth [16], Wolfgang Abenhardt [17], Christian Kurbacher [18], Rachel Wuerstlein [19], Christoph Thomssen [20], Michael Untch [21], Peter A. Fasching [1,*], Wolfgang Janni [3], Tanja N. Fehm [22], Diethelm Wallwiener [2], Andreas Schneeweiss [11,23,†] and Sara Y. Brucker [2,†]

1 Department of Gynecology and Obstetrics, Erlangen University Hospital, Comprehensive Cancer Center Erlangen-EMN, Friedrich-Alexander University of Erlangen–Nuremberg, Universitätsstrasse 21–23, 91054 Erlangen, Germany; michael.lux@uk-erlangen.de (M.P.L.); Naiba.Nabieva@uk-erlangen.de (N.N.); bernhard.volz@uk-erlangen.de (B.V.); lothar.haeberle@uk-erlangen.de (L.H.); matthias.beckmann@uk-erlangen.de (M.W.B.)

2 Department of Obstetrics and Gynecology, University of Tübingen, 72076 Tübingen, Germany; andreas.hartkopf@uni-tuebingen.de (A.D.H.); florin-andrei.taran@med.uni-tuebingen.de (F.-A.T.); diethelm.wallwiener@med.uni-tuebingen.de (D.W.); sara.brucker@med.uni-tuebingen.de (S.Y.B.)

3 Department of Gynecology and Obstetrics, Ulm University Hospital, 89070 Ulm, Germany; jens.huober@uniklinik-ulm.de (J.H.); wolfgang.janni@uniklinik-ulm.de (W.J.)

4 Oncologianova GmbH, 45657 Recklinghausen, Germany; overkamp@oncoconsult.onmicrosoft.com

5 Marienhospital Bottrop, 46236 Bottrop, Germany; hans-christian.kolberg@mhb-bottrop.de

6 Department of Bone Oncology, Nordwest Hospital, 60488 Frankfurt, Germany; hadji.peyman@khnw.de

7 Oncology Practice at Bethanien Hospital Frankfurt; 60389 Frankfurt, Germany; hans.tesch@chop-studien.de

8 Department of Gynecology and Obstetrics, Biostatistics Unit, Erlangen University Hospital, 91054 Erlangen, Germany

9 Department of Obstetrics and Gynecology, Klinikum rechts der Isar, Technical University of Munich, 81675 Munich, Germany; johannes.ettl@tum.de

10 Charité University Hospital, Berlin, Campus Benjamin Franklin, Department of Hematology, Oncology and Tumour Immunology, 12203 Berlin, Germany; diana.lueftner@charite.de

11 Department of Obstetrics and Gynecology, University of Heidelberg, 69120 Heidelberg, Germany; markus.wallwiener@gmail.com (M.W.); andreas.schneeweiss@med.uni-heidelberg.de (A.S.)

12 Department of Gynecology, Hamburg-Eppendorf University Medical Center, 20246 Hamburg, Germany; v.mueller@uke.de

13 ClinSol GmbH & Co KG, 97074 Würzburg, Germany; belleville@clin-sol.com

14 Department of Gynecology and Obstetrics, Dresden University Hospital, 01307 Dresden, Germany; pauline.wimberger@uniklinikum-dresden.de

15 gSUND Gynäkologie Kompetenzzentrum Stralsund, 18435 Stralsund, Germany; hielscher@gyn-stralsund.de

16 Gynäkologische Praxisklinik am Rosengarten, 68165 Mannheim, Germany; mail@mgeberth.de

17 Medizinischen Versorgungszentrum Onkologie, Onkologie im Elisenhof, 80335 Munich, Germany; abenhardt@t-online.de

18 Department of Gynecology and Obstetrics, Medizinisches Zentrum Bonn Friedensplatz, 53111 Bonn, Germany; kurbacher@web.de

19 Department of Gynecology and Obstetrics, Breast Center and Comprehensive Cancer Center Munich, Munich University Hospital, 80337 Munich, Germany; rachel.wuerstlein@med.uni-muenchen.de

20 Department of Gynecology, Martin Luther University of Halle-Wittenberg, 06120 Halle (Saale), Germany; christoph.thomssen@uk-halle.de

21 Department of Gynecology and Obstetrics, Helios Clinics Berlin Buch, 13125 Berlin, Germany; michael.untch@helios-gesundheit.de

22 Department of Gynecology and Obstetrics, Düsseldorf University Hospital, 40225 Düsseldorf, Germany; tanja.fehm@med.uni-duesseldorf.de
23 National Center for Tumor Diseases and Department of Gynecology and Obstetrics, Heidelberg University Hospital, 69120 Heidelberg, Germany
* Correspondence: peter.fasching@uk-erlangen.de
† These authors contributed equally to this study.

Abstract: This study presents comprehensive real-world data on the use of anti-human epidermal growth factor receptor 2 (HER2) therapies in patients with HER2-positive metastatic breast cancer (MBC). Specifically, it describes therapy patterns with trastuzumab (H), pertuzumab + trastuzumab (PH), lapatinib (L), and trastuzumab emtansine (T-DM1). The PRAEGNANT study is a real-time, real-world registry for MBC patients. All therapy lines are documented. This analysis describes the utilization of anti-HER2 therapies as well as therapy sequences. Among 1936 patients in PRAEGNANT, 451 were HER2-positive (23.3%). In the analysis set (417 patients), 53% of whom were included in PRAEGNANT in the first-line setting, 241 were treated with H, 237 with PH, 85 with L, and 125 with T-DM1 during the course of their therapies. The sequence PH → T-DM1 was administered in 51 patients. Higher Eastern Cooperative Oncology Group (ECOG) scores, negative hormone receptor status, and visceral or brain metastases were associated with more frequent use of this therapy sequence. Most patients received T-DM1 after treatment with pertuzumab. Both novel therapies (PH and T-DM1) are utilized in a high proportion of HER2-positive breast cancer patients. As most patients receive T-DM1 after PH, real-world data may help to clarify whether the efficacy of this sequence is similar to that in the approval study.

Keywords: advanced breast cancer; metastatic; chemotherapy; antihormone therapy; HER2 c-erbB2; HER2/neu; trastuzumab; pertuzumab; T-DM1; lapatinib

---

1. Introduction

Overexpression of human epidermal growth factor receptor 2 (HER2), or amplification of the *HER2* gene, is seen in approximately 15–25% of breast cancer (BC) patients [1]. Since the discovery in the late 1980s of HER2 amplifications and their prognostic relevance [2], treatment for HER2-positive BC in this subgroup of patients has greatly improved [3–6]. Adding the monoclonal anti-HER2 antibody trastuzumab to standard chemotherapy resulted in a significant improvement in the progression-free survival (PFS) and overall survival (OS) in patients with metastatic HER2-positive BC [7]. These results led to the approval of trastuzumab for the treatment of HER2-positive metastatic BC.

Later, the dual tyrosine kinase inhibitor lapatinib was also analyzed in this group of patients. Women whose cancers had progressed after treatment with an anthracycline, a taxane, and trastuzumab were randomly assigned to therapy with capecitabine plus lapatinib or capecitabine alone. In contrast to the monotherapy, the combination treatment led to a significantly longer PFS. Therefore, lapatinib also became the standard of care in the early 2000s [8,9].

The CLEOPATRA study demonstrated an additional improvement in survival outcomes in treatment-naïve (chemotherapy and biological therapy, one endocrine treatment was allowed) HER2-positive patients with metastatic BC. Patients who were receiving docetaxel and dual HER2 blockade with trastuzumab plus pertuzumab, another monoclonal HER2 antibody, were compared with patients receiving docetaxel plus trastuzumab alone. The improved survival results led to the approval of pertuzumab for the first-line treatment setting. The enrolled patients were allowed to have had (neo)adjuvant chemotherapy with or without trastuzumab. However, the observed benefit of the addition of palliative pertuzumab was independent of any previous (neo)adjuvant treatment with trastuzumab [10,11].

Another HER2-targeted approved drug is trastuzumab emtansine (T-DM1), which was designed as an antibody–drug conjugate to target specifically HER2-enriched tumor cells, and in this way, reduce side effects in nontargeted tissue. In the EMILIA trial, the efficacy of T-DM1 was analyzed in women with HER2-positive advanced or metastatic disease who had previously been treated with a taxane and trastuzumab in the advanced therapy setting and were randomly assigned to second-line or further treatment with T-DM1 versus capecitabine plus lapatinib. It was found that T-DM1 was clearly superior with regard to survival outcomes in comparison with the control arm [12].

After the approval of T-DM1 and pertuzumab, the question arose of whether a combination of the two might result in an additional benefit. However, the MARIANNE study showed in first-line HER2-positive metastatic BC patients that neither T-DM1 alone nor T-DM1 in combination with pertuzumab improved the PFS in comparison with trastuzumab plus a taxane [13]. Although the reason for this remains unclear, there are cell line data that suggest that the correct therapy sequence for the drugs might have an influence on the treatment response [14].

Moreover, novel substances are also being investigated to further improve outcomes for patients. For instance, neratinib, another tyrosine kinase inhibitor, was recently approved for the adjuvant treatment of patients with HER2-positive early BC, due to its significant improvement of five-year disease-free survival (DFS) [15], and is currently also being analyzed in the metastatic setting. Afatinib, however, did not show any improvement in the outcomes for patients with metastatic BC in comparison with trastuzumab [16]. Margetuximab has now made available a third novel HER2 antibody that appears to enhance antibody-dependent cellular toxicity (ADCC), while at the same time being well-tolerated [17]. Its efficacy and safety are currently being investigated in the phase III SOPHIA trial in patients with HER2-positive metastatic BC who were previously treated with trastuzumab, pertuzumab, and T-DM1 [14].

As more and more therapy options become available, it is possible that treatment sequences may no longer be following the same inclusion and exclusion criteria as those that applied in the respective clinical trials. Understanding current therapy practice may be helpful for estimating the extent to which results from clinical trials can be generalized for specific patient populations. Therefore, the objective of this study is to describe comprehensive real-world evidence on the use of trastuzumab, pertuzumab, lapatinib, and T-DM1 in first-line treatment in the metastatic setting.

2. Patients and Methods

2.1. The PRAEGNANT Research Network

The PRAEGNANT study (Prospective Academic Translational Research Network for the Optimization of the Oncological Health Care Quality in the Adjuvant and Advanced/Metastatic Setting; NCT02338167 [18]) is an ongoing, prospective BC registry with a documentation system similar to that of a clinical trial. The aims of PRAEGNANT are to assess treatment patterns and quality of life, and to identify patients who may be eligible for clinical trials or specific targeted treatments [18–21]. Patients can be included at any point in time during the course of their disease. All of the patients included in the present study provided informed consent, and the study was approved by the relevant ethics committees.

2.2. Patients

A total of 2379 patients with advanced or metastatic BC were registered in the PRAEGNANT study between July 2014 and March 2018 at 52 study sites. Patients were excluded in the following hierarchical order: 39 patients were excluded due to unknown HER2 status, as well as 53 patients due to unknown hormone receptor status. In 138 patients, the date of the first diagnosis of a metastasis or their birth date was missin. Therefore, these patients also had to be excluded. Male patients (n = 20) were also not included in the analysis. Treatment information was not available for an additional 193 women, leaving 1936 patients for whom the above-mentioned data were known. A total of 451 of these women had HER2-positive tumors (Figure 1). For analysis, patients were divided into distinct patient groups based on the documentation status concerning the therapy lines. Group 1 is defined as the patient population for which only the first therapy line is documented. Group 2 is the population for which the first and the second therapy lines are documented. Group 3 is the patient population for which only the first, seco, nd and third therapy lines are documented. Group 4 is the patient population for which at least the first to the forth therapy lines are documented. Each group cannot be part of the other groups. These groups are the natural consequence of patients being treated with more or less therapy lines in the metastatic setting.

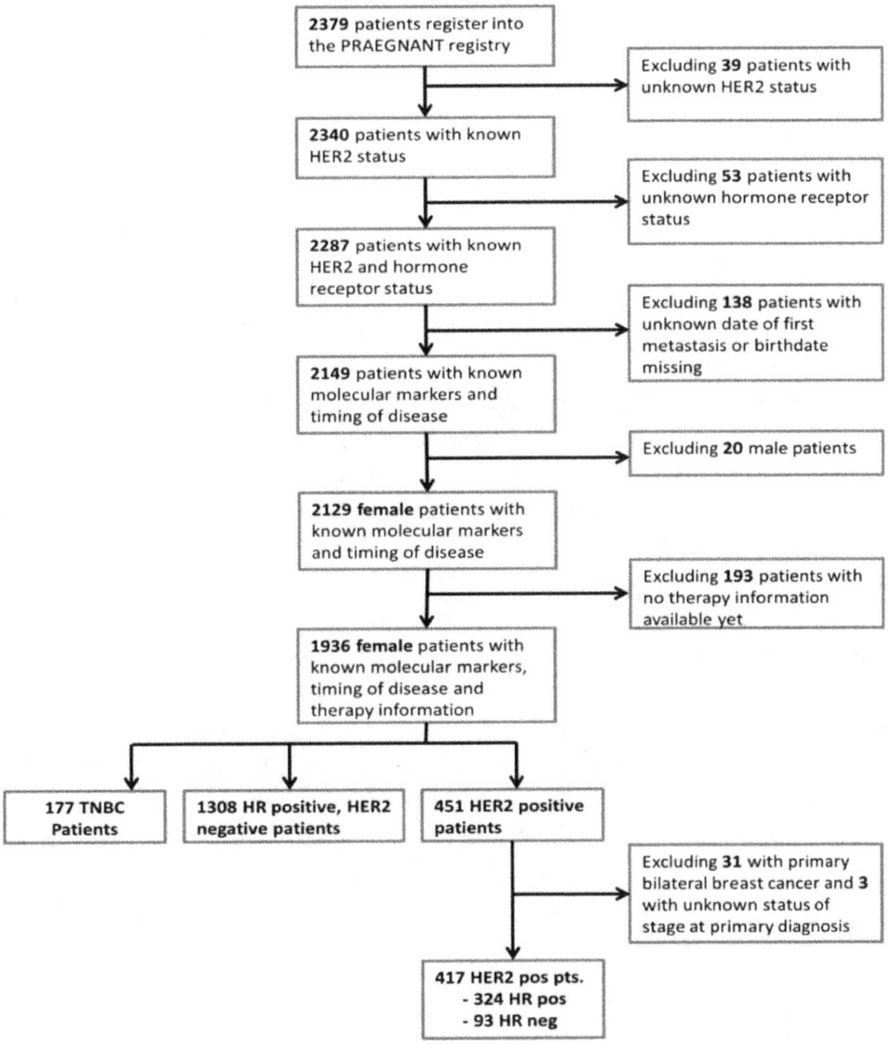

Figure 1. Patient flow chart and patient selection.

2.3. Data Collection

The data were collected by trained staff and documented in an electronic case report form [18]. The data were monitored using automated plausibility checks and on-site monitoring. Data that are not usually documented as part of routine clinical work are collected prospectively using structured questionnaires completed on paper. These consist of epidemiological data, such as family history, cancer risk factors, quality of life, nutrition and lifestyle items, and psychological health. Supplementary Table S1 provides an overview of the collected data.

2.4. Definition of Hormone Receptors, HER2 Status and Grading

The definition of hormone receptors, HER2 status, and grading was described previously [19]. Briefly, data about estrogen receptor status, progesterone receptor status, HER2 status, and grading were obtained for documentation purposes for each tumor that had been biopsied. Therefore, there could be several possible sources (right breast, left breast, local recurrence, metastatic site). Biomarker status for ER, PR, and HER2 were determined as follows: If a biomarker assessment of the metastatic site was available, this receptor status was used for the analysis. If there was no information available for metastases, the latest biomarker results from the primary tumor were used. Additionally, all patients who received estrogen therapy in the metastatic setting were assumed to be HR-positive, and all patients who had ever received anti-HER2 therapy were assumed to be HER2-positive. There was no central review of biomarkers. The study protocol recommended assessing ER and PR status as positive if $\geq$ 1% was stained. A positive HER2 status required an immunohistochemistry score of 3+ or positive fluorescence in situ hybridization/competitive in situ hybridization (FISH/CISH).

2.5. Statistical Considerations

The analysis and reporting of treatments are descriptive. The total number of treatments for each of the following four therapy lines are provided: Trastuzumab (H), trastuzumab and pertuzumab (PH), lapatinib (L), and trastuzumab emtansine (T-DM1). It was also analyzed whether patients who had already completed a specific number of therapy lines (1–4) received these four anti-HER2 therapies in any therapy line. For this purpose, the patients were categorized into four distinct groups, namely: Patients for whom only the first therapy line was documented, patients for whom the first two therapy lines were documented, patients for whom the first three therapy lines were documented, and patients for whom at least the first four therapy lines were documented. Similarly, the frequencies of usage of the PH $\rightarrow$ T-DM1 and T-DM1 $\rightarrow$ PH therapy sequences were analyzed, regardless of whether these therapies followed each other directly.

It was also analyzed whether the patients' characteristics were associated with the frequency of utilization of the PH $\rightarrow$ T-DM1 sequence in the first four therapy lines, again regardless of whether these therapies followed each other directly.

With regard to the year of therapy, the patients were also categorized in relation to their first four therapy lines. The first group consisted of patients who completed all documented therapy lines before 2013, the second group had to have had at least one treatment administered before 2013 and one in 2013 or after 2013. In the last group, all patients had to have received all treatments after 2013.

Calculations were performed using IBM SPSS Statistics, version 24 (Armonk, New York, NY, USA: IBM Corporation).

3. Results

3.1. Patient and Disease Characteristics

A total of 451 (23.3%) patients in the registry had HER2-positive metastatic breast cancer. Figure 2 shows the frequency of HER2-positive metastatic breast cancer patients over the years. Although the HER2 status was positive in 37% (95% CI: 26–47%) of all patients with metastases who were treated up to 2006, HER2 positivity was seen in 25% (95% CI: 21–28%) and 22% (95% CI: 19–24%) of patients diagnosed with metastases in 2007–2013 and after 2013, respectively (Figure 2). For further analyses, patients with bilateral breast cancer at diagnosis and those with missing information about the stage at initial diagnosis were excluded. The final study population comprised 417 patients, 324 of whom were hormone receptor–positive and 93 hormone receptor–negative (Figure 1).

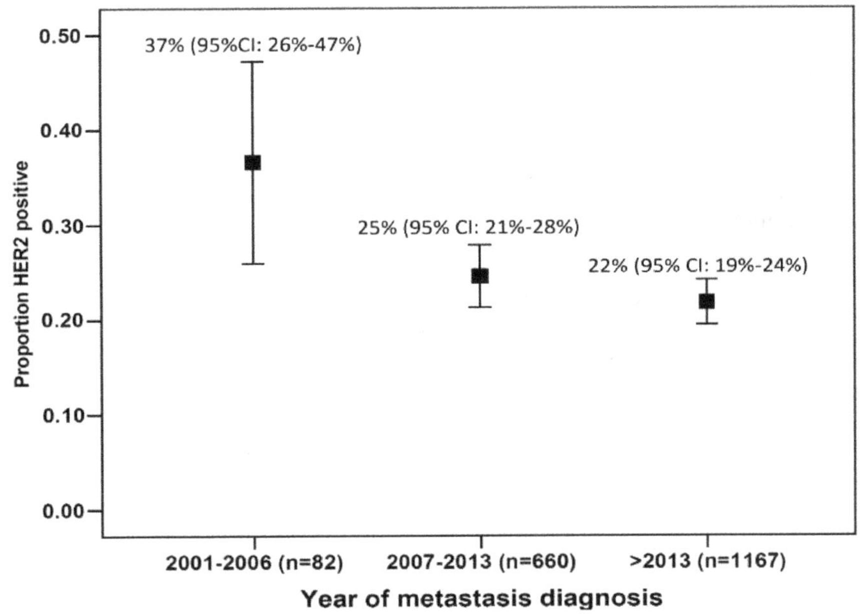

Figure 2. Proportion of human epidermal growth factor receptor 2 (HER2)-positive patients with 95% confidence intervals relative to the year in which the metastases were diagnosed.

The characteristics of the patients and diseases are listed in Table 1. Most patients entered the study in the first-line setting, had an Eastern Cooperative Oncology Group (ECOG) score of 0, and had visceral metastases. Approximately 40% of the patients had metastases at the time of diagnosis.

Table 1. Patient characteristics at baseline.

Characteristic	n or Mean	% or SD
Age at study entry	57.9	13.0
BMI	26.0	5.3
Time from diagnosis to metastasis (days)	1177.8	1743.0
Therapy situation at study entry		
First-line	223	53.5
Second-line	70	16.8
Third-line	53	12.7
Fourth-line	26	6.2
Fifth-line and higher	34	8.2
Therapy situation at database closure		
First-line	171	41.0
Second-line	82	19.7
Third-line	47	11.3
Fourth-line	17	4.1
Fifth-line and higher	59	14.1
Hormone receptor status		
Negative	93	22.3
Positive	324	77.7
ECOG		
0	196	47.0
1	155	37.2
2	35	8.4
3	12	2.9
4	2	0. 4

Table 1. *Cont.*

Characteristic	n or Mean	% or SD
	Metastasis site at study entry	
Brain [a]	79	18.9
Visceral [b]	222	53.2
Bone only	58	13.9
Other [c]	50	12.0
	Metastatic at time of diagnosis	
No	244	58.5
Yes	173	41.5

BMI (body mass index) ECOG (Eastern Cooperative Oncology Group) (score); SD (standard deviation). [a] Patients included in the "brain" group were allowed to have metastases at any other site. [b] Patients included in the "visceral" group were allowed to have metastases at any other site except the brain. [c] Patients included in this group were not allowed to have any brain, visceral, or bone metastases.

3.2. Therapies

Across all of the therapy lines (1 to 9+), 241 of the 417 patients were treated with H without additional anti-HER2 therapy, 237 with PH, 85 with L, and 125 with T-DM1. The respective figures up to therapy line four are 236 (H), 220 (PH), 79 (L), and 108 (T-DM1) patients.

Table 2 shows patterns of therapy utilization relative to patient groups with first-line therapy documented, with first- and second-line therapy documented, with first- to third-line therapy documented, and with first- to fourth-line therapy documented, relative to the treatment period. Trastuzumab, either as a single anti-HER2 therapy or together with pertuzumab, was already administered in over 80% of the patients for whom only the first-line was documented. PH utilization increased across the different time periods, with approximately 60–70% of all patients already receiving this treatment as first-line therapy. T-DM1 utilization also increased across the time periods, although patients with a larger number of documented therapy lines had a higher frequency (approximately 52% of patients had four therapy lines documented and approximately 33% of patients had only two therapy lines documented). Lapatinib use did not change across the time periods and was mainly administered in later therapy lines (Table 2).

Table 2. Frequencies of patients who received the respective treatments. The patients are categorized here into four mutually exclusive (distinct) patient groups according to the number of documented therapy lines. The percentages of patients treated are marked in bold. The numbers and percentages of treated patients refer to the cumulative number of patients treated up to the highest documented therapy line. For example, in the group of patients with three therapy lines documented and treated after 2013, 33 patients have been treated with trastuzumab in one of the first three therapy lines.

Therapy	Patients Treated Before 2012		Patients Treated Crossing 2013		Patients Treated After 2013	
	Not Treated	Treated	Not Treated	Treated	Not Treated	Treated
			Trastuzumab (H)			
treatments in patient group 1 [a]	4 (19)	17 (**80.9**)	0 (0)	6 (**100**)	28 (20.4)	109 (**79.5**)
treatments in patient group 2 [b]	0 (0)	6 (**100**)	2 (13.3)	13 (**86.6**)	11 (15)	62 (**84.9**)
treatments in patient group 3 [c]	0 (0)	4 (**100**)	3 (15.7)	16 (**84.2**)	6 (15.3)	33 (**84.6**)
treatments in patient group 4 [d]	3 (20)	12 (**80**)	8 (18.1)	36 (**81.8**)	7 (18.4)	31 (**81.5**)
			Trastuzumab + pertuzumab (PH)			
treatments in patient group 1 [a]	19 (90.4)	2 (**9.5**)	3 (50)	3 (**50**)	51 (37.2)	86 (**62.7**)
treatments in patient group 2 [b]	6 (100)	0 (**0**)	11 (73.3)	4 (**26.6**)	21 (28.7)	52 (**71.2**)
treatments in patient group 3 [c]	4 (100)	0 (**0**)	13 (68.4)	6 (**31.5**)	12 (30.7)	27 (**69.2**)
treatments in patient group 4 [d]	15 (100)	0 (**0**)	28 (63.6)	16 (**36.3**)	14 (36.8)	24 (**63.1**)

Table 2. *Cont.*

Therapy	Patients Treated Before 2012		Patients Treated Crossing 2013		Patients Treated After 2013	
	Not Treated	Treated	Not Treated	Treated	Not Treated	Treated
Lapatinib (L)						
treatments in patient group 1 [a]	20 (95.2)	1 (**4.7**)	5 (83.3)	1 (**16.6**)	134 (97.8)	3 (**2.1**)
treatments in patient group 2 [b]	6 (100)	0 (**0**)	12 (80)	3 (**20**)	65 (89)	8 (**10.9**)
treatments in patient group 3 [c]	3 (75)	1 (**25**)	15 (78.9)	4 (**21**)	30 (76.9)	9 (**23**)
treatments in patient group 4 [d]	8 (53.3)	7 (**46.6**)	22 (50)	22 (**50**)	18 (47.3)	20 (**52.6**)
Trastuzumab emtansine (T-DM1)						
treatments in patient group 1 [a]	21 (100)	0 (**0**)	6 (100)	0 (**0**)	131 (95.6)	6 (**4.3**)
treatments in patient group 2 [b]	6 (100)	0 (**0**)	10 (66.6)	5 (**33.3**)	49 (67.1)	24 (**32.8**)
treatments in patient group 3 [c]	4 (100)	0 (**0**)	8 (42.1)	11 (**57.8**)	21 (53.8)	18 (**46.1**)
treatments in patient group 4 [d]	14 (93.3)	1 (**6.6**)	21 (47.7)	23 (**52.2**)	18 (47.3)	20 (**52.6**)

[a] Group 1 is the patient population for which only the 1st therapy line is documented. These patients are not part of groups 2–4; [b] Group 2 is the patient population for which only the 1st and the 2nd therapy lines are documented. These patients are not part of the other groups. [c] Group 3 is the patient population for which only the 1st, 2nd and 3rd therapy lines are documented. These patients are not part of the other groups. [d] Group 4 is the patient population for which the 1st to the 4th therapy lines are documented. These patients are not part of the other groups.

The sequence of PH followed by T-DM1 (PH → T-DM1) was administered in 51 patients throughout all therapy lines and in 50 patients in lines one to four. Of those 50 patients, 48 patients were treated with the combination of PH and chemotherapy, and two with the combination of PH and endocrine therapy. Eleven patients received a sequence of T-DM1 → PH, eight of whom were treated within the first four therapy lines. This is equivalent to a utilization rate of PH → T-DM1 up to therapy line four after approval of about 42%, with an increase of approximately 10% from lines two to four per therapy line (Table 3).

Table 3. Frequencies of patients who were treated with the respective treatment sequences, irrespective of whether the sequences were administered directly after each other. The patients are categorized into four mutually exclusive patient groups according to the numbers of documented therapy lines. The percentages of patients treated are marked in bold.

Therapy	Patients Treated Before 2012		Patients Treated Crossing 2012		Patients Treated After 2012	
	Not Treated	Treated	Not Treated	Treated	Not Treated	Treated
Pertuzumab/trastuzumab → trastuzumab emtansine (PH → T-DM1)						
treatments in patient group 1 [a]	21 (100)	0 (**0**)	6 (100)	0 (**0**)	137 (100)	0 (**0**)
treatments in patient group 2 [b]	6 (100)	0 (**0**)	14 (93.3)	1 (**6.6**)	59 (80.8)	14 (**19.1**)
treatments in patient group 3 [c]	4 (100)	0 (**0**)	17 (89.4)	2 (**10.5**)	27 (69.2)	12 (**30.7**)
treatments in patient group 4 [d]	15 (100)	0 (**0**)	39 (88.6)	5 (**11.3**)	22 (57.8)	16 (**42.1**)
Trastuzumab emtansine → pertuzumab/trastuzumab (T-DM1 → PH)						
treatments in patient group 1 [a]	21 (100)	0 (**0**)	6 (100)	0 (**0**)	136 (99.2)	1 (**0.7**)
treatments in patient group 2 [b]	6 (100)	0 (**0**)	15 (100)	0 (**0**)	73 (100)	0 (**0**)
treatments in patient group 3 [c]	4 (100)	0 (**0**)	18 (94.7)	1 (**5.2**)	38 (97.4)	1 (**2.5**)
treatments in patient group 4 [d]	15 (100)	0 (**0**)	41 (93.1)	3 (**6.8**)	36 (94.7)	2 (**5.2**)

[a] Group 1 is the patient population for which only the 1st therapy line is documented. These patients are not part of groups 2–4; [b] Group 2 is the patient population for which only the 1st and the 2nd therapy lines are documented. These patients are not part of the other groups. [c] Group 3 is the patient population for which only the 1st, 2nd and 3rd therapy lines are documented. These patients are not part of the other groups. [d] Group 4 is the patient population for which the 1st to the 4th therapy lines are documented. These patients are not part of the other groups.

3.3. Predictors of the Use of a Therapy Sequence of PH Followed by T-DM1

Several patient and disease characteristics were analyzed in relation to their influence on the utilization of the therapy sequence PH → T-DM1 (Table 4). Age, grading, and stage at the initial diagnosis did not have any influence. Patients with higher ECOG scores appeared to be treated with this sequence more often, as well as patients with brain or visceral metastases. One patient with metastases only in the bone was treated with PH → T-DM1. Patients with a positive hormone receptor status were less frequently treated with the PH → T-DM1 sequence. Although only 23.7% of patients with a positive hormone receptor status received this sequence up to therapy line four, hormone receptor–negative patients were treated with this sequence in about 44% of cases.

Table 4. Frequency of patients who received the treatment sequence pertuzumab/trastuzumab → trastuzumab emtansine (PH → T-DM1), irrespective of whether the sequences were administered directly after each other. All patients who had at least two documented therapy lines and in whom all treatments started after 2013 are included.

Characteristic	PH → T-DM1	
	No	Yes
	Age	
<50	28 (65.1)	15 (34.9)
50–65	53 (72.6)	20 (27.4)
>65	27 (79.4)	7 (20.6)
	Eastern Cooperative Oncology Group (ECOG) score	
0	59 (79.7)	15 (20.3)
1	34 (63.0)	20 (37.0)
2	6 (60.0)	4 (40.0)
3	5 (100)	0 (0)
	Metastasis site at study entry	
Brain [a]	14 (58.3)	10 (41.7)
Visceral [b]	56 (68.3)	23 (31.7)
Bone only [c]	16 (94.1)	1 (5.9)
Other [d]	19 (82.6)	4 (14.7)
	Hormone receptor status	
Negative	18 (56.3)	14 (43.8)
Positive	90 (76.3)	28 (23.7)
	Grade	
1	2 (100)	0 (0)
2	45 (78.9)	12 (21.1)
3	50 (64.1)	28 (35.9)
	Primary metastatic	
No	68 (73.9)	24 (26.1)
Yes	40 (69.0)	42 (28.0)

[a] Patients included in the "brain" group were allowed to have metastases at any other site. [b] Patients included in the "visceral" group were allowed to have metastases at any other site except the brain. [c] Patients included in this group were not allowed to have any brain, visceral, or bone metastases.

4. Discussion

This analysis of a cohort from a real-world breast cancer registry shows how frequently anti-HER2 therapies are used. Although most patients received trastuzumab, the percentage of patients who received pertuzumab and trastuzumab, lapatinib, or T-DM1 was clearly lower. Most of the trastuzumab and pertuzumab therapies were administered in the first-line setting, but TDM-1 was administered in most cases between the second and fourth lines, and lapatinib more often in the third- and fourth-line setting. The sequence of TDM-1 after trastuzumab and pertuzumab was administered in up to 40% of patients with four therapy lines, while the sequence T-DM1 followed by pertuzumab was only administered in about 5% of the patients.

The analysis shows that HER2-positive metastatic breast cancer is a subgroup with a clinically relevant frequency. The frequency of HER2-positive patients in the present cohort of metastatic breast cancer patients was 23.3%, a rate similar to the initially described frequencies of 25–30% in primary breast cancer before the introduction of anti-HER2 therapies [2,22]. The frequency of triple-negative breast cancer was much lower in this cohort, at 9.1% of all cases. Looking at HER2 positivity over the years, it seems that HER2 positivity decreased over time. One possible explanation could be the introduction of trastuzumab in the adjuvant setting [23–25], possibly reducing the number of HER2 positive patients, who would develop a metastasis at a later timepoint. However, it should be noted that the PRAEGNANT study has been registering patients since 2014, and data from before that year are purely descriptive. Therefore, this trend might be the result of a bias.

Pertuzumab and T-DM1 were approved in Germany in 2013. These therapies were thus inevitably not prevalent in the cohort before that time. Few patients were treated in clinical trials before that, and it can be clearly seen that the use of pertuzumab and trastuzumab during the first four therapy lines increased from 27–36% around 2013 to 63–71% after 2013. Most of these treatments were administered as first-line therapy, which is in accordance with the current national therapy guidelines [26]. T-DM1, which is administered after tumor progression in the metastatic setting, was already used in 23–58% of patients around 2013 and continued to be administered in 33–53% of patients after 2013. This therapy pattern also matched the current national therapy guidelines [26]. Most patients received T-DM1 after pertuzumab—a sequence that is under discussion, since at the time when the EMILIA study was conducted, only previous trastuzumab therapy was available [12]. A recent retrospective study did not show any differences in the prognosis when patients who had been treated with T-DM1 after pertuzumab were compared with patients who had not received previous T-DM1 treatment [27]. However, analyses of differences between subgroups with earlier and later therapy lines in which T-DM1 was administered were inconclusive [27]. The use of lapatinib did not change much over time in the first four therapy lines, despite the introduction of pertuzumab and T-DM1.

With regard to possible predictive factors that may have influenced physicians in deciding to treat patients with the pertuzumab–trastuzumab sequence, it appears that patients with more advanced disease or a less favorable prognosis were more likely to be treated with the PH → T-DM1 therapy sequence. Parameters that were associated with a higher frequency of PH → T-DM1 use were poorer ECOG scores, brain and visceral metastases, negative hormone receptor status, and higher grading. The higher frequency of PH → T-DM1 therapy in patients with brain metastases could be the enrichment of patients with brain metastases in patients treated with anti-HER2 therapies, while in patients with positive hormone receptor status, the avoidance of chemotherapy could be a motivation behind not giving an anti-HER2 directed therapy. With regard to visceral metastasis, its more frequent use in patients with visceral metastases could be explained with the possible need for an effective therapy regimen including anti-HER2 treatments and chemotherapy. Moreover, in exploratory subgroup analyses of both studies, CLEOPATRA and EMILIA patients with visceral metastases had a larger benefit from PH or T-DM1 than the patients treated with the respective comparator therapies [10–12].

To the best of our knowledge, no comparable data concerning this healthcare research question was previously published. Hormone receptor status in particular appears to be of special interest, since a desire to avoid chemotherapy in this patient group is a possible reason why specific treatment regimens are not administered.

This study has several strengths and limitations. Although the PRAEGNANT breast cancer registry has registered more than 2300 patients with metastatic breast cancer, only 451 of the patients were HER2-positive. Although this is a large number in comparison with other publications reporting on prospective or retrospective cohorts, the sample size might be low for identifying treatment patterns and possible predictors of patient/tumor characteristics that are associated with specific therapy sequences and possible outcomes. Clinical cancer registries might be helpful for gathering data on larger patient populations [28], but the degree of detail in the information might be limited in such population-based registries. Data completeness and detail are certainly strengths in the PRAEGNANT registry, which documents therapy lines, side effects, progression, and mortality with an approach similar to that used in clinical trials. Another fact that needs to be taken into consideration when interpreting the data is that in real-world cohorts, not all patients enter the study or end the study at comparable time points. Patients in the first-line setting may therefore be overrepresented, as patients die during the course of the disease, or may be lost to follow-up. An attempt was made to account for this by categorizing the patients into groups for which documentation for all therapy lines up to a specific line was available, with treatment utilization being reported for each of these groups separately.

5. Conclusions

In conclusion, the utilization of trastuzumab appeared to be sufficiently high in this cohort of patients with metastatic breast cancer. The utilization of the PH $\rightarrow$ T-DM1 sequence appeared to be rather low, and the reasons for this should be analyzed in future studies.

Author Contributions: Conceptualization, P.A.F., N.N., M.P.L., S.Y.B. and E.B.; Methodology, P.A.F. and L.H..; Software, B.V., L.H. and P.A.F.; Validation, B.V., L.H. and P.A.F.; Formal Analysis, B.V., L.H. and P.A.F.; Investigation, all authors; Resources, all authors; Data Curation, all authors; Writing-Original Draft Preparation, M.P.L., N.N., P.A.F., A.S. and S.Y.B.; Writing-Review & Editing, all authors; Visualization, all authors; Supervision, P.A.F., D.W., H.T., A.S. and S.Y.B.; Project Administration, P.A.F., D.W., H.T., A.S. and S.Y.B., Funding Acquisition, S.Y.B.

Acknowledgments: We acknowledge support by Deutsche Forschungsgemeinschaft and Friedrich-Alexander-Universität Erlangen-Nürnberg (FAU) within the funding programme Open Access Publishing.

References

1. Wolff, A.C.; Hammond, M.E.H.; Hicks, D.G.; Dowsett, M.; McShane, L.M.; Allison, K.H.; Allred, D.C.; Bartlett, J.M.; Bilous, M.; Fitzgibbons, P.; et al. Recommendations for human epidermal growth factor receptor 2 testing in breast cancer: American Society of Clinical Oncology/College of American Pathologists clinical practice guideline update. *J. Clin. Oncol.* **2013**, *31*, 3997–4013. [CrossRef]
2. Slamon, D.J.; Clark, G.M.; Wong, S.G.; Levin, W.J.; Ullrich, A.; McGuire, W.L. Human breast cancer: Correlation of relapse and survival with amplification of the HER-2/neu oncogene. *Science* **1987**, *235*, 177–182. [CrossRef] [PubMed]
3. Schneeweiss, A.; Lux, M.P.; Janni, W.; Hartkopf, A.D.; Nabieva, N.; Taran, F.A.; Overkamp, F.; Kolberg, H.C.; Hadji, P.; Tesch, H.; et al. Update Breast Cancer 2018 (Part 2)—Advanced Breast Cancer, Quality of Life and Prevention. *Geburtshilfe Frauenheilkd* **2018**, *78*, 246–259. [CrossRef] [PubMed]
4. Taran, F.A.; Schneeweiss, A.; Lux, M.P.; Janni, W.; Hartkopf, A.D.; Nabieva, N.; Overkamp, F.; Kolberg, H.C.; Hadji, P.; Tesch, H.; et al. Update Breast Cancer 2018 (Part 1)—Primary Breast Cancer and Biomarkers. *Geburtshilfe Frauenheilkd* **2018**, *78*, 237–245. [CrossRef] [PubMed]
5. Lux, M.P.; Janni, W.; Hartkopf, A.D.; Nabieva, N.; Taran, F.A.; Overkamp, F.; Kolberg, H.C.; Hadji, P.; Tesch, H.; Ettl, J.; et al. Update Breast Cancer 2017—Implementation of Novel Therapies. *Geburtshilfe Frauenheilkd* **2017**, *77*, 1281–1290. [CrossRef] [PubMed]
6. Untch, M.; Huober, J.; Jackisch, C.; Schneeweiss, A.; Brucker, S.Y.; Dall, P.; Denkert, C.; Fasching, P.A.; Fehm, T.; Gerber, B.; et al. Initial Treatment of Patients with Primary Breast Cancer: Evidence, Controversies, Consensus: Spectrum of Opinion of German Specialists at the 15th International St. Gallen Breast Cancer Conference (Vienna 2017). *Geburtshilfe Frauenheilkd* **2017**, *77*, 633–644. [CrossRef] [PubMed]
7. Slamon, D.J.; Leyland-Jones, B.; Shak, S.; Fuchs, H.; Paton, V.; Bajamonde, A.; Fleming, T.; Eiermann, W.; Wolter, J.; Pegram, M.; et al. Use of chemotherapy plus a monoclonal antibody against HER2 for metastatic breast cancer that overexpresses HER2. *N. Engl. J. Med.* **2001**, *344*, 783–792. [CrossRef]
8. Geyer, C.E.; Forster, J.; Lindquist, D.; Chan, S.; Romieu, C.G.; Pienkowski, T.; Jagiello-Gruszfeld, A.; Crown, J.; Chan, A.; Kaufman, B.; et al. Lapatinib plus capecitabine for HER2-positive advanced breast cancer. *N. Engl. J. Med.* **2006**, *355*, 2733–2743. [CrossRef]

9. Cameron, D.; Casey, M.; Press, M.; Lindquist, D.; Pienkowski, T.; Romieu, C.G.; Chan, S.; Jagiello-Gruszfeld, A.; Kaufman, B.; Crown, J.; et al. A phase III randomized comparison of lapatinib plus capecitabine versus capecitabine alone in women with advanced breast cancer that has progressed on trastuzumab: Updated efficacy and biomarker analyses. *Breast Cancer Res. Treat.* **2008**, *112*, 533–543. [CrossRef]
10. Swain, S.M.; Kim, S.B.; Cortés, J.; Ro, J.; Semiglazov, V.; Campone, M.; Ciruelos, E.; Ferrero, J.M.; Schneeweiss, A.; Knott, A.; et al. Pertuzumab, trastuzumab, and docetaxel for HER2-positive metastatic breast cancer (CLEOPATRA study): Overall survival results from a randomised, double-blind, placebo-controlled, phase 3 study. *Lancet Oncol.* **2013**, *14*, 461–471. [CrossRef]
11. Swain, S.M.; Baselga, J.; Kim, S.B.; Ro, J.; Semiglazov, V.; Campone, M.; Ciruelos, E.; Ferrero, J.M.; Schneeweiss, A.; Heeson, S.; et al. Pertuzumab, trastuzumab, and docetaxel in HER2-positive metastatic breast cancer. *N. Engl. J. Med.* **2015**, *372*, 724–734. [CrossRef] [PubMed]
12. Verma, S.; Miles, D.; Gianni, L.; Krop, I.E.; Welslau, M.; Baselga, J.; Pegram, M.; Oh, D.Y.; Diéras, V.; Guardino, E.; et al. Trastuzumab emtansine for HER2-positive advanced breast cancer. *N. Engl. J. Med.* **2012**, *367*, 1783–1791. [CrossRef] [PubMed]
13. Perez, E.A.; Barrios, C.; Eiermann, W.; Toi, M.; Im, Y.H.; Conte, P.; Martin, M.; Pienkowski, T.; Pivot, X.; Burris, H., III; et al. Trastuzumab Emtansine With or Without Pertuzumab Versus Trastuzumab Plus Taxane for Human Epidermal Growth Factor Receptor 2-Positive, Advanced Breast Cancer: Primary Results From the Phase III MARIANNE Study. *J. Clin. Oncol.* **2017**, *35*, 141–148. [CrossRef] [PubMed]
14. Loibl, S.; Gianni, L. HER2-positive breast cancer. *Lancet* **2017**, *389*, 2415–2429. [CrossRef]
15. Deeks, E.D. Neratinib: First Global Approval. *Drugs* **2017**, *77*, 1695–1704. [CrossRef] [PubMed]
16. Harbeck, N.; Huang, C.S.; Hurvitz, S.; Yeh, D.C.; Shao, Z.; Im, S.A.; Jung, K.H.; Shen, K.; Ro, J.; Jassem, J.; et al. Afatinib plus vinorelbine versus trastuzumab plus vinorelbine in patients with HER2-overexpressing metastatic breast cancer who had progressed on one previous trastuzumab treatment (LUX-Breast 1): An open-label, randomised, phase 3 trial. *Lancet Oncol.* **2016**, *17*, 357–366. [CrossRef]
17. Bang, Y.J.; Giaccone, G.; Im, S.A.; Oh, D.Y.; Bauer, T.M.; Nordstrom, J.L.; Li, H.; Chichili, G.R.; Moore, P.A.; Hong, S.; et al. First-in-human phase 1 study of margetuximab (MGAH22), an Fc-modified chimeric monoclonal antibody, in patients with HER2-positive advanced solid tumors. *Ann. Oncol.* **2017**, *28*, 855–861. [CrossRef] [PubMed]
18. Fasching, P.A.; Brucker, S.Y.; Fehm, T.N.; Overkamp, F.; Janni, W.; Wallwiener, M.; Hadji, P.; Belleville, E.; Häberle, L.; Taran, F.A.; et al. Biomarkers in Patients with Metastatic Breast Cancer and the PRAEGNANT Study Network. *Geburtshilfe Frauenheilkd* **2015**, *75*, 41–50. [CrossRef]
19. Hartkopf, A.D.; Huober, J.; Volz, B.; Nabieva, N.; Taran, F.A.; Schwitulla, J.; Overkamp, F.; Kolberg, H.C.; Hadji, P.; Tesch, H.; et al. Treatment landscape of advanced breast cancer patients with hormone receptor positive HER2 negative tumors - Data from the German PRAEGNANT breast cancer registry. *Breast* **2018**, *37*, 42–51. [CrossRef]
20. Müller, V.; Nabieva, N.; Häberle, L.; Taran, F.A.; Hartkopf, A.D.; Volz, B.; Overkamp, F.; Brandl, A.L.; Kolberg, H.C.; Hadji, P.; et al. Impact of disease progression on health-related quality of life in patients with metastatic breast cancer in the PRAEGNANT breast cancer registry. *Breast* **2018**, *37*, 154–160. [CrossRef]
21. Hein, A.; Gass, P.; Walter, C.B.; Taran, F.A.; Hartkopf, A.; Overkamp, F.; Kolberg, H.C.; Hadji, P.; Tesch, H.; Ettl, J.; et al. Computerized patient identification for the EMBRACA clinical trial using real-time data from the PRAEGNANT network for metastatic breast cancer patients. *Breast Cancer Res. Treat.* **2016**, *158*, 59–65. [CrossRef]
22. Slamon, D.J.; Godolphin, W.; Jones, L.A.; Holt, J.A.; Wong, S.G.; Keith, D.E.; Levin, W.J.; Stuart, S.G.; Udove, J.; Ullrich, A.; et al. Studies of the HER-2/neu proto-oncogene in human breast and ovarian cancer. *Science* **1989**, *244*, 707–712. [CrossRef]
23. Perez, E.A.; Romond, E.H.; Suman, V.J.; Jeong, J.H.; Sledge, G.; Geyer, C.E., Jr.; Martino, S.; Rastogi, P.; Gralow, J.; Swain, S.M.; et al. Trastuzumab plus adjuvant chemotherapy for human epidermal growth factor receptor 2-positive breast cancer: Planned joint analysis of overall survival from NSABP B-31 and NCCTG N9831. *J. Clin. Oncol.* **2014**, *32*, 3744–3752. [CrossRef] [PubMed]
24. Slamon, D.; Eiermann, W.; Robert, N.; Pienkowski, T.; Martin, M.; Press, M.; Mackey, J.; Glaspy, J.; Chan, A.; Pawlicki, M.; et al. Adjuvant trastuzumab in HER2-positive breast cancer. *N. Engl. J. Med.* **2011**, *365*, 1273–1283. [CrossRef] [PubMed]

25. Piccart-Gebhart, M.J.; Procter, M.; Leyland-Jones, B.; Goldhirsch, A.; Untch, M.; Smith, I.; Gianni, L.; Baselga, J.; Bell, R.; Jackisch, C.; et al. Trastuzumab after adjuvant chemotherapy in HER2-positive breast cancer. *N. Engl. J. Med.* **2005**, *353*, 1659–1672. [CrossRef]
26. AGO Commission Breast. Diagnosis and Therapy of patients with primary and metastatic breast cancer. Available online: http://www.ago-online.de/fileadmin/downloads/leitlinien/mamma/2017-03/AGO_deutsch/PDF_Gesamtdatei_deutsch/Alle%20aktuellen%20Empfehlungen_2017.pdf (accessed on 20 March 2017).
27. Vici, P.; Pizzuti, L.; Michelotti, A.; Sperduti, I.; Natoli, C.; Mentuccia, L.; Di Lauro, L.; Sergi, D.; Marchetti, P.; Santini, D.; et al. A retrospective multicentric observational study of trastuzumab emtansine in HER2 positive metastatic breast cancer: A real-world experience. *Oncotarget* **2017**, *8*, 56921–56931. [CrossRef]
28. Pobiruchin, M.; Bochum, S.; Martens, U.M.; Schramm, W. Clinical Cancer Registries—Are They Up for Health Services Research? *Stud. Health Technol. Inform.* **2016**, *228*, 242–246. [PubMed]

6

Contralateral Prophylactic Mastectomy in Women with Unilateral Breast Cancer Who are Genetic Carriers, have a Strong Family History or are just Young at Presentation

Victoria Teoh *, Marios-Konstantinos Tasoulis and Gerald Gui

Department of Breast Surgery, Royal Marsden NHS Foundation Trust, Fulham Road, London SW36JJ, UK; marios.tasoulis@rmh.nhs.uk (M.-K.T.); Gerald.Gui@rmh.nhs.uk (G.G.)

* Correspondence: victoriateoh@doctors.org.uk

Abstract: The uptake of contralateral prophylactic mastectomy is rising with increasing trends that are possibly highest in the USA. Whilst its role is generally accepted in carriers of recognized high-risk predisposition genes such as *BRCA1* and *BRCA2* when the affected individual is premenopausal, controversy surrounds the benefit in less understood risk-profile clinical scenarios. This comprehensive review explores the current evidence underpinning the role of contralateral prophylactic mastectomy and its impact on contralateral breast cancer risk and survival in three distinct at-risk groups affected by unilateral breast cancer: known genetic carriers, those with strong familial risk but no demonstrable genetic mutation and women who are of young age at presentation. The review supports the role of contralateral prophylactic mastectomy in "high risk" groups where the evidence suggests a reduction in contralateral breast cancer risk. However, this benefit is less evident in women who are just young at presentation or those who have strong family history but no demonstrable genetic mutation. A multidisciplinary and personalized approach to support individuals in a shared-decision making process is recommended.

Keywords: contralateral prophylactic mastectomy; contralateral breast cancer; BRCA; CHEK2; PALB2; ATM; mutation carriers; family history; survival

---

1. Introduction

The incidence of women with breast cancer who elect to undergo contralateral prophylactic mastectomy is steadily increasing, with preponderance amongst Caucasians, young women, and those with a higher socioeconomic status [1,2]. A study of 496,488 women with unilateral Stage I–III breast cancer, from the Surveillance, Epidemiology, End Results (SEER) Program database demonstrated an increase in contralateral prophylactic mastectomy rates performed for unilateral invasive breast cancer from 3.9% in 2002 to 12.7% in 2012 [3]. This effect was reproduced in a National Cancer Database review of 553,593 patients, showing an increase in contralateral prophylactic mastectomies from 4.1% in 2003 to 9.7% in 2010. This finding was most marked in young women, where those <45 years (n = 73,888) showed an increase from 9.3% in 2003 to 26.4% in 2010 [4].

Factors that contribute to this decision include patient age, disease stage, previous breast biopsies, genetic predisposition or family history of breast cancer, fear of recurrence, concern with cosmetic symmetry and physician recommendation [1,5–8].

Patients tend to overestimate their risk of developing a contralateral breast cancer [9,10] as well as the extent of risk reduction conferred by contralateral prophylactic mastectomy [9,11]. Interestingly, whilst 43.9% of women with breast cancer considered contralateral prophylactic mastectomy, only 38.1% were aware that it did not improve survival, highlighting the importance of patient education [12].

Improvements in modern multidisciplinary management have led to a reduction in the incidence of contralateral breast cancer from approximately 0.6% to 0.2–0.5%/year [13]. Consequently, the role of contralateral prophylactic mastectomy and the context in which it is supported is debatable.

This comprehensive review explores the current evidence underpinning the role of contralateral prophylactic mastectomy and its impact on contralateral breast cancer risk and survival in three high-risk groups affected by breast cancer: (i) genetic carriers, (ii) strong family history with no demonstrable mutation, and (iii) young women.

2. Methods

A comprehensive literature review was performed, assessing all studies published in the English literature from 1974 to March 2019 across Embase and Medline search engines. Search terms "contralateral prophylactic mastectomy", "unilateral breast cancer", "*BRCA*", "*TP53*", "*PALB2*", "*CHEK2*", "*ATM*", "mutation carrier", "family history", "young women", "non-genetic carriers", "overall survival", "disease-free survival", "contralateral breast cancer" and "risk" were included. Relevant references from identified papers were also included.

3. *BRCA 1/2* Carriers with Breast Cancer

3.1. *BRCA 1/2* Carriers and Contralateral Breast Cancer Risk

BRCA carriers with breast cancer carry a higher risk of contralateral breast cancer, 23.7% (95% CI 17.6–30.5), compared with non-carriers, 6.8% (95% CI 4.2–10), respectively, (RR 3.56, 95% CI 2.50–5.08; $p < 0.001$). This risk was higher in *BRCA1* compared to *BRCA2* carriers (RR 1.42, 95% CI 1.01–1.99; $p = 0.04$) [14]. In a Dutch multicentre study of 6294 invasive breast cancer patients ≤50 years, the risk of contralateral breast cancer for *BRCA1/2* carriers at a median follow-up of 12.5 years was shown to be 2–3 times higher compared to non-carriers (HR 3.31, 95% CI 2.41–4.55; $p < 0.001$ and 2.17, 95% CI 1.22–3.85; $p = 0.01$ respectively). The 10-year cumulative contralateral breast cancer risk following the initial breast cancer diagnosis was 21.1% for *BRCA1*, 10.8% for *BRCA2* and 5.1% for non-carriers [15]. These findings were confirmed in a recent multicentre study where the 10-year cumulative risk was 25.1% (95% CI 19.6–31.9) for *BRCA1*, 13.5% (95% CI 9.2–19.1) for *BRCA2* and 3.6% (95% CI 2.2–5.7) for non-carriers [16].

The age of first breast cancer diagnosis is a significant predictor of contralateral breast cancer risk in *BRCA* carriers [17–19]. Risk estimates vary in the literature, ranging from 23.7–30.7% in young women (<40 years) across *BRCA1/2* carriers combined (*BRCA1*: 24–32%; *BRCA2*: 17–29%) [19–24]. This risk is lower in the >40 years age group, ranging from 8.4–21% (*BRCA1*: 11–52%; *BRCA2*: 7–18%) [15,17,19–22,24,25]. Similar results were shown in another study demonstrating a 10-year cumulative contralateral breast cancer risk of 23.9% (*BRCA1*: 25.5%; *BRCA2*: 17.2%) in patients <41 years, compared to 12.6% in the 41–49 year group (*BRCA1* 15.6%; *BRCA2* 7.2%) [15].

In a retrospective study of 1042 *BRCA1/2* carriers with breast cancer, Graeser demonstrated that the 25-year cumulative contralateral breast cancer risk for *BRCA1* carriers with the first breast cancer diagnosis at age <40years, 40–50 years and >50 years, was 62.9% (95% CI 50.4–75.4), 43.7% (95% CI 24.9–62.5) and 19.6% (95% CI 5.3–33.9) respectively. In *BRCA2* carriers, the corresponding rates were 63% (95% CI 32.8–93.2), 48.8% (95% CI 22.7–74.9) and 16.7% (95% CI 1.0–32.4) for the respective age groups [19].

3.2. Contralateral Prophylactic Mastectomy and Risk of Contralateral Breast Cancer

Contralateral prophylactic mastectomy reduces the risk of contralateral breast cancer in *BRCA* mutation carriers [14,26,27]. This risk reduction has been reported to be in the range of 91% [27]. This is further supported by a meta-analysis showing that contralateral prophylactic mastectomy resulted in a 93% reduction in contralateral breast cancer risk (RR 0.072; 95%CI 0.035–0.588) [26].

3.3. *Contralateral Prophylactic Mastectomy and Survival*

There is conflicting evidence on whether contralateral prophylactic mastectomy improves survival in *BRCA* carriers with breast cancer [14,26–31] (Table 1). In a multicenter, retrospective study of 242 *BRCA* carriers with breast cancer, contralateral prophylactic mastectomy was associated with improved overall survival on multivariate analysis, having adjusted for risk-reducing salpingo-oophorectomy (HR 0.49, 95% CI 0.29–0.82) [30]. Similar findings have been reported in other cohort studies [27,29–31].

Table 1. Studies looking at the impact of CPM on CBC risk and survival in *BRCA1/2* mutation carriers.

Author	Year	Study Type	Follow up	Patient	Findings
Li [26]	2016	Meta-analysis (2 RC/1 PC/1 RCC)	n/a	4/4574 studies (1672 individuals)	CPM significantly decreased CBC risk in *BRCA1/2* mutation carriers (RR 0.072; 95% CI, 0.035–0.148). CPM is associated with a decrease in "all–cause" mortality (HR 0.512; 95% CI 0.368–0.588)
Valachis [14]	2014	Meta-analysis (1 RCC/1 RC)	n/a	2/13 studies	CPM was not associated with a benefit in BCSS HR 0.78 (95% CI 0.44–1.39, $p = 0.40$)
Copson [32]	2018	Prospective cohort	Median 8.2 years	21 *BRCA* carriers/10 non-carriers, with TNBC	CPM conferred no difference in 5-year OS between *BRCA* carriers and non-carriers with TNBC 83% (95% CI 74–89) vs. 74% (95% CI 69–78) HR 0.98 (95% CI 0.58–1.65), $p = 0.94$
Heemskerk-Gerritsen [30]	2015	Multicentre retrospective cohort	Median 11.4 years	242/583(52%) carriers with BC who underwent CPM	CPM improved OS HR 0.49 (0.29–0.82)
Metcalfe [29]	2014	Retrospective observational	Median follow up 14.3 yrs (0.1–20.0)	390 *BRCA1/BRCA2* carriers with a positive family history	At 20 years follow up, CPM was associated with a 48% reduction in death from breast cancer (HR 0.52; $p = 0.03$). * Not significant on propensity score adjusted analysis
Evans [31]	2013	Retrospective case-control	Median 9.7 years	105/698 (15%) *BRCA 1/2* carriers with BC who underwent CPM	CPM improves OS 89% (CPM) vs. 71% (non-CPM) at 10 year follow up ($p < 0.001$)
Van Sprundel [27]	2005	Retrospective cohort	Mean 3.5 years	69/148 (47%) BRCA 1/2 carriers with BC who underwent CPM	CPM reduced the risk of CBC in BRCA1/2 carriers by 91% No significant difference in OS between CPM and non-CPM group HR 0.35, $p = 0.14$ (adjusted for prophylactic oophorectomy)
Brekelmans [28]	2007	Retrospective case-control	Median 4.3 years	260 BRCA 1/2 carriers with BC vs. 759 non-carriers	CPM conferred no difference in BCSS HR 0.98 (95% CI 0.5–0.91, $p = 0.96$)

RC: retrospective cohort; RCC: Retrospective case-control; PC: prospective cohort; BCCS: breast-cancer-specific; OS overall survival; CPM: contralateral prophylactic mastectomy; BC: breast cancer; CBC: contralateral breast cancer; TNBC: triple negative breast cancer; HR: hazard ratio.

In a retrospective study by Van Sprundel, contralateral prophylactic mastectomy was associated with superior overall survival compared to active surveillance at 5-year follow up (94% vs 77%, $p = 0.03$). However, this difference was not significant once adjusted for prophylactic oophorectomy (HR 0.35, $p = 0.14$) [27]. Notably, Metcalfe observed a survival benefit only in the second decade of follow-up following initial breast cancer diagnosis (HR 0.52, 95% CI 0.29–0.93) but not during the first 10 years of follow-up (HR 0.65, 95% CI 0.34–1.22) [29].

A meta-analysis by Valachis demonstrated no difference in breast-cancer-specific survival between *BRCA* carriers who underwent contralateral prophylactic mastectomy against those who did not (HR

0.78, 95% CI 0.44–1.39; $p = 0.40$) [14]. However, a meta-analysis including two additional studies demonstrated a decrease in "all-cause" mortality [26]. To further add to the ambiguity, a recent prospective study showed that contralateral prophylactic mastectomy conferred no benefit in 5-year overall survival between *BRCA* carriers and non-carriers with triple negative breast cancer [32]. The available findings should be interpreted with caution as they are mostly based on retrospective studies that may contain recognized and unrecognized biases.

4. "Other" Genetic Carriers (*CHEK2, TP53, ATM, PALB2, PTEN, CDH1*) with Breast Cancer

Mutations in *CHEK2, TP53, ATM, PALB2, PTEN,* and *CDH1* account for a small fraction of familial breast cancers. The available studies are sparse and primarily family-based, with potential ascertainment bias. It should be noted that the existing literature focusses mainly on relative rather than absolute risk estimates.

4.1. "Other" Genetic Carriers and Contralateral Breast Cancer Risk

4.1.1. CHEK2 Mutation Carriers and Contralateral Breast Cancer Risk

In a recent meta-analysis, Akdeniz demonstrated an increased contralateral breast cancer risk for *CHEK2* 1100d*elC carriers (RR 2.75, 95% CI 1.77–4.27) [33]. This mutation is associated with bilateral disease and an increased risk of bilateral breast cancer which varies between two to six-fold [15,34–40] (Table 2). It has been suggested that *CHEK2* carriers may be more sensitive to ionizing radiation that may contribute to contralateral breast cancer rates in patients receiving adjuvant radiotherapy following breast conserving surgery [40,41]. The true impact of radiation in this context is questionable as consistently increased contralateral breast cancer risk has been demonstrated in patients treated with or without radiotherapy (HR 4.12, 95% CI 2.49–6.83 and HR 3.17, 95% CI 1.36–7.35, respectively) [39,41].

4.1.2. TP53 Mutation Carriers and Contralateral Breast Cancer Risk

There are no studies estimating contralateral breast cancer risk in *TP53* carriers with breast cancer.

4.1.3. ATM Mutation Carriers and Contralateral Breast Cancer Risk

In a multicentre, population-based, case-control study, Concannon suggested that four common variants of *ATM (c.1899-55T>G; c.3161C>G; c.6348-54T>C and c.5558A>T)* were associated with a lower contralateral breast cancer risk (overall RR 0.8, 95% CI 0.6–0.9) compared to those with rare, missense *ATM* mutations. The protective mechanisms may occur through an alteration in *ATM* activity as an initiator of DNA damage response or through its role in TP53 regulation [42]. Bernstein suggested that common *ATM* variants may exert a protective effect and reduce contralateral breast cancer risk, while rare *ATM* missense, deleterious variants may act synergistically with radiation exposure to increase this risk [43]. In this study, the variants: *c.1899-55T>G* (RR 0.5, 95% CI 0.3–0.8), c.3161C>G (RR 0.5, 95% CI 0.3–0.9), *c.5558A>T* (RR 0.2, 95% CI 0.1–0.6), and *c.6348-54T>C* (RR 0.2, 95% CI 0.1–0.8) were associated with significantly reduced risk. On the other hand, female carriers of any rare missense *ATM* variant, who received radiation therapy for their first breast cancer, had a significantly elevated contralateral breast cancer risk compared to unexposed women (RR = 2.8 for <1.0 Gy dose and RR = 3.3 for ≥ 1.0 Gy dose to the contralateral breast).

The direct relationship between the presence of *ATM* variants and the overall risk of contralateral breast cancer remains controversial, although the combination of radiotherapy and certain *ATM* missense variants appears to accelerate tumour development [44].

Table 2. Studies looking at CBC risk and survival in *CHEK2* 1100delC* mutation carriers.

Author	Year	Study	Median Follow up	N	Findings
Akdeniz [33]	2019	Meta-analysis	N/A	68 studies	CBC risk by mutation carriers *BRCA1* RR 3.7 (95% CI, 2.8–4.9) *BRCA2* RR 2.8 (95% CI, 1.8–4.3) *CHEK2* 1100delC* RR 2.7 (95% CI, 2.0–3.7)
Kriege [39]	2014	Retrospective, multicentre cohort study	6.8 years	193/4722 (4.1%) BC patients with *CHEK2* 1100delC* mutation	Higher risk of CBC HR 3.97 (95% CI 2.59–6.07) 10-year risk of CBC is 28.9%
Weischer [37]	2012	Meta-analysis	6 years	459/25571 (1.8%) BC patients with *CHEK2* 1100delC* mutation	20-year cumulative risk of developing BC is 25–30% (HR 3.52) No comment on CBC rates
Mellemkjaer [40]	2008	Population based, multicentre cohort study	N/A	17/2103 (0.8%) BC patients with *CHEK2* 1100delC*	No significant association between *CHEK2* 1100delC* mutation and CBC
Broeks [41]	2004	Case study	N/A	15/233 (6.4%) *CHEK2* 1100delC* mutation carriers with BBC 2/191 (1%) *CHEK2* 1100delC* mutation carriers with UBC	Increased risk of CBC in carriers OR 6.5 (95% CI 1.5–28.8, $p = 0.005$)
Schmidt [36]	2007	Retrospective cohort study	Median 10.1 years	54/1479 (3.7%) pre-menopausal BC patients with CHEK2* 1100delC mutation	*CHEK2* 1100delC mutation* carriers: Increased risk of ipsilateral second breast cancer HR 2.1 (95% CI 1.0–4.3; $p = 0.049$) Increased risk of CBC HR 1.7 (95% CI 1.2–2.4) Worse breast-cancer-specific survival HR 1.4 (95% CI 1.0–2.1; $p = 0.072$) Worse recurrence- free survival HR 1.7 (95% CI 1.2–2.4; $p = 0.06$)
De Bock [45]	2004	Prospective cohort	Median 3.8 years	34 BC patients with *CHEK2* 1100delC* mutation; 102 BC patients with no mutation	Compared to non-carriers, *CHEK2* 1100delC* mutation carriers: Increased risk of CBC compared RR = 5.74 (95% CI 1.67–19.65) Increased risk of distant metastasis RR 2.81 (95% CI 1.2–6.58) Worse DFS RR = 3.86 (1.91–7.78) No difference in overall survival. Mutation carriers more frequently had a 1st or 2nd degree female relative with breast cancer ($p = 0.03$)

BC: breast cancer; CBC: contralateral breast cancer; BBC: bilateral breast cancer; UBC: unilateral breast cancer; RR: relative risk; DFS: disease-free survival; ER: oestrogen receptor; HR: hazard ratio.

4.1.4. PALB2 Mutation Carriers and Contralateral Breast Cancer Risk

There are no studies estimating contralateral breast cancer risk in *PALB2* carriers with breast cancer.

4.1.5. CDH1 Mutation Carriers and Contralateral Breast Cancer Risk

There are no studies on the risk of contralateral breast cancer in *CDH1* carriers.

4.1.6. PTEN Mutation Carriers and Contralateral Breast Cancer Risk

There are no studies estimating contralateral breast cancer risk in *PTEN* carriers with breast cancer.

4.2. Contralateral Prophylactic Mastectomy and Risk of Contralateral Breast Cancer

No studies have investigated the role of contralateral prophylactic mastectomy in the risk reduction of contralateral breast cancer in patients with a diagnosis of breast cancer that harbor a genetic mutation in non-*BRCA1/2* genes (*CHEK2, TP53, ATM, PALB2, CDH1* and *PTEN*).

4.3. Contralateral Prophylactic Mastectomy and Survival

There is no data to support any survival benefit from contralateral prophylactic mastectomy in this group of patients ("other" genetic carriers). This would be even more challenging in those with *TP53, CDH1 and PTEN* mutations because of the additional competing cancer risk. In view of the limited evidence, no further comment can be made, except to reinforce that contralateral prophylactic mastectomy should be considered on an individual basis for women with unilateral breast cancer in this group.

5. Familial Breast Cancers with no Demonstrable Genetic Mutations

5.1. Familial Breast Cancers with No Demonstrable Genetic Mutation and Contralateral Breast Cancer Risk

A positive family history remains a strong risk factor for contralateral breast cancer, even after excluding mutation carriers [46–48]. Table 3 summarizes the current literature on the impact of positive family history on contralateral breast cancer risk and survival. In a multicentre, population-based, case-control study of 1521 contralateral breast cancer cases against 2212 matched controls of unilateral breast cancer, Reiner demonstrated that non-mutation carriers with any 1st or 2nd degree relative of breast cancer had a nearly two-fold increased contralateral breast cancer risk (RR 1.8, 95% CI 1.3–2.4), compared to individuals without a family history. This risk is similar to that shown in previous studies [49,50]. In this non-mutation carrier group, a 1st degree family history of bilateral breast cancer increased the contralateral breast cancer risk by more than three-fold (RR 3.4, 95% CI 1.5–7.4). Where there is only an affected 2nd degree relative, the individual is at a 40% increased risk compared to an individual without a family history. The 10-year absolute contralateral breast cancer risk in non-mutation carriers with a 1st or 2nd degree family history is 8.3% (95% CI 5.5–12.6) and 6.6% (95% CI 4.4–10) respectively [46].

Table 3. Studies looking at the impact of positive FH of breast cancer on CBC rates, disease-free and overall survival.

The Impact of Positive FH of Breast Cancer on CBC Rates, Disease-Free and Overall Survival					
Author	**Year**	**Study Type**	**Follow up**	**Patients**	**Findings**
Reiner [46]	2018	Multicentre, population-based, case-control study	Not stated	1521 CBC cases with 2212 UBC controls	A 1st degree relative with BC confers increased risk of CBC RR 1.9 (95% CI 1.6–2.3) A 1st degree relative with BBC confers the highest risk of CBC RR 3.4 (95% CI 2.4–5) A 2nd degree relative increases the risk of CBC RR 1.4 (95% CI 1.2–1.7) Any 1st degree relative with breast cancer confers a 10-year AR of developing CBC of 8.1% (95% CI 6.7–9.8). The 10-year AR increases to 13.5% (95% CI 8.8–20.8) if this relative was <40 years at age of diagnosis. The 10-year AR is highest at 36% (95% CI 14.5–90.5) if the first degree relative was diagnosed with BBC at age <40 years. On subgroup analysis and exclusion of mutation carriers i.e., *BRCA*, *ATM*, *PALB2* and *CHEK2*, the increased 10-year AR associated with a 1st degree relative and a 1st degree relative with BBC remained significant similar to above-reported.
Kuchenbaecker [20]	2017	Prospective, multicentre, cohort study	Median 4 years (2–7)	3886 eligible for breast cancer analysis *BRCA1* (n = 2276); *BRCA2* (n = 1610)	Increased risk if ≥two 1st or 2nd degree relatives with breast cancer compared to no family history of BC; HR 1.99 Did not evaluate the effect of FH on CBC risk
Bernstein [51]	1992	Prospective cohort study	Mean 52 months	136/4550 (2.9%) patients with CBC and varying familial risk	Compared with no FH of breast cancer: Increased risk of CBC ~2x with a 1st degree relative with BC Increased risk of CBC ~3x if 1st degree relative was diagnosed at a young age (<35 years)
Ji [52]	2007	Population based, national database study	Not stated	56190 invasive and 6841 in situ BC patients	The risk of metachronous CBC measured by SIRs was higher with primary in situ disease compared to invasive cancer. SIR for metachronous CBC in women diagnosed with invasive BC: <45 years: 5.12 (95% CI 4.47–5.85) 45–55 years: 1.95 (95% CI 1.76–2.16) >55 years: 1.49 (95% CI 1.37–1.61) SIR for metachronous CBC in women diagnosed with 1st invasive BC and have: A positive FH 2.74 (95% CI 2.3–3.23) No FH 1.85 (95% CI 1.75–1.96) SIR for metachronous CBC in women diagnosed with in situ disease: <45 years: 5.12 (95% CI 4.47–5.85) 45–55 years: 1.95 (95% CI 1.76–2.16) >55 years: 1.49 (95% CI 1.37–1.61)

Table 3. *Cont.*

The Impact of Positive FH of Breast Cancer on CBC Rates, Disease-Free and Overall Survival					
Author	**Year**	**Study Type**	**Follow up**	**Patients**	**Findings**
Narod [53]	2016	Population based, national database study	Not stated	4839 CBC patients out of 84819 patients with BC * (5.7%)	Young age at 1st BC diagnosis and a maternal cancer history increases the risk of CBC The 15-year cumulative risk of CBC was: 8.8% (95% CI 8.5–9.1) in the general population (regardless of maternal BC status) 12% (95% CI 11–13) in maternal UBC 13% (95% CI 9.5–17) in maternal BBC A maternal cancer history of UBC at an early age conferred the daughter a lifetime CBC risk of 35% (95% CI 25–46) * Mutation carriers not excluded as information not available from cancer registry
Vaittinen [54]	2000	Population based, national database study	Not stated	2529/72,092 (3.5%) CBC patients. 147 (5.8%) of CBC cases with 1st degree relative	Modest elevation in CBC risk for women with an affected 1st degree relative RR of 1.53
Boughey [55]	2010	Retrospective cohort	Median 17.3 years	385 patients with a positive FH; 385 matched controls	Patients with stage I or II BC and a positive family history who underwent CPM had: A 95% reduction in CBC rates; adjusted HR 0.05 (95% CI 0.01–0.19, $p < 0.0001$)

CPM: contralateral prophylactic mastectomy; BC: breast cancer; BBC: bilateral breast cancer; CBC: contralateral breast cancer; UBC: unilateral breast cancer; AR: absolute risk; SIR: Standardized incidence ratio; FH: family history; RD: risk difference; HR: hazard ratio.

In a retrospective study of 6230 women from high risk families, with or without a known *BRCA1/2* mutation, Rhiem observed a cumulative contralateral breast cancer risk, 25 years after a first breast cancer diagnosis of 44.1% (95% CI 37.6–50.6) in *BRCA1* positive families, 33.5% (95% CI 22.4–44.7) in *BRCA2* positive families and 17.2% (95% CI 14.5–19.9) in *BRCA1/2* negative families [56]. This effect was previously demonstrated in smaller cohort studies linking a higher contralateral breast cancer risk with a family history with and without a young age of first breast cancer diagnosis [51,53].

The age at which the affected relative is diagnosed with their first breast cancer and the presence of bilateral disease impacts on contralateral breast cancer risk. Rhiem further observes that patients diagnosed with breast cancer at age <40 years had a cumulative risk 25 years from primary diagnosis of 55.1% and 38.4% for *BRCA1* and *BRCA2*-positive family history, respectively. The corresponding risk was 28.4% in patients from non-*BRCA* families [56].

The highest risk lies with women who have relatives with early-onset, bilateral breast cancer [52–54,57]. The 10-year absolute risk in individuals whose 1st degree relative received a unilateral breast cancer diagnosis at a young age (<40 years) is similar to that of an individual with a 1st degree relative diagnosed with bilateral breast cancer (13.5% and 14.1% respectively). When there was a combination of a family history of a 1st degree relative, an affected relative with bilateral breast cancer or at a young age (<40 years), the 10-year contralateral breast cancer risk increased significantly to 36% [46]. A similar cumulative risk of contralateral breast cancer by the age of 80 (32%, 95% CI 13–66) was observed in a study of 78,775 breast cancer patients, with a maternal history of bilateral breast cancer [53].

5.2. Contralateral Prophylactic Mastectomy and Risk of Contralateral Breast Cancer

Contralateral prophylactic mastectomy may reduce the risk of contralateral breast cancer in women with an elevated genetic or familial risk [21]. This meta-analysis demonstrated a risk reduction in women with *BRCA*-positive families (HR 0.03; $p = 0.0005$). However, only 4% (19/430) of the cohort were non-carriers, with the remaining 96% representing mutation carriers. Fayanju reported a significant reduction in pooled relative (RR 0.04, 95% CI 0.02–0.09) and absolute risk (−24%, 95% CI (−35)–(−12.4)) of metachronous contralateral breast cancer amongst recipients of contralateral prophylactic mastectomy [58]. This analysis included studies with a significant proportion of BRCA carriers which may lead to an overestimation of risk. A case-control study of women with stage I/II breast cancer and a positive family history reported a 95% decreased risk (HR 0.05, 95% CI 0.01–0.19; $p < 0.0001$) of contralateral breast cancer following contralateral prophylactic mastectomy, at a median follow-up of 17.3 years, compared to a matched cohort of women who did not receive mastectomy. However, this cohort, with either an affected 1st or 2nd degree relative was not screened for mutation status [55].

McDonnell also demonstrated a contralateral breast cancer risk reduction following contralateral prophylactic mastectomy in pre- and postmenopausal women with a strong family history of breast/ovarian cancer i.e., 94.4% (95% CI 87.7–97.9) and 96% (95% CI 85.6–99.5) respectively, at a median follow up of 10 years using the Anderson model [59] to predict the risk [60]. Although the cohort had a strong family history, the patients had not been screened for mutations. Similar to studies with undefined gene carriers within the study population, this data should be interpreted with caution as the effect from contralateral prophylactic mastectomy may be overestimated from competing risks conferred by mutation carriers.

5.3. Contralateral Prophylactic Mastectomy and Survival

The evidence on the effect of contralateral prophylactic mastectomy on disease-free and overall survival is conflicting (Table 4).

A Cochrane review of 1708 women with variable familial risk, who underwent contralateral prophylactic mastectomy, concluded that although this decreased the incidence of contralateral breast cancer, there was no association with survival improvement [61]. The meta-analysis conducted by Fayanju demonstrated no association with breast-cancer-specific and overall survival, despite a reduction in the risk of distant metastases or recurrence [58]. The lack of survival benefit from contralateral prophylactic mastectomy in breast cancer patients with elevated familial risk is also reported in smaller, retrospective cohort studies [27,62,63] but with notable exceptions. Boughey reported improved overall (HR 0.77, 95% CI 0.60–0.98; $p = 0.03$) and disease-free survival (HR 0.67, 95% CI 0.54–0.84) on multivariate analysis [55]. In a review of 908 patients receiving against 46,368 not receiving contralateral prophylactic mastectomy, Herrinton demonstrated that mastectomy reduced breast cancer mortality (HR 0.57, 95% CI 0.45–0.72) and overall mortality (HR 0.6, 95% CI 0.5–0.72) across all levels of familial risk [64]. Furthermore, Davies demonstrated that young women (<40 years) with unilateral, stage I disease and a 1st degree relative with bilateral breast cancer, were the only group to have a quality-adjusted life year benefit from contralateral prophylactic mastectomy, which was similar to that of a *BRCA1/2* carrier [63].

Table 4. Studies looking at the impact of CPM on CBC and survival in BC patients with elevated familial risk.

Author	Year	Study Type	Follow up	Patients	Findings
Akdeniz [33]	2019	Meta-analysis	N/A	68 studies	A positive FH of BC was associated with increased CBC risk RR = 1.72 (95% CI 1.15–2.57)
Engel [16]	2019	Multicentre, prospective cohort study	Median 2.9 years	667 *BRCA1* carriers, 402 *BRCA2* carriers 1924 *BRCA1/2* noncarriers (*BRCA1/2*-negative families)	10-year cumulative CBC risk for *BRCA1/2* non carriers 3.6% (95 CI 2.2–5.7) Women with ≥2 relatives with BC had an increased risk of CBC, compared to women without any relative affected by BC HR 2.35 (95% CI 1.21–4.55) ER-negativity was not associated with an increased CBC risk in *BRCA1/2* non-carriers
Fayanju [58]	2014	Meta-analysis	N/A	14/79 studies	Patients with an elevated familial/genetic risk who had CPM (vs no CPM): Reduction in pooled RR of mCBC; RR 0.04 (95% CI 0.02–0.09; $p < 0.001$)) Reduction in pooled AR of mCBC; RD of −24% (95% CI −35.6 to −12.4; $p = 0.013$) Significant reduction in rates of distant/metastatic recurrence. CPM was not associated with improved OS or BCSS
Boughey [55]	2010	Retrospective cohort	Median 17.3 years	385 patients with a positive FH; 385 matched controls (parent, sibling or 2nd degree relative with BC) * no genetic screening	Patients with stage I/II BC and a positive family history who underwent CPM had: A 95% reduction in CBC rates; adjusted HR 0.05 (95% CI 0.01–0.19, $p < 0.0001$) Improved OS (HR 0.77 (95% CI 0.60–0.98, $p = 0.03$)) Improved DFS (HR 0.67 (95% CI 0.54–0.84))
McDonnell [60]	2001	Retrospective cohort	Median 10 years	745 BC patients (388 premenopausal (<50 yrs); 357 postmenopausal with a positive FH	CPM conferred a CBC risk-reduction: In premenopausal women of 94.4% (95% CI 87.7–97.9) In postmenopausal women of 96% (95% CI 85.6–99.5)
Herrinton [64]	2005	Retrospective cohort	Median 5.7 years	1072/50,000 BC patients undergoing CPM	Across all levels of familial risk, CPM: Reduces breast cancer mortality (HR = 0.57; 95% CI 0.45–0.72) Reduces overall mortality (HR = 0.6; 95% CI 0.5–0.72)

Table 4. *Cont.*

Author	Year	Study Type	Follow up	Patients	Findings
Peralta [65]	2001	Retrospective cohort	Mean 6.8 years	23/64 (36%) BC patients undergoing CPM and with ≥one affected 1st degree relative (not screened for mutations)	None of the patients undergoing CPM developed a subsequent CBC
Kiely [62]	2010	Retrospective cohort	Median 8 years	154/1018 women who underwent CPM, with FH of BC ± BRCA mutations	Reduced rate of CBC in women who underwent CPM with no apparent benefit in survival

CPM: contralateral prophylactic mastectomy; BC: breast cancer; CBC: contralateral breast cancer; mCBC: metachronous contralateral breast cancer; BBC: bilateral breast cancer; UBC: unilateral breast cancer; FH: Family history; RR: relative risk; AR: absolute risk; DFS: disease-free survival; OS: overall survival; BCSS: breast cancer-specific survival' ER: oestrogen receptor; HR: hazard ratio.

6. Young Women with Breast Cancer

6.1. Young Women with Breast Cancer and Contralateral Breast Cancer Risk

The definition of 'young' age group in the literature, varies from the "under-35"- to 50 years. Young age at first primary breast cancer diagnosis is associated with an increased contralateral breast cancer risk, poor prognosis and serves as an independent predictor of recurrence and breast-cancer-related death [66–71] (Table 5). Older studies did not account for *BRCA* mutation carriers, which may confound contralateral breast cancer risk and survival. Furthermore, they do not consider risk-reducing adjuvant therapies. In a retrospective study of 652 patients ≤35 years compared to 2608 women >35 years, the relative risk of contralateral breast cancer was 2.48 in the younger, compared to the older group [70]. This finding is supported by Li, who demonstrated an increased HR of 2.8 (95% CI 1.1–6.9), 2.1 (95% CI 1.1–4.4) and 1.9 (95% CI 1.1–3.5) in the ≤29 years, 30–34 years and 35–39 years age groups, compared to women diagnosed at age ≥40 [67]. The contralateral breast cancer risk is further elevated in HER2-overexpressing and triple negative subtypes [70].

Table 5. Studies looking at the impact of CPM on CBC and survival in young women with breast cancer.

Author	Year	Study Type	Median Follow up	Patient Demographics (Age, CPM Status)	Findings
Chen [2]	2019	Retrospective cohort	113 months	<35 years and CPM 811/3083 (26.3%) 35–39 years and CPM 1243/5961 (20.9%)	No difference in BCSS from CPM HR 1.209 (95% CI 0.908–1.610, $p = 0.194$) No difference in OS from CPM HR 1.179 (95% CI 0.902–1.540, $p = 0.228$)
Yu [72]	2018	Retrospective cohort	6.9 years	910/1806 young patients (18–50 years) with CPM	No difference in OS in women with a young age (18–50 years) who had CPM HR 0.93 (95% CI 0.70–1.24; $p = 0.627$)
Pesce [73]	2014	Retrospective cohort	6.1 years	4338/10,289 (29.7%) young women (<45 years) with Stage I/II cancer with CPM	CPM provides no survival benefit in young women (<45 years) Compared to unilateral mastectomy HR 0.93; $p = 0.39$ With early-stage (T1N0) breast cancer HR 0.85; $p = 0.37$ With ER-negative breast cancer HR 1.12; $p = 0.32$
Bedrosian [74]	2010	Population based cohort study	47 months	3731/27,336 (13.6%) young women (18–49 years) with CPM	CPM offers benefit in BCSS for young women (18–49 years) with early stage, ER-negative breast cancer HR 0.68 (95% CI 0.53–0.69), $p < 0.001$

Table 5. *Cont.*

Author	Year	Study Type	Median Follow up	Patient Demographics (Age, CPM Status)	Findings
Bouchard-Fortier [75]	2018	Population-based cohort	11 years	81/614 (13.2%) young women (≤35 years) with CPM	Risk of recurrence (breast/distant) was lower in the CPM group HR 0.61, $p = 0.02$ No difference in breast cancer-specific mortality from CPM HR 0.73 (95% CI 0.47–1.21)
Zeichner [71]	2014	Retrospective cohort	68 months	42/481 (8.73%) young women (<40 years) with CPM	CPM provides a benefit in 10-year overall survival * HR 2.35 (95% CI 1.02–5.41, $p = 0.046$) * effect not seen at 5-year overall survival
Lazow [76]	2018	Population-based cohort	Mean 62 months	4139/11,859 (34.9%) young women (<40 years) with CPM	CPM improves 10-year overall survival HR 0.75 (95% CI, 0.59–0.96) $p = 0.023$]
Park [77]	2017	Population based, national database study	Not stated	3648 DCIS patients <40 years (25.8% UM; 15.8% CPM)	No overall survival benefit from CPM compared to UM in the <40 years group

OS: overall survival; CPM: contralateral prophylactic mastectomy; unilateral mastectomy: BCSS: breast-cancer-specific survival.

6.2. Contralateral Prophylactic Mastectomy and Risk of Contralateral Breast Cancer

The younger age group is generally underrepresented in studies evaluating the role of contralateral prophylactic mastectomy. Using a Surveillance, Epidemiology, End Results database analysis of 107,106 women, of whom 8902 (8.3%) underwent contralateral prophylactic mastectomy, Bedrosian conducted a subgroup analysis of young women (<50 years) and the risk of contralateral breast cancer after contralateral prophylactic mastectomy, in both ER-negative and ER-positive, early-stage breast cancer. In ER-positive disease, the cumulative incidence of contralateral breast cancer during the 6-year study period was 0.13% vs. 0.46% ($p = 0.07$) in the contralateral prophylactic mastectomy vs. non-mastectomy group, and in ER-negative disease, 0.16% vs. 0.90% ($p = 0.05$) respectively [74]. These results should be interpreted with caution though as the study population was not screened for genetic carriers and also patients with a strong family history were not excluded.

6.3. Contralateral Prophylactic Mastectomy and Survival

There is conflicting data on the impact of contralateral prophylactic mastectomy on survival in this patient group. In a population-based study of 614 women <35 years, 81 (13.2%) of whom were elected for contralateral prophylactic mastectomy, Bouchard-Fortier demonstrated that recurrences, defined as local, regional or distant, were significantly fewer for patients with contralateral prophylactic mastectomy than without (32.1% vs. 52.9%, $p < 0.001$; HR 0.61; $p = 0.02$). However, this did not translate to an improvement in breast cancer-specific survival [75].

In an analysis of the National Cancer Database between 2004 and 2014, Lazow demonstrated that after controlling for patient demographics, tumor grade and use of adjuvant therapies, bilateral mastectomy in women < 40 years was associated with increased 10-year overall survival (HR 0.75, 95% CI 0.59–0.96; $p = 0.023$), compared to the unilateral mastectomy group [76]. This trend was also observed in a preceding National Cancer Database review from 1998–2002, demonstrating a 5-year overall survival benefit of 2% in young patients (adjusted HR 0.88, 95% CI 0.83–0.93; $p < 0.001$) between these two groups [78]. In a retrospective study of 42/481 (8.73%) young women <40 years, who were elected for contralateral prophylactic mastectomy, Zeicher reported that this was associated with improved 10-year overall survival (HR 2.35, 95% CI 1.02–5.41; $p = 0.046$), although this effect was not demonstrable for 5-year overall survival [71].

There is a suggestion that contralateral prophylactic mastectomy may confer benefit in young women with early-stage, ER-negative breast cancer. In a population-based study of 107,106 breast cancer patients, 3731 (3.48%) of whom were young (18–49 years), contralateral prophylactic mastectomy was associated with improved disease-specific mortality (HR 0.68, 95% CI 0.53–0.88; $p = 0.004$). This effect was not reproduced in young women with early-stage, ER-positive breast cancer [74].

Other retrospective cohort or population-based studies refute the survival benefit of contralateral prophylactic mastectomy in young women [72,73,75,77]. In a review of 9044 young women (<40 years) with breast cancer, Chen demonstrated no improvement in overall or breast cancer-specific survival [2]. This was supported in a retrospective study of 10,226 patients with invasive lobular carcinoma, demonstrating no overall survival benefit from contralateral prophylactic mastectomy in the 18–50 years group, at a median follow up of 6.9 years [72]. Moreover, in a review of 14,627 women and at median follow-up of 6.1 years, having matched for tumour size/grade, ER status and nodal status, Pesce demonstrated that contralateral prophylactic mastectomy offered no overall survival benefit, in women aged <45 years, with stage I/II breast cancer (HR 0.93, $p = 0.39$) [73].

Overall, these findings should be interpreted with caution as the quality of the data does not allow for definitive conclusions to be drawn.

7. Discussion

Contralateral prophylactic mastectomy is increasingly being performed despite an ambiguity of evidence to support an oncological benefit. In 2007 and 2009, two studies reported that contralateral prophylactic mastectomy rate had increased 148% and 150% among all patients diagnosed with non-invasive and invasive breast cancer respectively [79,80]. Current trends in the U.S.A show an absolute percentage increase in the range of 25% [81]. This trend is modest in European studies suggesting a difference in practice and healthcare environments [82–84]. Nonetheless, this increased utilization of contralateral prophylactic mastectomy is a cause of concern for clinicians because of the associated surgical risks, complications, and psychological and financial burden in the absence of robust evidence to support significant oncological benefits.

Although intuitively it is expected that contralateral prophylactic mastectomy would decrease the risk of contralateral breast cancer, the available data only support this in patients with *BRCA1/2* gene mutations [14,26,27]. In women with strong family history or young age at diagnosis, the effect of contralateral prophylactic mastectomy is less well studied and the existing literature should be interpreted with caution because of the potential biases. At present, there are no models that allow for calculation of contralateral breast cancer risk in a polyfactorial model. Such a model might be useful in stratifying risk and aiding physicians to provide precise and unbiased estimation of risk, in order to offer individualized counselling to patients, inform decision-making and mitigate patient overestimation of cancer risk which may drive unnecessary surgery.

Despite the potential decrease in contralateral breast cancer, the effect of contralateral prophylactic mastectomy on oncological outcomes is debatable as studies suggest that this reduction is not translated into survival benefit. Moreover, the role of contralateral prophylactic mastectomy per se as a contributing factor for improved outcomes in women with unilateral breast cancer is difficult to accurately define, as the majority of the available data is of limited quality. Meta-analyses are only as strong as the independent studies they comprise. The majority of studies are retrospective cohorts and based on population/family studies. Therefore, the results should be interpreted with caution because of potential uncontrolled biases. The way to address these issues is with higher quality data but it is unlikely that the future will harbour randomized clinical trials investigating the impact of contralateral prophylactic mastectomy on contralateral breast cancer risk and survival due to patient preference and ethical considerations. One proposal is to set up robust prospective registries to help enhance our knowledge in the field. The majority of existing studies do not account for the significant role conferred by improved systemic therapies and its effect on contralateral breast cancer risk and improved oncological outcomes, factors that merit future research.

Recently, and in order to aid clinicians approach this controversial topic, both the American Society of Breast Surgeons and Association of Breast Surgery published consensus statements on the utilization of contralateral prophylactic mastectomy. Both were aligned on supporting its use in women with significant contralateral breast cancer risk i.e., *BRCA1/2* mutations, patients with a history of mantle field radiation to the chest before age 30 years [85,86]. However, a multidisciplinary, individualised approach is required to help women in their informed decision-making process.

8. Conclusions

In conclusion, contralateral prophylactic mastectomy may be supported in 'high-risk' groups as evidence indicates a possible reduction in contralateral breast cancer risk and also potentially improved oncological outcomes. The evidence to demonstrate that this may confer benefit in the other risk groups or in older patients is less established. It is therefore imperative to follow a multidisciplinary, personalised approach, to educate women on the best available evidence and to support individuals in a shared-decision making process.

Acknowledgments: The authors acknowledge the David Adams library, The Royal Marsden NHS Foundation Trust and The National Institute for Health Research Biomedical Research Centre (NIHR-BRC) for supporting this study.

References

1. Bhat, S.; Orucevic, A.; Woody, C.; Heidel, R.E.; Bell, J.L. Evolving Trends and Influencing Factors in Mastectomy Decisions. *Am. Surg.* **2017**, *83*, 233–238. [PubMed]
2. Chen, H.; Zhang, P.; Zhang, M.; Wang, M.; Bai, F.; Wu, K. Growing Trends of Contralateral Prophylactic Mastectomy and Reconstruction in Young Breast Cancer. *J. Surg. Res.* **2019**, *239*, 224–232. [CrossRef] [PubMed]
3. Wong, S.M.; Freedman, R.A.; Sagara, Y.; Aydogan, F.; Barry, W.T.; Golshan, M. Growing Use of Contralateral Prophylactic Mastectomy Despite no Improvement in Long-term Survival for Invasive Breast Cancer. *Ann. Surg.* **2017**, *265*, 581–589. [CrossRef] [PubMed]
4. Pesce, C.E.; Liederbach, E.; Czechura, T.; Winchester, D.J.; Yao, K. Changing surgical trends in young patients with early stage breast cancer, 2003 to 2010: A report from the National Cancer Data Base. *J. Am. Coll. Surg.* **2014**, *219*, 19–28. [CrossRef] [PubMed]
5. Arrington, A.K.; Jarosek, S.L.; Virnig, B.A.; Habermann, E.B.; Tuttle, T.M. Patient and surgeon characteristics associated with increased use of contralateral prophylactic mastectomy in patients with breast cancer. *Ann. Surg. Oncol.* **2009**, *16*, 2697–2704. [CrossRef]
6. Buchanan, P.J.; Abdulghani, M.; Waljee, J.F.; Kozlow, J.H.; Sabel, M.S.; Newman, L.A.; Chung, K.C.; Momoh, A.O. An Analysis of the Decisions Made for Contralateral Prophylactic Mastectomy and Breast Reconstruction. *Plast. Reconstr. Surg.* **2016**, *138*, 29–40. [CrossRef]
7. Brewster, A.M.; Parker, P.A. Current knowledge on contralateral prophylactic mastectomy among women with sporadic breast cancer. *Oncologist* **2011**, *16*, 935–941. [CrossRef]
8. Chung, A.; Huynh, K.; Lawrence, C.; Sim, M.S.; Giuliano, A. Comparison of patient characteristics and outcomes of contralateral prophylactic mastectomy and unilateral total mastectomy in breast cancer patients. *Ann. Surg. Oncol.* **2012**, *19*, 2600–2606. [CrossRef]
9. Ager, B.; Butow, P.; Jansen, J.; Phillips, K.A.; Porter, D. Contralateral prophylactic mastectomy (CPM): A systematic review of patient reported factors and psychological predictors influencing choice and satisfaction. *Breast* **2016**, *28*, 107–120. [CrossRef]
10. Patient Request for Contralateral Prophylactic Mastectomy Is Due to A False Perception of Increased Risk at the Time of Initial Diagnosis. Available online: https://www.ecco-org.eu/ecco_content/EBCC7_abstractbook/files/assets/seo/page134.html (accessed on 2 February 2019).
11. Butow, P. Applying social-cognition models to understand women's hypothetical intentions for contralateral prophylactic mastectomy. *Proc. Asia Pac. J. Clin. Oncol.* **2014**, *10*, 189.
12. Jagsi, R.; Hawley, S.T.; Griffith, K.A.; Janz, N.K.; Kurian, A.W.; Ward, K.C.; Hamilton, A.S.; Morrow, M.; Katz, S.J. Contralateral Prophylactic Mastectomy Decisions in a Population-Based Sample of Patients With Early-Stage Breast Cancer. *JAMA Surg.* **2017**, *152*, 274–282. [CrossRef] [PubMed]

13. Lizarraga, I.M.; Sugg, S.L.; Weigel, R.J.; Scott-Conner, C.E. Review of risk factors for the development of contralateral breast cancer. *Am. J. Surg.* **2013**, *206*, 704–708. [CrossRef] [PubMed]
14. Valachis, A.; Nearchou, A.D.; Lind, P. Surgical management of breast cancer in BRCA-mutation carriers: A systematic review and meta-analysis. *Breast Cancer Res. Treat.* **2014**, *144*, 443–455. [CrossRef] [PubMed]
15. Van den Broek, A.J.; van't Veer, L.J.; Hooning, M.J.; Cornelissen, S.; Broeks, A.; Rutgers, E.J.; Smit, V.T.; Cornelisse, C.J.; van Beek, M.; Janssen-Heijnen, M.L.; et al. Impact of Age at Primary Breast Cancer on Contralateral Breast Cancer Risk in BRCA1/2 Mutation Carriers. *J. Clin. Oncol. Off. J. Am. Soc. Clin. Oncol.* **2016**, *34*, 409–418. [CrossRef] [PubMed]
16. Engel, C.; Fischer, C.; Zachariae, S.; Bucksch, K.; Rhiem, K.; Giesecke, J.; Herold, N.; Wappenschmidt, B.; Hubbel, V.; Maringa, M.; et al. Breast cancer risk in BRCA1/2 mutation carriers and noncarriers under prospective intensified surveillance. *Int. J. Cancer* **2019**. [CrossRef] [PubMed]
17. Verhoog, L.C.; Brekelmans, C.T.; Seynaeve, C.; Meijers-Heijboer, E.J.; Klijn, J.G. Contralateral breast cancer risk is influenced by the age at onset in BRCA1-associated breast cancer. *Br. J. Cancer* **2000**, *83*, 384–386. [CrossRef]
18. Malone, K.E.; Daling, J.R.; Doody, D.R.; Hsu, L.; Bernstein, L.; Coates, R.J.; Marchbanks, P.A.; Simon, M.S.; McDonald, J.A.; Norman, S.A.; et al. Prevalence and predictors of BRCA1 and BRCA2 mutations in a population-based study of breast cancer in white and black American women ages 35 to 64 years. *Cancer Res.* **2006**, *66*, 8297–8308. [CrossRef]
19. Graeser, M.K.; Engel, C.; Rhiem, K.; Gadzicki, D.; Bick, U.; Kast, K.; Froster, U.G.; Schlehe, B.; Bechtold, A.; Arnold, N.; et al. Contralateral breast cancer risk in BRCA1 and BRCA2 mutation carriers. *J. Clin. Oncol. Off. J. Am. Soc. Clin. Oncol.* **2009**, *27*, 5887–5892. [CrossRef]
20. Kuchenbaecker, K.B.; Hopper, J.L.; Barnes, D.R.; Phillips, K.A.; Mooij, T.M.; Roos-Blom, M.J.; Jervis, S.; van Leeuwen, F.E.; Milne, R.L.; Andrieu, N.; et al. Risks of Breast, Ovarian, and Contralateral Breast Cancer for BRCA1 and BRCA2 Mutation Carriers. *JAMA* **2017**, *317*, 2402–2416. [CrossRef]
21. Metcalfe, K.; Lynch, H.T.; Ghadirian, P.; Tung, N.; Olivotto, I.; Warner, E.; Olopade, O.I.; Eisen, A.; Weber, B.; McLennan, J.; et al. Contralateral breast cancer in BRCA1 and BRCA2 mutation carriers. *J. Clin. Oncol. Off. J. Am. Soc. Clin. Oncol.* **2004**, *22*, 2328–2335. [CrossRef]
22. Pierce, L.J.; Haffty, B.G. Radiotherapy in the treatment of hereditary breast cancer. *Semin. Radiat. Oncol.* **2011**, *21*, 43–50. [CrossRef] [PubMed]
23. Robson, M.; Gilewski, T.; Haas, B.; Levin, D.; Borgen, P.; Rajan, P.; Hirschaut, Y.; Pressman, P.; Rosen, P.P.; Lesser, M.L.; et al. BRCA-associated breast cancer in young women. *J. Clin. Oncol. Off. J. Am. Soc. Clin. Oncol.* **1998**, *16*, 1642–1649. [CrossRef] [PubMed]
24. Mavaddat, N.; Peock, S.; Frost, D.; Ellis, S.; Platte, R.; Fineberg, E.; Evans, D.G.; Izatt, L.; Eeles, R.A.; Adlard, J.; et al. Cancer risks for BRCA1 and BRCA2 mutation carriers: Results from prospective analysis of EMBRACE. *J. Natl. Cancer Inst.* **2013**, *105*, 812–822. [CrossRef] [PubMed]
25. Robson, M.E.; Chappuis, P.O.; Satagopan, J.; Wong, N.; Boyd, J.; Goffin, J.R.; Hudis, C.; Roberge, D.; Norton, L.; Begin, L.R.; et al. A combined analysis of outcome following breast cancer: Differences in survival based on BRCA1/BRCA2 mutation status and administration of adjuvant treatment. *Breast Cancer Res.* **2004**, *6*, R8–R17. [CrossRef] [PubMed]
26. Li, X.; You, R.; Wang, X.; Liu, C.; Xu, Z.; Zhou, J.; Yu, B.; Xu, T.; Cai, H.; Zou, Q. Effectiveness of Prophylactic Surgeries in BRCA1 or BRCA2 Mutation Carriers: A Meta-analysis and Systematic Review. *Clin. Cancer Res.* **2016**, *22*, 3971–3981. [CrossRef] [PubMed]
27. Van Sprundel, T.C.; Schmidt, M.K.; Rookus, M.A.; Brohet, R.; van Asperen, C.J.; Rutgers, E.J.; Van't Veer, L.J.; Tollenaar, R.A. Risk reduction of contralateral breast cancer and survival after contralateral prophylactic mastectomy in BRCA1 or BRCA2 mutation carriers. *Br. J. Cancer* **2005**, *93*, 287–292. [CrossRef] [PubMed]
28. Brekelmans, C.T.; Tilanus-Linthorst, M.M.; Seynaeve, C.; vd Ouweland, A.; Menke-Pluymers, M.B.; Bartels, C.C.; Kriege, M.; van Geel, A.N.; Burger, C.W.; Eggermont, A.M.; et al. Tumour characteristics, survival and prognostic factors of hereditary breast cancer from BRCA2-, BRCA1- and non-BRCA1/2 families as compared to sporadic breast cancer cases. *Eur. J. Cancer* **2007**, *43*, 867–876. [CrossRef]
29. Metcalfe, K.; Gershman, S.; Ghadirian, P.; Lynch, H.T.; Snyder, C.; Tung, N.; Kim-Sing, C.; Eisen, A.; Foulkes, W.D.; Rosen, B.; et al. Contralateral mastectomy and survival after breast cancer in carriers of BRCA1 and BRCA2 mutations: Retrospective analysis. *BMJ (Clin. Res. Ed.)* **2014**, *348*, g226. [CrossRef]

30. Heemskerk-Gerritsen, B.A.; Rookus, M.A.; Aalfs, C.M.; Ausems, M.G.; Collee, J.M.; Jansen, L.; Kets, C.M.; Keymeulen, K.B.; Koppert, L.B.; Meijers-Heijboer, H.E.; et al. Improved overall survival after contralateral risk-reducing mastectomy in BRCA1/2 mutation carriers with a history of unilateral breast cancer: A prospective analysis. *Int. J. Cancer* **2015**, *136*, 668–677. [CrossRef]
31. Evans, D.G.; Ingham, S.L.; Baildam, A.; Ross, G.L.; Lalloo, F.; Buchan, I.; Howell, A. Contralateral mastectomy improves survival in women with BRCA1/2-associated breast cancer. *Breast Cancer Res. Treat.* **2013**, *140*, 135–142. [CrossRef]
32. Copson, E.R.; Maishman, T.C.; Tapper, W.J.; Cutress, R.I.; Greville-Heygate, S.; Altman, D.G.; Eccles, B.; Gerty, S.; Durcan, L.T.; Jones, L.; et al. Germline BRCA mutation and outcome in young-onset breast cancer (POSH): A prospective cohort study. *Lancet Oncol.* **2018**, *19*, 169–180. [CrossRef]
33. Akdeniz, D.; Schmidt, M.K.; Seynaeve, C.M.; McCool, D.; Giardiello, D.; van den Broek, A.J.; Hauptmann, M.; Steyerberg, E.W.; Hooning, M.J. Risk factors for metachronous contralateral breast cancer: A systematic review and meta-analysis. *Breast* **2019**, *44*, 1–14. [CrossRef] [PubMed]
34. Fletcher, O.; Johnson, N.; Dos Santos Silva, I.; Kilpivaara, O.; Aittomäki, K.; Blomqvist, C.; Nevanlinna, H.; Wasielewski, M.; Meijers-Heijerboer, H.; Broeks, A.; et al. Family history, genetic testing, and clinical risk prediction: Pooled analysis of CHEK2 1100delC in 1828 bilateral breast cancers and 7030 controls. *Cancer Epidemiol. Biomark. Prev.* **2009**, *18*, 230–234. [CrossRef] [PubMed]
35. Schmidt, M.K.; Hogervorst, F.; van Hien, R.; Cornelissen, S.; Broeks, A.; Adank, M.A.; Meijers, H.; Waisfisz, Q.; Hollestelle, A.; Schutte, M.; et al. Age- and Tumor Subtype-Specific Breast Cancer Risk Estimates for CHEK2*1100delC Carriers. *J. Clin. Oncol. Off. J. Am. Soc. Clin. Oncol.* **2016**, *34*, 2750–2760. [CrossRef] [PubMed]
36. Schmidt, M.K.; Tollenaar, R.A.; de Kemp, S.R.; Broeks, A.; Cornelisse, C.J.; Smit, V.T.; Peterse, J.L.; van Leeuwen, F.E.; Van't Veer, L.J. Breast cancer survival and tumor characteristics in premenopausal women carrying the CHEK2*1100delC germline mutation. *J. Clin. Oncol. Off. J. Am. Soc. Clin. Oncol.* **2007**, *25*, 64–69. [CrossRef] [PubMed]
37. Weischer, M.; Nordestgaard, B.G.; Pharoah, P.; Bolla, M.K.; Nevanlinna, H.; Van't Veer, L.J.; Garcia-Closas, M.; Hopper, J.L.; Hall, P.; Andrulis, I.L.; et al. CHEK2*1100delC heterozygosity in women with breast cancer associated with early death, breast cancer-specific death, and increased risk of a second breast cancer. *J. Clin. Oncol. Off. J. Am. Soc. Clin. Oncol.* **2012**, *30*, 4308–4316. [CrossRef] [PubMed]
38. Meyer, A.; Dork, T.; Sohn, C.; Karstens, J.H.; Bremer, M. Breast cancer in patients carrying a germ-line CHEK2 mutation: Outcome after breast conserving surgery and adjuvant radiotherapy. *Radiother. Oncol. J. Eur. Soc. Ther. Radiol. Oncol.* **2007**, *82*, 349–353. [CrossRef]
39. Kriege, M.; Hollestelle, A.; Jager, A.; Huijts, P.E.; Berns, E.M.; Sieuwerts, A.M.; Meijer-van Gelder, M.E.; Collee, J.M.; Devilee, P.; Hooning, M.J.; et al. Survival and contralateral breast cancer in CHEK2 1100delC breast cancer patients: Impact of adjuvant chemotherapy. *Br. J. Cancer* **2014**, *111*, 1004–1013. [CrossRef]
40. Mellemkjaer, L.; Dahl, C.; Olsen, J.H.; Bertelsen, L.; Guldberg, P.; Christensen, J.; Børresen-Dale, A.L.; Stovall, M.; Langholz, B.; Bernstein, L.; et al. Risk for contralateral breast cancer among carriers of the CHEK2*1100delC mutation in the WECARE Study. *Br. J. Cancer* **2008**, *98*, 728–733. [CrossRef]
41. Broeks, A.; de Witte, L.; Nooijen, A.; Huseinovic, A.; Klijn, J.G.; van Leeuwen, F.E.; Russell, N.S.; van't Veer, L.J. Excess risk for contralateral breast cancer in CHEK2*1100delC germline mutation carriers. *Breast Cancer Res. Treat.* **2004**, *83*, 91–93. [CrossRef]
42. Concannon, P.; Haile, R.W.; Borresen-Dale, A.L.; Rosenstein, B.S.; Gatti, R.A.; Teraoka, S.N.; Diep, T.A.; Jansen, L.; Atencio, D.P.; Langholz, B.; et al. Variants in the ATM gene associated with a reduced risk of contralateral breast cancer. *Cancer Res.* **2008**, *68*, 6486–6491. [CrossRef]
43. Bernstein, J.L.; Concannon, P. ATM, radiation, and the risk of second primary breast cancer. *Int. J. Radiat. Biol.* **2017**, *93*, 1121–1127. [CrossRef] [PubMed]
44. Broeks, A.; Braaf, L.M.; Huseinovic, A.; Schmidt, M.K.; Russell, N.S.; van Leeuwen, F.E.; Hogervorst, F.B.; Van't Veer, L.J. The spectrum of ATM missense variants and their contribution to contralateral breast cancer. *Breast Cancer Res. Treat.* **2008**, *107*, 243–248. [CrossRef] [PubMed]
45. De Bock, G.H.; Schutte, M.; Krol-Warmerdam, E.M.; Seynaeve, C.; Blom, J.; Brekelmans, C.T.; Meijers-Heijboer, H.; Van Asperen, C.J.; Cornelisse, C.J.; Devilee, P.; et al. Tumour characteristics and prognosis of breast cancer patients carryting the germline CHEK2*1100delC variant. *J. Med. Genet.* **2004**, *41*, 731–735. [CrossRef] [PubMed]

46. Reiner, A.S.; Sisti, J.; John, E.M.; Lynch, C.F.; Brooks, J.D.; Mellemkjaer, L.; Boice, J.D.; Knight, J.A.; Concannon, P.; Capanu, M.; et al. Breast Cancer Family History and Contralateral Breast Cancer Risk in Young Women: An Update From the Women's Environmental Cancer and Radiation Epidemiology Study. *J. Clin. Oncol. Off. J. Am. Soc. Clin. Oncol.* **2018**, *36*, 1513–1520. [CrossRef] [PubMed]
47. Begg, C.B.; Haile, R.W.; Borg, A.; Malone, K.E.; Concannon, P.; Thomas, D.C.; Langholz, B.; Bernstein, L.; Olsen, J.H.; Lynch, C.F.; et al. Variation of breast cancer risk among BRCA1/2 carriers. *JAMA* **2008**, *299*, 194–201. [CrossRef] [PubMed]
48. Reiner, A.S.; John, E.M.; Brooks, J.D.; Lynch, C.F.; Bernstein, L.; Mellemkjaer, L.; Malone, K.E.; Knight, J.A.; Capanu, M.; Teraoka, S.N.; et al. Risk of asynchronous contralateral breast cancer in noncarriers of BRCA1 and BRCA2 mutations with a family history of breast cancer: A report from the Women's Environmental Cancer and Radiation Epidemiology Study. *J. Clin. Oncol. Off. J. Am. Soc. Clin. Oncol.* **2013**, *31*, 433–439. [CrossRef] [PubMed]
49. Bernstein, J.L.; Thomas, D.C.; Shore, R.E.; Robson, M.; Boice, J.D., Jr.; Stovall, M.; Andersson, M.; Bernstein, L.; Malone, K.E.; Reiner, A.S.; et al. Contralateral breast cancer after radiotherapy among BRCA1 and BRCA2 mutation carriers: A WECARE study report. *Eur. J. Cancer* **2013**, *49*, 2979–2985. [CrossRef]
50. Pharoah, P. Family history and the risk of breast cancer: A systematic review and meta-analysis. *Int. J. Cancer* **1997**, *71*, 800–809. [CrossRef]
51. Bernstein, J.L.; Thompson, W.D.; Risch, N.; Holford, T.R. Risk factors predicting the incidence of second primary breast cancer among women diagnosed with a first primary breast cancer. *Am. J. Epidemiol.* **1992**, *136*, 925–936. [CrossRef]
52. Ji, J.; Hemminki, K. Risk for contralateral breast cancers in a population covered by mammography: Effects of family history, age at diagnosis and histology. *Breast Cancer Res. Treat.* **2007**, *105*, 229–236. [CrossRef]
53. Narod, S.A.; Kharazmi, E.; Fallah, M.; Sundquist, K.; Hemminki, K. The risk of contralateral breast cancer in daughters of women with and without breast cancer. *Clin. Genet.* **2016**, *89*, 332–335. [CrossRef] [PubMed]
54. Vaittinen, P.; Hemminki, K. Risk factors and age-incidence relationships for contralateral breast cancer. *Int. J. Cancer* **2000**, *88*, 998–1002. [CrossRef]
55. Boughey, J.C.; Hoskin, T.L.; Degnim, A.C.; Sellers, T.A.; Johnson, J.L.; Kasner, M.J.; Hartmann, L.C.; Frost, M.H. Contralateral prophylactic mastectomy is associated with a survival advantage in high-risk women with a personal history of breast cancer. *Ann. Surg. Oncol.* **2010**, *17*, 2702–2709. [CrossRef] [PubMed]
56. Rhiem, K.; Engel, C.; Graeser, M.; Zachariae, S.; Kast, K.; Kiechle, M.; Ditsch, N.; Janni, W.; Mundhenke, C.; Golatta, M.; et al. The risk of contralateral breast cancer in patients from BRCA1/2 negative high risk families as compared to patients from BRCA1 or BRCA2 positive families: A retrospective cohort study. *Breast Cancer Res.* **2012**, *14*, R156. [CrossRef] [PubMed]
57. Bernstein, J.L.; Thompson, W.D.; Risch, N.; Holford, T.R. The genetic epidemiology of second primary breast cancer. *Am. J. Epidemiol.* **1992**, *136*, 937–948. [CrossRef]
58. Fayanju, O.M.; Stoll, C.R.; Fowler, S.; Colditz, G.A.; Margenthaler, J.A. Contralateral prophylactic mastectomy after unilateral breast cancer: A systematic review and meta-analysis. *Ann. Surg.* **2014**, *260*, 1000–1010. [CrossRef]
59. Anderson, D.E.; Badzioch, M.D. Risk of familial breast cancer. *Cancer* **1985**, *56*, 383–387. [CrossRef]
60. McDonnell, S.K.; Schaid, D.J.; Myers, J.L.; Grant, C.S.; Donohue, J.H.; Woods, J.E.; Frost, M.H.; Johnson, J.L.; Sitta, D.L.; Slezak, J.M.; et al. Efficacy of contralateral prophylactic mastectomy in women with a personal and family history of breast cancer. *J. Clin. Oncol. Off. J. Am. Soc. Clin. Oncol.* **2001**, *19*, 3938–3943. [CrossRef]
61. Lostumbo, L.; Carbine, N.E.; Wallace, J. Prophylactic mastectomy for the prevention of breast cancer. *Cochrane Database Syst. Rev.* **2010**, CD002748. [CrossRef]
62. Kiely, B.E.; Jenkins, M.A.; McKinley, J.M.; Friedlander, M.L.; Weideman, P.; Milne, R.L.; McLachlan, S.A.; Hopper, J.L.; Phillips, K.A. Contralateral risk-reducing mastectomy in BRCA1 and BRCA2 mutation carriers and other high-risk women in the Kathleen Cuningham Foundation Consortium for Research into Familial Breast Cancer (kConFab). *Breast Cancer Res. Treat.* **2010**, *120*, 715–723. [CrossRef]
63. Davies, K.R.; Brewster, A.M.; Bedrosian, I.; Parker, P.A.; Crosby, M.A.; Peterson, S.K.; Shen, Y.; Volk, R.J.; Cantor, S.B. Outcomes of contralateral prophylactic mastectomy in relation to familial history: A decision analysis (BRCR-D-16-00033). *Breast Cancer Res.* **2016**, *18*, 93. [CrossRef] [PubMed]

64. Herrinton, L.J.; Barlow, W.E.; Yu, O.; Geiger, A.M.; Elmore, J.G.; Barton, M.B.; Harris, E.L.; Rolnick, S.; Pardee, R.; Husson, G.; et al. Efficacy of prophylactic mastectomy in women with unilateral breast cancer: A cancer research network project. *J. Clin. Oncol. Off. J. Am. Soc. Clin. Oncol.* **2005**, *23*, 4275–4286. [CrossRef] [PubMed]
65. Peralta, E.A.; Ellenhorn, J.D.; Wagman, L.D.; Dagis, A.; Andersen, J.S.; Chu, D.Z. Contralateral prophylactic mastectomy improves the outcome of selected patients undergoing mastectomy for breast cancer. *Am. J. Surg.* **2000**, *180*, 439–445. [CrossRef]
66. Kurian, A.W.; McClure, L.A.; John, E.M.; Horn-Ross, P.L.; Ford, J.M.; Clarke, C.A. Second primary breast cancer occurrence according to hormone receptor status. *J. Natl. Cancer Inst.* **2009**, *101*, 1058–1065. [CrossRef]
67. Li, C.I.; Malone, K.E.; Porter, P.L.; Daling, J.R. Epidemiologic and molecular risk factors for contralateral breast cancer among young women. *Br. J. Cancer* **2003**, *89*, 513–518. [CrossRef]
68. Healey, E.A.; Cook, E.F.; Orav, E.J.; Schnitt, S.J.; Connolly, J.L.; Harris, J.R. Contralateral breast cancer: Clinical characteristics and impact on prognosis. *J. Clin. Oncol. Off. J. Am. Soc. Clin. Oncol.* **1993**, *11*, 1545–1552. [CrossRef]
69. Vichapat, V.; Gillett, C.; Fentiman, I.S.; Tutt, A.; Holmberg, L.; Luchtenborg, M. Risk factors for metachronous contralateral breast cancer suggest two aetiological pathways. *Eur. J. Cancer* **2011**, *47*, 1919–1927. [CrossRef]
70. Yoon, T.I.; Kwak, B.S.; Yi, O.V.; Kim, S.; Um, E.; Yun, K.W.; Shin, H.N.; Lee, S.; Sohn, G.; Chung, I.Y.; et al. Age-related risk factors associated with primary contralateral breast cancer among younger women versus older women. *Breast Cancer Res. Treat.* **2019**, *173*, 657–665. [CrossRef]
71. Zeichner, S.B.; Zeichner, S.B.; Ruiz, A.L.; Markward, N.J.; Rodriguez, E. Improved long-term survival with contralateral prophylactic mastectomy among young women. *Asian Pac. J. Cancer Prev.* **2014**, *15*, 1155–1162. [CrossRef]
72. Yu, T.J.; Liu, Y.Y.; Hu, X.; Di, G.H. No survival improvement of contralateral prophylactic mastectomy among women with invasive lobular carcinoma. *J. Surg. Oncol.* **2018**, *118*, 928–935. [CrossRef] [PubMed]
73. Pesce, C.; Liederbach, E.; Wang, C.; Lapin, B.; Winchester, D.J.; Yao, K. Contralateral prophylactic mastectomy provides no survival benefit in young women with estrogen receptor-negative breast cancer. *Ann. Surg. Oncol.* **2014**, *21*, 3231–3239. [CrossRef]
74. Bedrosian, I.; Hu, C.Y.; Chang, G.J. Population-based study of contralateral prophylactic mastectomy and survival outcomes of breast cancer patients. *J. Natl. Cancer Inst.* **2010**, *102*, 401–409. [CrossRef] [PubMed]
75. Bouchard-Fortier, A.; Baxter, N.N.; Sutradhar, R.; Fernandes, K.; Camacho, X.; Graham, P.; Quan, M.L. Contralateral prophylactic mastectomy in young women with breast cancer: A population-based analysis of predictive factors and clinical impact. *Curr. Oncol.* **2018**, *25*, e562–e568. [CrossRef] [PubMed]
76. Lazow, S.P.; Riba, L.; Alapati, A.; James, T.A. Comparison of breast-conserving therapy vs mastectomy in women under age 40: National trends and potential survival implications. *Breast J.* **2019**, *25*, 578–584. [CrossRef]
77. Park, H.L.; Chang, J.; Lal, G.; Lal, K.; Ziogas, A.; Anton-Culver, H. Trends in Treatment Patterns and Clinical Outcomes in Young Women Diagnosed With Ductal Carcinoma In Situ. *Clin. Breast Cancer* **2018**, *18*, e179–e185. [CrossRef]
78. Yao, K.; Winchester, D.J.; Czechura, T.; Huo, D. Contralateral prophylactic mastectomy and survival: Report from the National Cancer Data Base, 1998–2002. *Breast Cancer Res. Treat.* **2013**, *142*, 465–476. [CrossRef]
79. Tuttle, T.M.; Habermann, E.B.; Grund, E.H.; Morris, T.J.; Virnig, B.A. Increasing use of contralateral prophylactic mastectomy for breast cancer patients: A trend toward more aggressive surgical treatment. *J. Clin. Oncol. Off. J. Am. Soc. Clin. Oncol.* **2007**, *25*, 5203–5209. [CrossRef]
80. Tuttle, T.M.; Jarosek, S.; Habermann, E.B.; Arrington, A.; Abraham, A.; Morris, T.J.; Virnig, B.A. Increasing rates of contralateral prophylactic mastectomy among patients with ductal carcinoma in situ. *J. Clin. Oncol. Off. J. Am. Soc. Clin. Oncol.* **2009**, *27*, 1362–1367. [CrossRef]
81. Kummerow, K.L.; Du, L.; Penson, D.F.; Shyr, Y.; Hooks, M.A. Nationwide trends in mastectomy for early-stage breast cancer. *JAMA Surg.* **2015**, *150*, 9–16. [CrossRef]
82. Guth, U.; Myrick, M.E.; Viehl, C.T.; Weber, W.P.; Lardi, A.M.; Schmid, S.M. Increasing rates of contralateral prophylactic mastectomy—A trend made in USA? *Eur. J. Surg. Oncol. J. Eur. Soc. Surg. Oncol. Br. Assoc. Surg. Oncol.* **2012**, *38*, 296–301. [CrossRef] [PubMed]

83. Fancellu, A.; Sanna, V.; Cottu, P.; Feo, C.F.; Scanu, A.M.; Farina, G.; Bulla, A.; Spanu, A.; Paliogiannis, P.; Porcu, A. Mastectomy patterns, but not rates, are changing in the treatment of early breast cancer. Experience of a single European institution on 2315 consecutive patients. *Breast* **2018**, *39*, 1–7. [CrossRef] [PubMed]
84. Neuburger, J.; Macneill, F.; Jeevan, R.; van der Meulen, J.H.; Cromwell, D.A. Trends in the use of bilateral mastectomy in England from 2002 to 2011: Retrospective analysis of hospital episode statistics. *BMJ Open* **2013**, 3. [CrossRef] [PubMed]
85. Boughey, J.C.; Attai, D.J.; Chen, S.L.; Cody, H.S.; Dietz, J.R.; Feldman, S.M.; Greenberg, C.C.; Kass, R.B.; Landercasper, J.; Lemaine, V.; et al. Contralateral Prophylactic Mastectomy Consensus Statement from the American Society of Breast Surgeons: Additional Considerations and a Framework for Shared Decision Making. *Ann. Surg. Oncol.* **2016**, *23*, 3106–3111. [CrossRef]
86. ABS Summary Statement Contralateral Mastectomy for Unilateral Breast Cancer. Available online: https://associationofbreastsurgery.org.uk/media/63462/contralateral-mastectomy-abs-summary-documen.pdf (accessed on 15 February 2019).

Dasatinib Treatment Increases Sensitivity to c-Met Inhibition in Triple-Negative Breast Cancer Cells

Patricia Gaule [1], Nupur Mukherjee [1], Brendan Corkery [1], Alex J. Eustace [1,*], Kathy Gately [2], Sandra Roche [1], Robert O'Connor [1], Kenneth J. O'Byrne [3], Naomi Walsh [1], Michael J. Duffy [4,5], John Crown [1,6] and Norma O'Donovan [1]

1 Molecular Therapeutics for Cancer Ireland, National Institute for Cellular Biotechnology, Dublin City University, Dublin D09 NR58, Ireland; Patricia.gaule@yale.edu (P.G.); mukherjeen@nirrh.res.in (N.M.); bcorkery@svhg.ie (B.C.); sandra.roche@dcu.ie (S.R.); roconnor@irishcancer.ie (R.O.); Naomi.walsh@dcu.ie (N.W.); john.crown@ccrt.ie (J.C.); normaodonov@gmail.com (N.O.)
2 Trinity Translational Medicine Institute, St. James's Hospital Dublin, Dublin 8, Ireland; gatelyk@tcd.ie
3 Institute of Health and Biomedical Innovation, Queensland University of Technology, Translational Research Institute, Woolloongabba QLD 4059, Australia; k.obyrne@qut.edu.au
4 UCD School of Medicine, UCD Conway Institute of Biomolecular and Biomedical Research, University College Dublin, Dublin 4, Ireland; michael.J.Duffy@ucd.ie
5 UCD Clinical Research Centre, St. Vincent's University Hospital, Dublin 4, Ireland
6 Department of Medical Oncology, St Vincent's University Hospital, Dublin 4, Ireland
* Correspondence: alex.eustace@dcu.ie

Abstract: In pre-clinical studies, triple-negative breast cancer (TNBC) cells have demonstrated sensitivity to the multi-targeted kinase inhibitor dasatinib; however, clinical trials with single-agent dasatinib showed limited efficacy in unselected populations of breast cancer, including TNBC. To study potential mechanisms of resistance to dasatinib in TNBC, we established a cell line model of acquired dasatinib resistance (231-DasB). Following an approximately three-month exposure to incrementally increasing concentrations of dasatinib (200 nM to 500 nM) dasatinib, 231-DasB cells were resistant to the agent with a dasatinib IC_{50} value greater than 5 μM compared to 0.04 ± 0.001 μM in the parental MDA-MB-231 cells. 231-DasB cells also showed resistance (2.2-fold) to the Src kinase inhibitor PD180970. Treatment of 231-DasB cells with dasatinib did not inhibit phosphorylation of Src kinase. The 231-DasB cells also had significantly increased levels of p-Met compared to the parental MDA-MB-231 cells, as measured by luminex, and resistant cells demonstrated a significant increase in sensitivity to the c-Met inhibitor, CpdA, with an IC_{50} value of 1.4 ± 0.5 μM compared to an IC_{50} of 6.8 ± 0.2 μM in the parental MDA-MB-231 cells. Treatment with CpdA decreased p-Met and p-Src in both 231-DasB and MDA-MB-231 cells. Combined treatment with dasatinib and CpdA significantly inhibited the growth of MDA-MB-231 parental cells and prevented the emergence of dasatinib resistance. If these in vitro findings can be extrapolated to human cancer treatment, combined treatment with dasatinib and a c-Met inhibitor may block the development of acquired resistance and improve response rates to dasatinib treatment in TNBC.

Keywords: Src kinase; basal-like breast cancer; cMet

---

1. Introduction

Triple-negative breast cancer (TNBC) lacks expression of estrogen receptor (ER) and progesterone receptor (PR) and exhibits overexpression of human epidermal growth factor receptor 2 (HER2). It accounts for approximately 15% of all breast cancer cases and patients with this form demonstrate higher rates of recurrence and shorter disease progression than those with luminal or HER2-positive tumours [1]. Treatment of TNBC predominantly relies on the use of cytotoxic chemotherapies due to a lack of proven molecular targets [2].

We have previously shown that Proto-oncogene tyrosine-protein kinase Src (Src kinase) is frequently expressed in TNBC and may be a rational therapeutic target for TNBC [3]. Src is a proto-oncogene and a member of the Src family kinases (SFKs). SFKs are non-membrane-bound tyrosine kinases consisting of nine members. Src, Yes, Fyn and Fgr belong to the Src A family subtype. Lck, Hck, Blk and Lyn belong to Src B family subtype, with Frk in its own subfamily [4]. The SFKs display high levels of homology to one another and are involved in propagating downstream cell signalling to effect cellular biological functions including cell proliferation, cell migration, angiogenesis and cell survival [5–7].

Dasatinib is a multi-targeted tyrosine kinase inhibitor whose targets include BCR/Abl and Src family kinases. Pre-clinical studies suggested that basal-like TNBC cell lines show higher sensitivity to dasatinib than luminal cell lines, supporting dasatinib as a potential targeted treatment for TNBC [3,8,9]. Additionally, when TNBC was further sub-classified into six molecular types, cell line models of the mesenchymal and mesenchymal stem-like group showed greater sensitivity to dasatinib than other cell line models [3,9,10]. However, in a phase II clinical trial, dasatinib showed limited single-agent activity in patients with metastatic breast cancer [11] or in patients with locally advanced or metastatic TNBC [12].

Several potential predictive biomarkers of response to dasatinib treatment have been identified [13], and a prospective phase II trial was designed to test three predictive gene signatures, whereby patients with metastatic breast cancer whose metastatic tumour biopsies were positive for one of the gene signatures were treated with dasatinib [13]. However, no significant clinical benefit was observed despite selecting patients having the highest scores for the three predictive signatures.

Thus, despite promising activity in preclinical studies, dasatinib has so far failed to produce clinical benefits in TNBC patients. One of the limitations of the preclinical studies that showed activity in TNBC cells, including our own [3], is that they were limited to short-term proliferation assays. Therefore, we examined the effects of longer exposure to dasatinib on TNBC cells that are highly sensitive to dasatinib in short-term proliferation assays. The overall aim was to identify novel combinatorial approaches that may block the development of acquired resistance to dasatinib and improve response rates to dasatinib treatment in TNBC.

2. Materials and Methods

2.1. Cell Lines and Reagents

MDA-MB-231 cells were obtained from the American Type Culture Collection (ATCC). 231-DasB was developed by continuous exposure to dasatinib (Sequoia Research Products, Berkshire, UK) with a starting concentration of 200 nM, increasing incrementally to a maximum of 500 nM dasatinib over a period of 13 weeks. Untreated (parental) MDA-MB-231 cells were cultured in a similar manner in the absence of drug to create an aged-matched control. Both cell lines were cultured in RPMI 1640 with 10% Foetal Bovine Serum, plus 10 nM dasatinib for 231DasB. Stock solutions (10 mM) of PD180970 (Merck, Dublin, Ireland), elacridar (Sequoia Research Products, Berkshire, UK) and Compound A (CpdA, Amgen, Thousand Oaks, CA, USA) were prepared in DMSO.

2.2. Proliferation Assays

Proliferation was measured in triplicate biological assays using an acid phosphatase assay or viable cell count. For acid phosphatase assays, 1×10^3 cells/well were seeded in 96-well plates. Plates were incubated overnight at 37 °C followed by the addition of the drug at the appropriate concentrations and incubated for a further five days until wells were 80–90% confluent. All media were removed and the wells were washed once with phosphate buffered solution (PBS). Paranitrophenol phosphate (PNP) substrate (Sigma-Aldrich, Dublin, Ireland) (10 mM of PNP in sodium acetate buffer, pH 5.5) was added to each well and incubated at 37 °C for 1 h. Fifty microliters of 1 M NaOH were added and the absorbance was read at 405 nM (reference: 620 nM). For viable cell counts, cells were trypsined and combined in a 1:1 ratio with Viacount Flex reagent and counted using a Guava Easycyte (Merck, Dublin, Ireland).

2.3. Doubling Time Assays

Next 2×10^3 cells were seeded in 24-well plates in 1 mL of serum-containing medium. Fresh medium (control) or drug-containing medium was added to the cells. Assays were conducted in triplicate. Duplicate wells per cell line for each condition (control and drug treatments) were seeded for each time point: day 0, day 4, and day 7. Cell counts were measured using the Guava Viacount method. Doubling times were calculated between days 4 and 7 using the formula

$$\text{Doubling time (hours)} = 24 \times \frac{\log 2x(\text{Tt} - \text{T0})}{(\text{logNt} - \text{logN0})},$$

where Tt is the end time point and T0 is the beginning time point (days), which in this case were 7 and 4, respectively, and N is the average cell count on each day.

2.4. Short-Term Resistance Assay

For the short-term resistance assays, 1.5×10^4 MDA-MB-231 cells per well were seeded in two identical 12-well plates (Plate-1 and Plate-2) in 1 mL of medium with 10% foetal bovine serum (day 1) and allowed to adhere overnight. The cells were treated with 2.5 µM compound A and/or 50 nM dasatinib. In addition, in plate 1, three wells were untreated as a control. In plate 2, the cells were similarly treated with 2.5 µM compound A and/or 50 nM dasatinib. Treatment was repeated twice weekly. After seven days, when the untreated control cells achieved confluency, the medium was removed from the cells in plate 1 and the cells were fixed with 3:1, v:v, methanol:acetic acid, (1 min), then washed with PBS and stained with 0.05%, w:v, crystal violet (5 min). The cells were allowed to air dry overnight, the crystal violet was eluted in 10% acetic acid and absorbance was measured at 590 nM. After 21 days, when the dasatinib-treated cells achieved confluency, cells in plate 2 were fixed and stained as for plate 1.

2.5. Invasion/Migration Assays

Invasion and migration assays were carried out using 5×10^4 cells in Matrigel (Corning)-coated 24-well invasion inserts (BD Biosciences) for invasion assays and uncoated inserts for migration assays. Cells were seeded in reduced serum medium (5% foetal calf serum in RPMI-1640) and incubated for 6 h to allow cell attachment, and then treated with 100 nM dasatinib for 18 h. Cells were stained with crystal violet and the number of invading/migrating cells was estimated by counting 10 fields of view at 200× magnification. The average count was multiplied by the conversion factor 140 (growth area of membrane divided by field of view area, viewed at 200× magnification) to determine the total number of invading/migrating cells. Invasion and migration assays were carried out in triplicate.

2.6. Dasatinib Accumulation Assays

Cells were seeded at the specified numbers in T25-cm^2 cell culture flasks (Thermo Fisher, Dublin, Ireland). After 24 h, the cell culture medium was removed and cells were treated with medium (control) or medium containing 2 µM dasatinib for 2 h. Non-adherent cells were collected and combined with adherent cells after trypsinisation, then centrifuged at 300 *g* for 3 min. The supernatant was removed and the cells were resuspended in 1 mL of ice-cold PBS. Fifty microliters of the cell suspension were removed for cell counting using the Guava Viacount method. The cell suspension was centrifuged as before, and the supernatant was removed. The cell pellet was stored at −20 °C.

Quantification of the mass of dasatinib present in the cells collected was performed using liquid chromatography tandem mass spectrometry (LC-MS/MS), as previously described [14]. Briefly, the drug was extracted using a liquid-liquid extraction procedure. One hundred microliters of 500 ng/mL lapatinib were added to an extraction tube (internal standard), along with 200 μL of 1 M Ammonium Formate pH 3.5 buffer and 1.6 mL of extraction solvent tert-Butyl Methyl Ether (tBME)/ acetonitrile (ACN) (3:1 v:v). The extraction tubes were vortexed and mixed on a blood tube mixer for 15 min. The samples were centrifuged at 6500 *g* for 5 min; the organic layer was removed and 1.1 mL of solvent was transferred to conical bottomed glass LC autosampler vials (Sigma-Aldrich, Dublin, Ireland). The vials were evaporated to dryness using a Genevac EZ-2 (Ipswich, UK) evaporator at ambient temperature, without light. The samples were reconstituted in 40 μL of acetonitrile with 20 μL injected automatically by the autosampler. The LC-MS was run in isocratic mobile phase (54% ACN:10 mM ammonium formate, pH 4) on a Hyperclone BDS C18 column, in multi-reaction monitoring (MRM) positive ion mode. Analysis was performed using MRM mode with the following transitions: m/z 581→m/z 365 for lapatinib, and m/z 488→m/z (231 and 401) for dasatinib, with a dwell time of 200 ms. Quantification was based on the integrated peak area determined by the Masshunter Quantification Analysis software, which quantitates the peak areas of the MRM transitions of each analyte. Results are reported as mean and standard deviation (SD) of the mass per million cells in triplicate flasks.

2.7. Protein Extraction and Western Blotting

RIPA buffer with 1× protease inhibitors, 2 mM PMSF and 1 mM sodium orthovanadate (Sigma-Aldrich) was added to cells and incubated on ice for 20 min. Following centrifugation at 10,000 rpm for 10 min at 4 °C, the resulting lysate was stored at −80 °C. Protein quantification was performed using the bicinchoninic acid (BCA) assay (Pierce). Thirty micrograms of protein in sample buffer were heated to 95 °C for 5 min and proteins were separated on 7.5% gels (Lonza) or 4–12% gels (Thermo-Fischer, Dublin, Ireland). The protein was transferred to a nitrocellulose membrane. The membrane was blocked with a blocking solution (PBS + 0.1% Tween + 5% skimmed milk powder (BioRad, Dublin, Ireland) or a 1× NET solution buffer (0.5 M NaCl, 0.05 M EDTA, 0.1 M Tris pH 7.8) at room temperature for 1 h, then incubated overnight at 4 °C in a blocking solution with a 1:1000 antibody dilution of total Src, c-Met, p-Met Y1234/1235 (Cell Signalling Technology, Leiden, Netherlands) or 1:500 p-Src Y419 (Merck-Millipore). The membrane was washed three times with PBS-Tween or 1× NET, then incubated at room temperature with anti-mouse secondary antibody (Sigma-Aldrich) at 1:1000 dilution or anti-rabbit secondary antibody (Sigma-Aldrich) at a 1:1000 dilution in blocking solution for 1 h. The membrane was washed three times with PBS-Tween/1× NET followed by one PBS wash. Detection was performed using Luminol (Santa Cruz Biotechnology, Heidelberg, Germany).

2.8. Luminex Magnetic Bead Assays

Magnetic bead assays were performed on the Luminex® MagPix® System (Merck Millipore (80-073), Dublin, Ireland) using Milliplex Map Phospho Mitogenesis RTK Magnetic Bead 7-Plex Kit (Merck Millipore 48-672 Mag) and Milliplex Map phospho Human Src Family Kinase Magnetic Bead 8-Plex kit (Merck Millipore 48-650 Mag). Protein extractions were prepared as described above. Protein (1–10 μg) was diluted in appropriate volume of assay buffer (final volume: 25 μL/well) and the assay was performed as per the manufacturer's instructions.

2.9. DNA Extraction and Nested PCR Amplification of Src Exons 9–12

DNA was extracted from the parent MDA-MB-231 and the resistant 231DasB cell lines using the QIAamp® DNA mini kit (Qiagen, Hilden, Germany). Exons 9–12 of the *Src* gene were amplified using the primer sets in Table S1. The forward outer primer and the reverse primer were used in the first PCR reaction and the forward inner primer and the reverse primer were used in the second PCR reaction. The following PCR conditions were used for the first reaction: 5 μL 10× Amplitaq Gold Buffer

(Thermo-Fischer, Dublin, Ireland), 3 μL 25 mM $MgCl_2$, 1 μL 10 mM dNTPs, 5 μM each of forward and reverse primer, 0.25 μL Amplitaq Gold DNA Polymerase (Applied Biosystems, Foster City, CA, USA) and 50 ng of DNA made up to a volume of 50 μL with dH_2O. A pre-PCR heat step of 95 °C for 5 min was carried out to activate the enzyme and the DNA was amplified for 35 cycles at 95 °C (1 min), 56 °C (1 min) and 72 °C (1 min) and at 72 °C (10 min) after the last cycle. The second PCR was carried out as above with 1 μL of the first PCR reaction replacing the DNA. Ten microliters of the PCR product were electrophoresed on 1% agarose gel to verify product integrity. PCR products were purified using a QIAquick PCR purification kit (Qiagen). The DNA concentration was measured using the Nanodrop 1000 spectrophotometer (Thermo Fischer, Dublin, Ireland).

2.10. *Cycle Sequencing of PCR Products*

Cycle sequencing reactions were set up as follows: 2 μL of BigDye® Terminator Mix v3.1, 20 ng amplicon DNA, 3.2 pmol of forward or reverse primer, 2 μL sequencing buffer and diluted to 20 μL with water. A positive control was also set up to ensure the efficiency of the sequencing reaction (1 μL pGem, 2 μL M13 primer, 2 μL of BigDye® Terminator Mix v3.1 and 2 μL sequencing buffer). The pGem and BigDye® Terminator v3.1 mix were both sourced from Applied Biosystems (Warrington, UK). Initial denaturation was carried out by a rapid thermal ramp to 96 °C (1 min), followed by 25 cycles of: rapid thermal ramp to 96 °C (10 s), rapid thermal ramp to 50 °C (5 s), rapid thermal ramp to 60 °C (4 min). Unincorporated dye terminators were removed before performing capillary electrophoresis using the DyeEx 2.0 Spinkit (Qiagen). Sequencing was performed on a 3130xl genetic analyser (Thermo-Ficsher, Ireland, and sequencing files were analysed using the BioEdit v 7.0.8 (Tom Hall, Ibis Biosciences, Carlsbad, CA, USA).

2.11. *Statistical Analysis*

Alterations in doubling times of cell lines, changes in the invasive and migratory potential of cell lines, and alterations in proteomic signalling were measured using the Student's t-test. Error bars represent the standard deviation of triplicate experiments, where '*'/'**'indicates a p-value of $\leq 0.05/0.01$, respectively, where a p-value < 0.05 was considered statistically significant.

3. Results

3.1. *Dasatinib Exposure Induces a Resistant Phenotype*

MDA-MB-231 cells are very sensitive to growth inhibition by dasatinib ($IC_{50} = 40 \pm 1$ nM) [3]. A cell line model of acquired resistance to dasatinib, MDA-MB-231 cells, was developed by continuous exposure to dasatinib for approximately three months. Following this treatment the IC_{50} value for dasatinib increased to greater than 5 μM, confirming acquired resistance to dasatinib ($IC_{50} > 1$ μM) (8) compared to MDA-MB-231 cells (Figure 1A). The MDA-MB-231 cells that developed acquired resistance to dasatinib were referred to as 231 DasB.

No significant difference in growth rate was observed between the MDA-MB-231 parental cells and the 231-DasB cells. MDA-MB-231 cells show a significant dose dependent increase in doubling time in the presence of dasatinib, whereas the 231-DasB cells show no significant change in doubling time in response to dasatinib (Table 1).

Table 1. Doubling time in hours (± standard deviation) of MDA-MB-231 and MDA-MB-231-Das cells with and without dasatinib treatment. * indicates $p < 0.05$ calculated using the Student's t-test.

Cell Line	Control	D 50 nM	D 100 nM
MDA-MB-231	17.6 ± 1.2	32.2 ± 3.3*	46.8 ± 5.1*
231 DasB	19.1 ± 2.4	21.0 ± 0.2	21.2 ± 3.1

We have previously shown that dasatinib treatment significantly decreases migration and invasion of MDA-MB-231 cells [3]. Migration, but not invasion, was significantly increased in the 231-DasB variant compared to the parental cell line ($p = 0.009$) (Figure 1B). In the 231-DasB-resistant variant, dasatinib did not inhibit invasion ($p = 0.772$) (Figure 1C) or migration ($p = 0.340$) (Figure 1D).

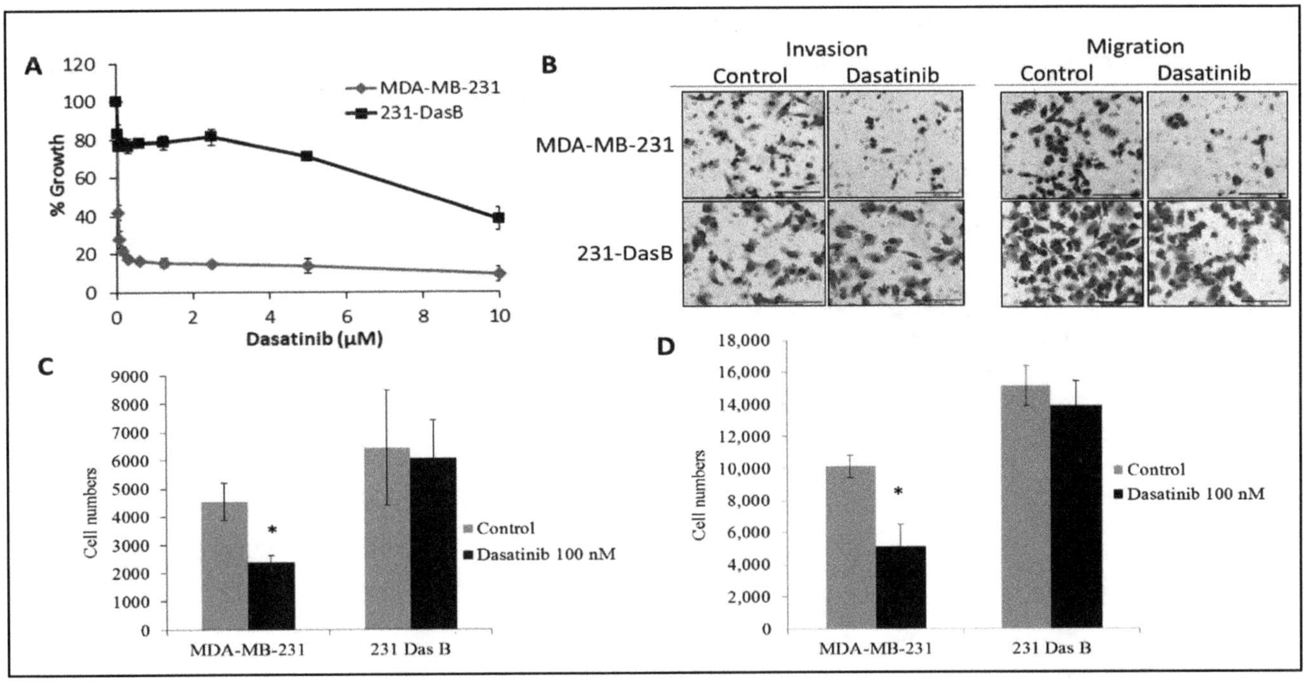

Figure 1. Characterisation of the 231DasB cell line: (**A**) Proliferation assays of MDA-MB-231 and 231-DasB with serially decreasing concentrations of dasatinib from 10 μM; (**B**) representative images of MDA-MB-231 and 231-DasB post-18 h 100 nM dasatinib treatment in invasion and migration assays; (**C**) invasion assays and (**D**) migration assays of MDA-MB-231 and 231-DasB post-18 h 100 nM dasatinib treatment. Error bars represent the standard deviation of triplicate experiments. * $p \leq 0.05$. p values were calculated using the Student's t-test.

Dasatinib is a substrate for the drug efflux pumps BCRP and MDR-1 [15]. Therefore, in order to determine if drug efflux pumps were involved in the resistance to dasatinib in 231-DasB cells, we assessed the uptake of dasatinib in the parental MDA-MB-231 cells and the resistant variant, 231-DasB. Initially, dasatinib accumulation was measured using 2 μM dasatinib across a range of cell seeding numbers. While the relative mass of drug measured increased with decreasing cell density, no significant difference in accumulation between parental and variant cells was observed, suggesting drug pumps do not influence resistance to dasatinib in the 231-DasB cell line (Figure S1). To confirm this, we tested growth inhibition with dasatinib combined with the potent BCRP and MDR-1 inhibitor, elacridar [16]. Proliferation was measured in the parental and variant cell lines treated with dasatinib alone or in combination with a concentration of elacridar sufficient to inhibit BCRP [17] and MDR-1 [18]. The addition of elacridar did not cause a significant increase in dasatinib-induced growth inhibition in either the parental or the variant cell line (Figure S2).

3.2. Phosphorylation of Src Is Altered in Dasatinib-Resistant Cells

The 231-DasB cells were tested for cross-resistance to the Src kinase inhibitor PD180970. The 231-DasB cells showed a 2.2-fold increase in the PD180970 IC_{50} compared to the MDA-MB-231 cells (876.1 ± 74.4 versus 400.2 ± 35.6 nM, $p = 0.003$), implicating Src in the resistant phenotype. Therefore, we examined phosphorylation of Src in the resistant cells. As expected, dasatinib treatment reduced the levels of p-Src (Y419) in MDA-MB-231 cells but no reduction in p-Src (Y419) was observed in the 231-DasB cells following dasatinib treatment (25–200 nM) (Figure 2A). The Src family kinases

(SFKs) consist of nine family members with high conservation between family members at tyrosine 419 (Y419). We examined the phosphorylation of seven of these proteins using magnetic multiplex assays. Consistent with the Western blot results, MDA-MB-231 showed a significant reduction in p-Src in response to dasatinib treatment (Figure 2B). p-FYN, p-YES and p-LYN were also significantly reduced after treatment with dasatinib. In the 231-DasB cells, treatment with dasatinib did not decrease the level of any of the phospho-SFK proteins examined (Figure 2B).

To determine if a mutation in the active site of Src kinase may be causing constitutive activation of p-Src, in the presence of dasatinib, we sequenced exons 9–12 of the *Src* gene, which encompass tyrosine 419 and the regulatory site at tyrosine 530 [19,20], in both the MDA-MB-231 parental and 231DasB cells. No alteration in the Src sequence was detected in the 231DasB cells (Figure S3).

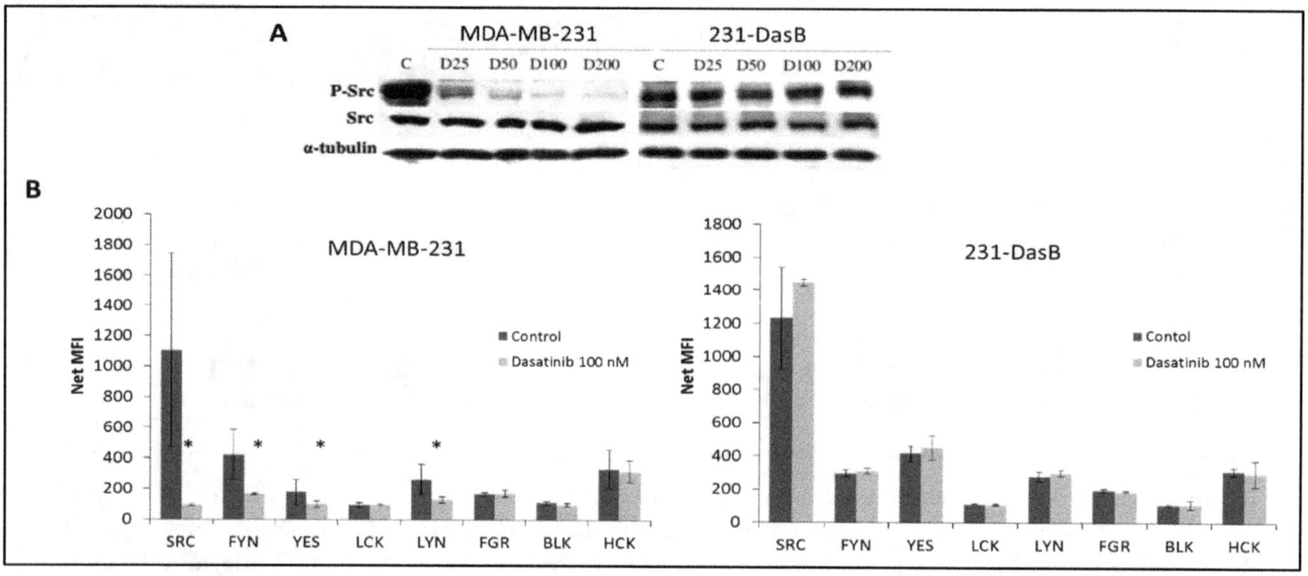

Figure 2. (**A**) Levels of total Src and phosphorylated Src [pY419] in MDA-MB-231 (parental and 231-DasB cells treated with dasatinib for 6 h. (P-: phospho-; C: control (untreated); D: dasatinib (nM)). (**B**) Phosphorylation of Src family kinases as determined by multiplex bead assay in MDA-MB-231 and 231-DasB cell lines with and without 6-h dasatinib treatment (100 nM). NET MFI is net median fluorescence intensity. Error bars represent the standard deviations of triplicate independent experiments. * indicates $p < 0.05$ calculated using the Student's t-test.

3.3. cMet Signalling Is Increased in Dasatinib-Resistant Cells

To investigate the possible role of upstream receptor tyrosine kinases (RTKs) in activation of Src kinase in the 231DasB cells, we examined the phosphorylation of a panel of RTKs using a multiplex assay. c-Met (panTYR) was the only RTK of the five tested that was altered in the 231-DasB cells. 231-DasB cells show significantly higher levels of p-Met ($p = 0.004$) as determined by ELISA, compared to the MDA-MB-231 cells (Figure 3A). We then demonstrated a non-significant 1.4-fold increase ($p = 0.08$) in phosphorylation of c-Met at its activation site (Y1234/Y1235) (Figure 3B). The difference in results between ELISA and Western blotting is likely due to the ELISA assay detecting all changes in p-Met activation, whilst we only analysed changes in p-Met (Y1234/1235) using Western blotting.

Based on the increased levels of p-Met in the 231-DasB cells, we examined sensitivity to a c-Met inhibitor, compound A (CpdA). The 231-DasB cells are more sensitive to CpdA, with an IC_{50} of 1.4 ± 0.5 μM, compared to the MDA-MB-231 cells where the CpdA IC_{50} is 6.8 ± 0.2 μM (Figure 3C).

Combined treatment with CpdA and dasatinib resulted in significantly decreased growth in MDA-MB-231 ($p = 0.02$) (Figure 3D). In the 231-DasB cells, the combination did not enhance growth inhibition compared to CpdA alone (Figure 3D).

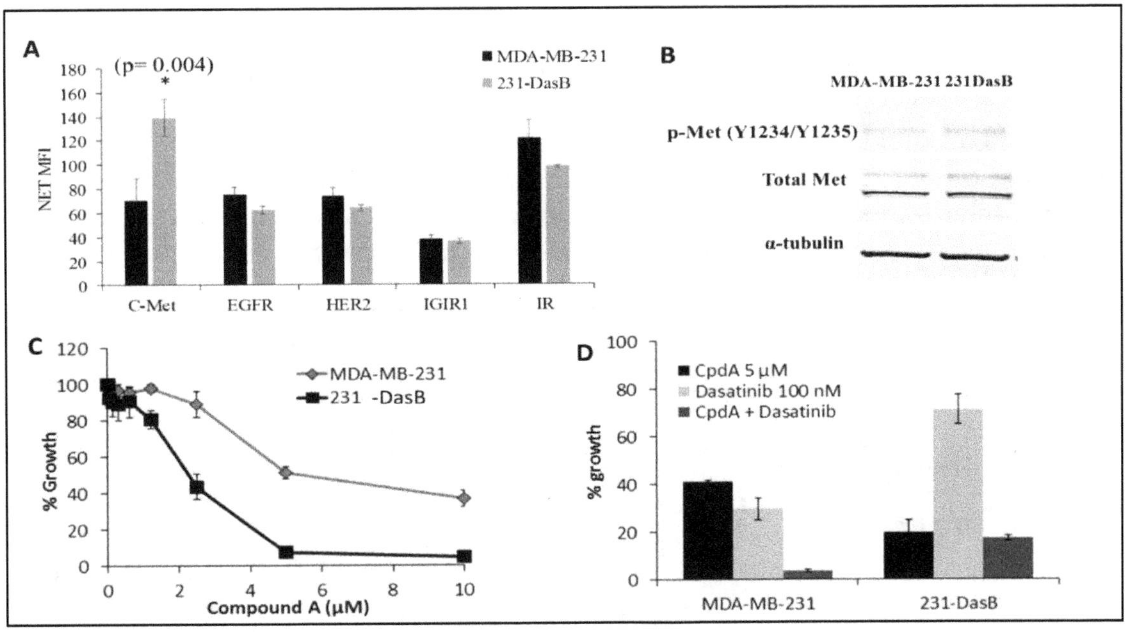

Figure 3. (**A**) Phosphorylation of five RTKs in the MDA-MB-231 and 231-DasB cell lines, where NET MFI is net median fluorescence. Error bars represent the standard deviations of triplicate independent experiments. * indicates $p < 0.05$. p values were calculated using the Student's t-test. (**B**) Immunoblots for p-Met (Y1234/Y1235) and total Met in MDA-MB-231 and 231-DasB cells. α-tubulin was used a loading control. (**C**) MDA-MB-231 and 231-DasB dose-response curves with serially decreasing concentrations of CpdA from 10 μM; (**D**) Fixed concentration proliferation assays with 100 nM dasatinib and 5 μM CpdA in MDA-MB-231 and 231-DasB cells.

The combined treatment also significantly reduced invasion in the MDA-MB-231 cells ($p = 0.002$), but not in the 231-DasB cells (Figure 4A). We examined the effects of CpdA on the phosphorylation of the SFKs. No significant change was observed in the parental MDA-MB-231 cells following treatment with CpdA; however, in 231-DasB cells six of the eight p-SFKs show a significant reduction in phosphorylation. FYN, YES, LCK, LYN, FGR and BLK all show significant reductions in phosphorylation in response to CpdA treatment (5 μM) (Figure 4B).

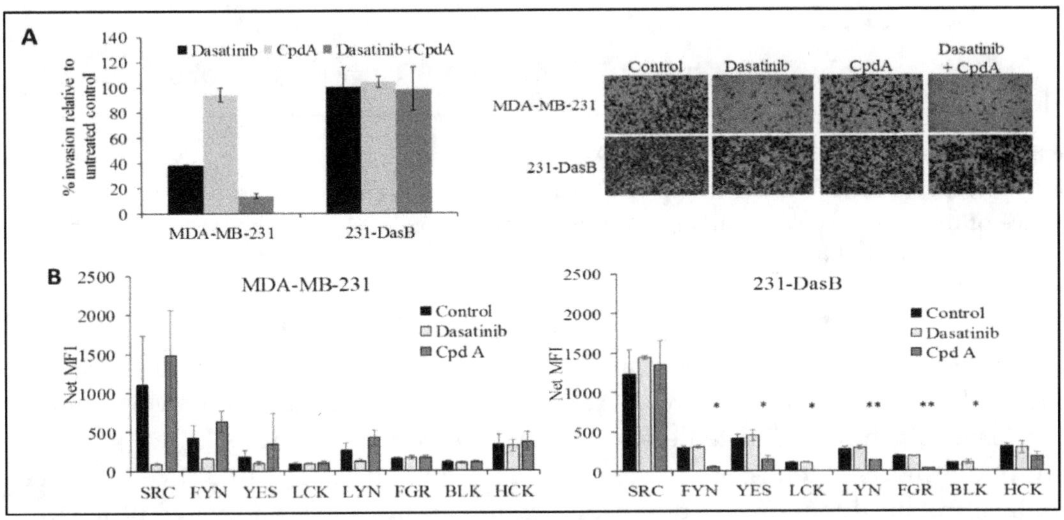

Figure 4. (**A**) Invasion assays in MDA-MB-231 and 231-DasB cells with/without dasatinib (100 nM) and/or CpdA (5 μM); (**B**) phosphorylation of SFKs in MDA-MB-231 and 231-DasB in response to dasatinib 100 nM and CpdA (5 μM) where NET MFI is net median fluorescence intensity. * $p < 0.05$, ** $p < 0.01$. Error bars represent the standard deviations of triplicate independent experiments. p values were calculated using the Student's t-test.

3.4. cMET Inhibition Blocks Dasatinib Resistance

To determine if cMET inhibition may prevent the emergence of resistance to dasatinib in TNBC cells, the MDA-MB-231 cells were treated with CpdA alone (2.5 μM), dasatinib alone (50 nM) or dasatinib plus CpdA. After seven days of treatment, both CpdA and dasatinib as single agents showed significant inhibition of growth (Figure 5). However, by day 21 cells treated with either CpdA or dasatinib started to grow again, suggesting the emergence of resistance, whereas the cells treated with CpdA combined with dasatinib showed no evidence of significant regrowth (Figure 5).

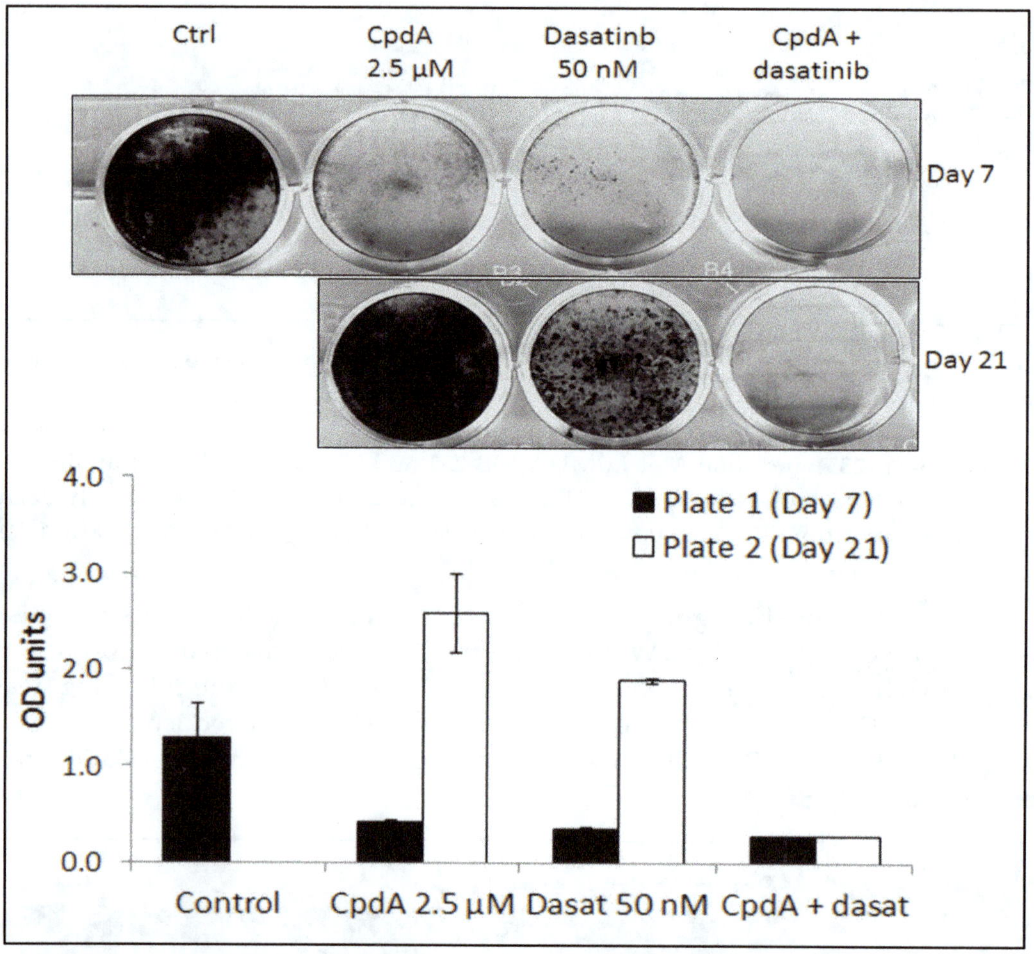

Figure 5. Short-term resistance assay in MDA-MB-231 cells treated with 2.5 μM CpdA and/or 50 nM dasatinib for seven days and 21 days. Optical density (OD) was determined by measuring the absorbance of the crystal violet eluted from stained cells, at 590 nM. Error bars represent the standard deviation of triplicate experiments.

4. Discussion

Pre-clinical models of TNBC demonstrated significant sensitivity to the multi-targeted Src kinase inhibitor dasatinib (with specificity for BCR/Abl and Src family kinases); however, clinical trials with single-agent dasatinib showed limited efficacy in unselected populations [3,8,12]. In this study we sought to study the effects of long-term exposure to dasatinib on MDA-MB-231 cells, which are highly sensitive to dasatinib in three- or five-day proliferation assays [3,8]. Clinical studies indicated that significant resistance emerged within three months of continuous exposure to physiologically relevant concentrations of dasatinib [21,22]. Interestingly, we also demonstrated that resistance to dasatinib developed very quickly in the MDA-MB-231 cells. In HER2 positive breast cancer cell lines, we have found that resistance to HER2 targeted therapies generally emerges after approximately six months of continuous exposure [23,24]. This rapid development of dasatinib resistance may contribute to the lack of clinical activity observed in the single-agent phase II clinical trials.

As dasatinib is a substrate for the drug efflux pumps BCRP and MDR-1 [15], we performed accumulation assays to determine if the concentration of dasatinib achieved in the resistant cells was lower than in the parental cells. No difference in dasatinib accumulation was observed in the resistant cells and inhibition of MDR-1 and BCRP by elacridar did not enhance response to dasatinib in the resistant cells. Taken together, these results suggest that neither altered drug uptake nor efflux plays a role in the acquired dasatinib-resistant phenotype in these cells.

In the 231-DasB cells phosphorylation of Src at Y419 is not inhibited by dasatinib. This site is highly conserved across the SFKs. Therefore, to examine if specific SFKs are altered in the resistant cells we performed a multiplex assay for seven SFK members. Src was the only member of the SFK family that showed increased phosphorylation in the resistant cells. While dasatinib inhibited phosphorylation of several of the SFKs in MDA-MB-231 cells, it did not inhibit phosphorylation of any of the SFKs in the resistant cells.

Activation of Src kinase has been documented in a number of cancer types; however, activating mutations are rare. A truncating mutation in Src at Y530 has been identified in small subsets of colon and endometrial cancers [20,25]. To determine if a mutation in Src could cause constitutive Src phosphorylation in 231-DasB cells, we sequenced exons 9–12 of the *Src* gene, which encompass the kinase domain and the regulatory site at tyrosine 530 [19]. No mutations were detected in the *Src* gene the 231-DasB cell line.

Altered receptor tyrosine kinase signalling, in particular EGFR and c-Met signalling have been implicated in increased pSrc signalling in cancer, particularly in lung cancer but also in breast cancer [26,27]. Therefore, we examined whether altered RTK signalling might play a role in the dasatinib-resistant phenotype. Of the five RTKs examined, only c-MET showed an increase in phosphorylation in the resistant cells. Although EGFR has been implicated in cross-talk with both Src and MET, pEGFR levels were unaltered in the 231-DasB cells suggesting that EGFR is not a mediator of the dasatinib-resistant phenotype.

Recently another TNBC model of dasatinib resistance has been described, using the BT20 cell line. Pinedo-Carpio et al. found that chronic exposure to dasatinib resulted in increased expression of TGFβ2 and increased resistance to a TGFβ inhibitor, with a shift towards non-canonical TGFβ signalling [28]. Zhang et al. have previously shown that non-canonical TGFβ signalling can stimulate phosphorylation of Src at Tyr419 in a lung cancer cell line [29]. Thus, it is possible that non-canonical TGFβ signalling may also play a role in the dasatinib resistance in our 231-DasB model. The MDA-MB-231 cell line used in our analysis represents a post-EMT cell line [1], whilst the BT20 dasatinib-resistant model [2] is not an epithelial-mesenchymal transition (EMT) cell line. Finn et al. reported that the majority of post-EMT TNBC cell lines are highly sensitive to dasatinib, similar to MDA-MB-231. Pinedo-Carpio et al. [2] did not report any changes in cMET expression as a result of acquired dasatinib resistance, indicating that the changes we observed in cMet in the 231 DasB cells may be unique to post-EMT cells in response to dasatinib treatment. Consistent, however, with the increased p-Met levels, the 231-DasB cells also showed increased sensitivity to the Met inhibitor CpdA. Interestingly, the combination of CpdA and dasatinib resulted in significantly enhanced growth inhibition in the parental cell line but not in the 231-DasB cells. Furthermore, short-term resistance assays in the MDA-MB-231 cells showed that, in the presence of compound A, dasatinib resistance did not emerge, suggesting that c-Met inhibition may sensitise the cells to dasatinib and prevent the delay or block the development of dasatinib resistance. CpdA also enhanced dasatinib-mediated inhibition of invasion in the parental cells but not in the resistant cells. In 231-DasB cells, CpdA inhibits phosphorylation of several members of the SFK family—FYN, YES, LCK, LYN, FGR and BLK—but did not inhibit phosphorylation of Src. Our results suggest that pSrc signalling may be critical in the development of the aggressive phenotype of TNBC, and that the inhibition of p-Src may be required to overcome established resistance to dasatinib and possibly the aggressive, invasive behaviour of TNBC.

c-Met has previously been implicated in other models of acquired resistance to other small molecule inhibitors, chemotherapy and radiotherapies. Cabozantinib, a small-molecule c-Met inhibitor, has been shown to overcome gemcitabine resistance in pancreatic cancer and, quite encouragingly, displayed only a very low level of acquired resistance despite long-term treatment [30]. A similar situation was observed in two primary multiple myeloma cell lines that show increased p-Met at the development of resistance compared to the sensitive cell lines [31]. In the MDA-MB-231 cell line, ionising radiation increases the activation of c-Met and targeting the cells with a c-Met inhibitor sensitises the cells to radiation therapy [32]. Met has also been implicated in the resistance to the antiangiogenic therapy bevacizumab in glioblastomas [33]. Upregulation of c-Met was noted after exposure to bevacizumab. Our results suggest that, while c-Met may be a potential target in the acquired resistance setting, it may also be appropriate to target c-Met in combination with other therapies to prevent the development of resistance.

Dasatinib has been previously tested and has failed clinical trials in breast cancer; however, combining dasatinib with a c-Met inhibitor may be a rational therapeutic strategy to test in TNBC. Further evaluation in preclinical models of TNBC, including in vivo, would be required to support the progression of this combination into clinical trials. Furthermore, the evaluation of changes in the phosphorylation of c-Met following dasatinib treatment in tumours from patients enrolled on previous dasatinib clinical trials would be important. These trials, which included sample collection for biomarker studies ([11], NCT00817531), would elucidate whether the increase in p-Met levels that we observed in vitro following dasatinib treatment also occurs in TNBC cells in patients following dasatinib exposure. If increases in p-Met were detected in dasatinib-treated tumours, it would support clinical testing of dasatinib plus a c-Met inhibitor to block the development of dasatinib resistance.

5. Conclusions

In conclusion, our results suggest that cMet may be a rational target in triple-negative tumours that have developed acquired resistance to dasatinib; or, perhaps a better approach may be to combine dasatinib and cMet inhibition before metastasis occurs to improve the response to dasatinib and potentially block the emergence of resistant cells.

Author Contributions: Conceptualization: N.O., J.C., M.J.D.; Methodology: P.G., N.M., B.C., A.J.E., K.G., S.R., N.O.; Formal analysis: P.G., N.M., B.C., A.J.E., K.G., S.R., N.O.; Investigation: P.G., N.M., B.C., A.J.E., K.G., S.R.; Data curation: P.G., N.M., B.C., A.J.E., K.G., S.R., N.O.; Writing—original draft preparation: P.G., N.M., B.C., S.R.; Writing—review and editing: K.G., R.O., K.J.O., N.W., M.J.D., J.C., N.O.; Supervision: R.O., K.J.O., N.W., M.J.D., J.C., N.O.; Funding acquisition: N.O., J.C.

Acknowledgments: We would like to acknowledge Amgen, who kindly gave us access to the c-Met inhibitor Compound-A used in our studies.

References

1. Pogoda, K.; Niwińska, A.; Murawska, M.; Pieńkowski, T. Analysis of pattern, time and risk factors influencing recurrence in triple-negative breast cancer patients. *Med. Oncol.* **2013**, *30*, 388. [CrossRef]
2. Narod, S.A.; Dent, R.A.; Foulkes, W.D. CCR 20thanniversary commentary: Triple-negative breast cancer in 2015—Still in the ballpark. *Clin. Cancer Res.* **2015**, *21*, 3813–3814. [CrossRef]
3. Tryfonopoulos, D.; Walsh, S.; Collins, D.M.; Flanagan, L.; Quinn, C.; Corkery, B.; McDermott, E.W.; Evoy, D.; Pierce, A.; O'Donovan, N.; et al. Src: A potential target for the treatment of triple-negative breast cancer. *Ann. Oncol.* **2011**, *22*, 2234–2240. [CrossRef] [PubMed]
4. Parsons, S.J.; Parsons, J.T. Src family kinases, key regulators of signal transduction. *Oncogene* **2004**, *23*, 7906–7909. [CrossRef]

5. Kim, M.P.; Park, S.I.; Kopetz, S.; Gallick, G.E. Src family kinases as mediators of endothelial permeability: Effects on inflammation and metastasis. *Cell Tissue Res.* **2009**, *335*, 249. [CrossRef]
6. Wheeler, D.L.; Iida, M.; Kruser, T.J.; Nechrebecki, M.M.; Dunn, E.F.; Armstrong, E.A.; Huang, S.; Harari, P.M. Epidermal growth factor receptor cooperates with Src family kinases in acquired resistance to cetuximab. *Cancer Biol. Ther.* **2009**, *8*, 696–703. [CrossRef] [PubMed]
7. Finn, R.S. Targeting Src in breast cancer. *Ann. Oncol.* **2008**, *19*, 1379–1386. [CrossRef] [PubMed]
8. Finn, R.S.; Dering, J.; Ginther, C.; Wilson, C.A.; Glaspy, P.; Tchekmedyian, N.; Slamon, D.J. Dasatinib, an orally active small molecule inhibitor of both the src and abl kinases, selectively inhibits growth of basal-type/"triple-negative" breast cancer cell lines growing in vitro. *Breast Cancer Res. Treat.* **2007**, *105*, 319–326. [CrossRef]
9. Huang, F.; Reeves, K.; Han, X.; Fairchild, C.; Platero, S.; Wong, T.W.; Lee, F.; Shaw, P.; Clark, E. Identification of candidate molecular markers predicting sensitivity in solid tumors to dasatinib: Rationale for patient selection. *Cancer Res.* **2007**, *67*, 2226–2238. [CrossRef]
10. Lehmann, B.D.; Bauer, J.A.; Chen, X.; Sanders, M.E.; Chakravarthy, A.B.; Shyr, Y.; Pietenpol, J.A. Identification of human triple-negative breast cancer subtypes and preclinical models for selection of targeted therapies. *J. Clin. Investig.* **2011**, *121*, 2750–2767. [CrossRef]
11. Herold, C.I.; Chadaram, V.; Peterson, B.L.; Marcom, P.K.; Hopkins, J.; Kimmick, G.G.; Favaro, J.; Hamilton, E.; Welch, R.A.; Bacus, S.; et al. Phase II trial of dasatinib in patients with metastatic breast cancer using real-time pharmacodynamic tissue biomarkers of Src inhibition to escalate dosing. *Clin. Res.* **2011**, *17*, 6061–6070. [CrossRef] [PubMed]
12. Finn, R.; Bengala, C.; Ibrahim, N.; Strauss, L.; Fairchild, J.; Sy, O.; Roche, H.; Sparano, J.; Goldstein, L. Phase II trial of dasatinib in triple-negative breast cancer: Results of study CA180059. *Cancer Res.* **2009**, *69*, 3118. [CrossRef]
13. Pusztai, L.; Moulder, S.; Altan, M.; Kwiatkowski, D.; Valero, V.; Ueno, N.T.; Esteva, F.J.; Avritscher, R.; Qi, Y.; Strauss, L.; et al. Gene signature-guided dasatinib therapy in metastatic breast cancer. *Clin. Cancer Res.* **2014**, *20*, 5265–5271. [CrossRef]
14. Roche, S.; McMahon, G.; Clynes, M.; O'Connor, R. Development of a high-performance liquid chromatographic-mass spectrometric method for the determination of cellular levels of the tyrosine kinase inhibitors lapatinib and dasatinib. *J. Chromatogr. B Anal. Technol. Biomed. Life Sci.* **2009**, *877*, 3982–3990. [CrossRef]
15. Hiwase, D.K.; Saunders, V.; Hewett, D.; Frede, A.; Zrim, S.; Dang, P.; Eadie, L.; To, L.B.; Melo, J.; Kumar, S.; et al. Dasatinib cellular uptake and efflux in chronic myeloid leukemia cells: Therapeutic implications. *Clin. Cancer Res.* **2008**, *14*, 3881–3888. [CrossRef] [PubMed]
16. Collins, D.M.; Crown, J.; O'Donovan, N.; Devery, A.; O'Sullivan, F.; O'Driscoll, L.; Clynes, M.; O'Connor, R. Tyrosine kinase inhibitors potentiate the cytotoxicity of MDR-substrate anticancer agents independent of growth factor receptor status in lung cancer cell lines. *Investig. New Drugs* **2010**, *28*, 433–444. [CrossRef] [PubMed]
17. Maliepaard, M.; Van Gastelen, M.A.; Tohgo, A.; Hausheer, F.H.; Van Waardenburg, R.C.A.M.; De Jong, L.A.; Pluim, D.; Beijnen, J.H.; Schellens, J.H.M. Circumvention of breast cancer resistance protein (BCRP)-mediated resistance to camptothecins in vitro using non-substrate drugs or the BCRP inhibitor GF120918. *Clin. Cancer Res.* **2001**, *7*, 935–941. [PubMed]
18. Hyafil, F.; Vergely, C.; Vignaud, P.; Du Grand-Perret, T. In Vitro and in Vivo Reversal of Multidrug Resistance by GF120918, an Acridonecarboxamide Derivative. *Cancer Res.* **1993**, *53*, 4595–4602. [PubMed]
19. Anderson, S.K.; Gibbs, C.P.; Tanaka, A.; Kung, H.J.; Fujita, D.J. Human Cellular src Gene: Nucleotide Sequence and Derived Amino Acid Sequence of the Region Coding for the Carboxy-Terminal Two-Thirds of pp6Oc-src. *Mol. Cell Biol.* **1985**, *5*, 1122–1129. [CrossRef] [PubMed]
20. Irby, R.B.; Mao, W.; Coppola, D.; Kang, J.; Loubeau, J.M.; Trudeau, W.; Karl, R.; Fujita, D.J.; Jove, R.; Yeatman, T.J. Activating SRC mutation in a subset of advanced human colon cancers. *Nat. Genet.* **1999**, *21*, 187–190. [CrossRef]
21. Takahashi, S.; Miyazaki, M.; Okamoto, I.; Ito, Y.; Ueda, K.; Seriu, T.; Nakagawa, K.; Hatake, K. Phase I study of dasatinib (BMS-354825) in Japanese patients with solid tumors. *Cancer Sci.* **2011**, *102*, 2058–2064. [CrossRef]
22. Haura, E.B.; Tanvetyanon, T.; Chiappori, A.; Williams, C.; Simon, G.; Antonia, S.; Gray, J.; Litschauer, S.; Tetteh, L.; Neuger, A.; et al. Phase I/II study of the Src inhibitor dasatinib in combination with erlotinib in advanced non-small-cell lung cancer. *J. Clin. Oncol.* **2010**, *28*, 1387–1394. [CrossRef]

23. McDermott, M.; Eustace, A.J.; Busschots, S.; Breen, L.; Crown, J.; Clynes, M.; O'Donovan, N.; Stordal, B. In vitro Development of Chemotherapy and Targeted Therapy Drug-Resistant Cancer Cell Lines: A Practical Guide with Case Studies. *Front. Oncol.* **2014**, *4*, 4. [CrossRef] [PubMed]
24. McDermott, M.S.J.; Browne, B.C.; Conlon, N.T.; O'Brien, N.A.; Slamon, D.J.; Henry, M.; Meleady, P.; Clynes, M.; Dowling, P.; Crown, J.; et al. PP2A inhibition overcomes acquired resistance to HER2 targeted therapy. *Mol. Cancer* **2014**, *13*, 157. [CrossRef] [PubMed]
25. Sugimura, M.; Kobayashi, K.; Sagae, S.; Nishioka, Y.; Ishioka, S.I.; Terasawa, K.; Tokino, T.; Kudo, R. Mutation of the SRC gene in endometrial carcinoma. *Jpn. J. Cancer Res.* **2000**, *91*, 395–398. [CrossRef] [PubMed]
26. Yoshida, T.; Okamoto, I.; Okamoto, W.; Hatashita, E.; Yamada, Y.; Kuwata, K.; Nishio, K.; Fukuoka, M.; Jänne, P.A.; Nakagawa, K. Effects of Src inhibitors on cell growth and epidermal growth factor receptor and MET signaling in gefitinib-resistant non-small cell lung cancer cells with acquired MET amplification. *Cancer Sci.* **2010**, *101*, 167–172. [CrossRef] [PubMed]
27. Formisano, L.; Nappi, L.; Rosa, R.; Marciano, R.; D'Amato, C.; D'Amato, V.; Damiano, V.; Raimondo, L.; Iommelli, F.; Scorziello, A.; et al. Epidermal growth factor-receptor activation modulates Src-dependent resistance to lapatinib in breast cancer models. *Breast Cancer Res.* **2014**, *16*, R45. [CrossRef] [PubMed]
28. Pinedo-Carpio, E.; Davidson, D.; Marignac, V.L.M.; Panasci, J.; Aloyz, R. Adaptive metabolic rewiring to chronic SFK inhibition. *Oncotarget* **2017**, *8*, 66758. [CrossRef] [PubMed]
29. Zhang, H.; Davies, K.J.A.; Forman, H.J. TGFβ1 rapidly activates Src through a non-canonical redox signaling mechanism. *Arch. Biochem. Biophys.* **2015**, *568*, 1–7. [CrossRef] [PubMed]
30. Hage, C.; Rausch, V.; Giese, N.; Giese, T.; Schönsiegel, F.; Labsch, S.; Nwaeburu, C.; Mattern, J.; Gladkich, J.; Herr, I. The novel c-Met inhibitor cabozantinib overcomes gemcitabine resistance and stem cell signaling in pancreatic cancer. *Cell Death Dis.* **2013**, *4*, e627. [CrossRef]
31. Moschetta, M.; Basile, A.; Ferrucci, A.; Frassanito, M.A.; Rao, L.; Ria, R.; Solimando, A.G.; Giuliani, N.; Boccarelli, A.; Fumarola, F.; et al. Novel targeting of phospho-cMET overcomes drug resistance and induces antitumor activity in multiple myeloma. *Clin. Cancer Res.* **2013**, *19*, 4371–4382. [CrossRef] [PubMed]
32. De Bacco, F.; Luraghi, P.; Medico, E.; Reato, G.; Girolami, F.; Perera, T.; Gabriele, P.; Comoglio, P.M.; Boccaccio, C. Induction of MET by ionizing radiation and its role in radioresistance and invasive growth of cancer. *J. Natl. Cancer Inst.* **2011**, *103*, 645–661. [CrossRef] [PubMed]
33. Jahangiri, A.; De Lay, M.; Miller, L.M.; Shawn Carbonell, W.; Hu, Y.L.; Lu, K.; Tom, M.W.; Paquette, J.; Tokuyasu, T.A.; Tsao, S.; et al. Gene expression profile identifies tyrosine kinase c-Met as a targetable mediator of antiangiogenic therapy resistance. *Clin. Cancer Res.* **2013**, *19*, 1773–1783. [CrossRef] [PubMed]

8

Mastectomy or Breast-Conserving Therapy for Early Breast Cancer in Real-Life Clinical Practice: Outcome Comparison of 7565 Cases

Stefanie Corradini [1,*], Daniel Reitz [1], Montserrat Pazos [1], Stephan Schönecker [1], Michael Braun [2], Nadia Harbeck [3], Christiane Matuschek [4], Edwin Bölke [4], Ute Ganswindt [5], Filippo Alongi [6], Maximilian Niyazi [1] and Claus Belka [1]

1 Department of Radiation Oncology, LMU University, 81377 Munich, Germany; daniel.reitz@med.uni-muenchen.de (D.R.); montserrat.pazos@med.uni-muenchen.de (M.P.); stephan.schoenecker@med.uni-muenchen.de (S.S.); maximilian.niyazi@med.uni-muenchen.de (M.N.); claus.belka@med.uni-muenchen.de (C.B.)
2 Department of Gynecology and Obstetrics, Red Cross Hospital, 80637 Munich, Germany; michael.braun@swmbrk.de
3 Breast Center, Department of Gynecology and Obstetrics, LMU University, 81377 Munich, Germany; nadia.harbeck@med.uni-muenchen.de
4 Department of Radiation Oncology, Heinrich Heine University, Medical faculty, 40225 Düsseldorf, Germany; matuschek@med.uni-duesseldorf.de (C.M.); boelke@med.uni-duesseldorf.de (E.B.)
5 Department of Radiation Oncology, Medical University, 6020 Innsbruck, Austria; ute.ganswindt@i-med.ac.at
6 Department of Radiation Oncology, Sacro Cuore Don Calabria Hospital, 37024 Negrar-Verona, University of Brescia, 25121 Brescia, Italy; filippo.alongi@sacrocuore.it
* Correspondence: stefanie.corradini@med.uni-muenchen.de

Abstract: Although the organ preservation strategy by breast-conserving surgery (BCS) followed by radiation therapy (BCT) has revolutionized the treatment approach of early stage breast cancer (BC), the choice between treatment options in this setting can still vary according to patient preferences. The aim of the present study was to compare the oncological outcome of mastectomy versus breast-conserving therapy in patients treated in a modern clinical setting outside of clinical trials. 7565 women diagnosed with early invasive BC (pT1/2pN0/1) between 1998 and 2014 were included in this study (median follow-up: 95.2 months). In order to reduce selection bias and confounding, a subgroup analysis of a matched 1:1 case-control cohort consisting of 1802 patients was performed (median follow-up 109.4 months). After adjusting for age, tumor characteristics and therapies, multivariable analysis for local recurrence-free survival identified BCT as an independent predictor for improved local control (hazard ratio [HR]:1.517; 95%confidence interval:1.092–2.108, $p = 0.013$) as compared to mastectomy alone in the matched cohort. Ten-year cumulative incidence (CI) of lymph node recurrences was 2.0% following BCT, compared to 5.8% in patients receiving mastectomy ($p < 0.001$). Similarly, 10-year distant-metastasis-free survival (89.4% vs. 85.5%, $p = 0.013$) was impaired in patients undergoing mastectomy alone. This translated into improved survival in patients treated with BCT (10-year overall survival (OS) estimates 85.3% vs. 79.3%, $p < 0.001$), which was also significant on multivariable analysis ($p = 0.011$). In conclusion, the present study showed that patients treated with BCS followed by radiotherapy had an improved outcome compared to radical mastectomy alone. Specifically, local control, distant control, and overall survival were significantly better using the conservative approach. Thus, as a result of the present study, physicians should encourage patients to receive BCS with radiotherapy rather than mastectomy, whenever it is medically feasible and appropriate.

Keywords: breast cancer; breast-conserving therapy; mastectomy; outcome; comparative effectiveness

1. Introduction

In the early 1980s, large randomized studies first proved that breast-conserving surgery (BCS) followed by postoperative radiotherapy (breast-conserving therapy, BCT) was a valid therapeutic alternative to radical mastectomy in women with early breast cancer (BC) [1,2]. Nowadays, in this setting, breast organ preservation by BCT has become the treatment of choice, due to the excellent outcome and optimal tolerability. Nevertheless, various population-based studies showed that mastectomy is still considered a concrete treatment option and continues to be chosen by several patients with BC in daily clinical practice [3–6].

Treatment of early-stage breast cancer can be considered as a preference-sensitive setting, where decision-making between treatment options can change according to patient preferences [7]. Typical factors able to influence the therapeutic choice in favor of mastectomy include: (i) concerns regarding cancer recurrence, (ii) perception that health outweighs breast retention [8], or (iii) perceived consequences of BCT, including potential adverse effects of radiation therapy [7,9]. Moreover, a renewed interest and trend towards mastectomy has recently emerged, with an increased use of skin-sparing or nipple-sparing mastectomies with immediate breast reconstruction [10–12]. This treatment strategy provides superior aesthetic and quality-of-life outcomes when compared to radical mastectomy. Nevertheless, long-term oncologic outcomes of these new surgical approaches are currently not provided and only retrospective studies were available as evidence. Moreover, the demand for more radical surgical therapies has recently gained wide public attention, as prophylactic mastectomy in BRCA gene mutation positive celebrities attracted notable media interest [13]. The prominence of this issue in the media might also have influenced oncologic patient´s preferences regarding their choice of surgical management. In fact, shared decision-making in daily clinical practice is strongly influenced by a number of confounding factors, including clinician preferences and trade-offs regarding toxicity risks or comorbidities [14].

BC management has changed dramatically over time, and local recurrence rates after BCT have decreased significantly [15]. The impact of mammography screening in downward stage migration resulted in smaller tumor sizes and less extensive nodal involvement and is accompanied by improvements in adjuvant treatments, tailored to disease biology.

Therefore, the aim of the present study was to compare the oncological outcome of mastectomy versus breast-conserving therapy in patients treated in "real life", in a modern clinical setting outside of clinical trials.

2. Results

2.1. Baseline Patient Characteristics

The final study cohort consisted of 7565 women and the subgroup analysis of the matched cohort included 1802 patients. Patient and treatment characteristics for both cohorts are summarized in Table 1. Overall, 84.8% (6412/7565) of patients were treated with BCS and postoperative RT, while 15.2% (1153/7565) a received mastectomy. A significant decrease of mastectomy was documented over time. While in 1998 approximately 21% of patients received a mastectomy, the proportion decreased to 12% in 2014.

Patients treated with BCT were significantly younger, with a median age at diagnosis of 58.2 years in the BCT group, as compared to 59.3 years in the mastectomy group ($p < 0.001$). Furthermore, patients treated with mastectomy presented with more high-risk features such as tumor size $\geq$20 mm (43.1%), positive lymph nodes (31.4%), high tumor grade (27.3%) and negative hormone receptor status (12.0%) than patients receiving BCT. Moreover, mastectomy patients received less adjuvant endocrine therapy (52.0% vs. 43.5%, $p < 0.001$). In the matched cohort, we controlled for all these imbalances.

Table 1. Patient and tumor characteristics for the entire cohort and the case control cohort.

Variable	Entire Cohort (n = 7565)					Case Control Cohort (n = 1802)				
	BCS + RT		Mastectomy		p-Value	BCS + RT		Mastectomy		p-Value
	n	(%) *	n	(%) *		n	(%) *	n	(%) *	
All	6412	(84.8)	1153	(15.2)		929	(50.0)	929	(50.0)	
Age at diagnosis					<0.001					n.s.
<40 years	353	(5.5)	102	(8.8)		68	(7.5)	62	(6.9)	
40–49 years	1193	(18.6)	221	(19.2)		201	(22.3)	184	(20.4)	
50–59 years	1880	(29.3)	282	(24.5)		241	(26.7)	234	(26.0)	
60–69 years	2043	(31.9)	258	(22.4)		215	(23.9)	225	(25.0)	
>70 years	943	(14.7)	290	(25.2)		176	(19.5)	196	(21.8)	
median (years)	58.2		59.3			58.6		58.8		
Lateralisation					0.007					n.s.
right	3181	(49.6)	522	(45.3)		414	(45.9)	414	(45.9)	
left	3231	(50.4)	631	(54.7)		487	(54.1)	487	(54.1)	
Tumour size					<0.001					n.s.
pT1	4790	(74.7)	656	(56.9)		514	(57.0)	514	(57.0)	
pT2	1622	(25.3)	497	(43.1)		387	(43.0)	387	(43.0)	
Nodal status					<0.001					n.s.
pN0	4904	(76.5)	791	(68.6)		646	(71.7)	646	(71.7)	
pN+ (1–3 LN)	1508	(23.5)	362	(31.4)		255	(28.3)	255	(28.3)	
Tumor stage					<0.001					n.s.
T1N0	3860	(60.2)	492	(42.7)		395	(43.8)	395	(43.8)	
T2N0	1044	(16.3)	299	(25.9)		251	(27.9)	251	(27.9)	
T1N1	930	(14.5)	164	(14.2)		119	(13.2)	119	(13.2)	
T2N1	578	(9.0)	198	(17.2)		136	(15.1)	136	(15.1)	
Resection status					n.s.					n.s.
R0	5769	(98.1)	922	(98.2)		812	(98.5)	740	(98.5)	
R1/R2	112	(1.9)	17	(1.8)		12	(1.5)	11	(1.5)	
[unknown]	531	(8.2)	214	(18.5)		77	(8.5)	150	(16.6)	
Grade					<0.001					n.s.
G1	1248	(19.9)	98	(9.1)		77	(8.5)	77	(8.5)	
G2	3610	(57.6)	684	(63.6)		599	(66.5)	599	(66.5)	
G3/4	1411	(22.5)	294	(27.3)		225	(25.0)	225	(25.0)	
[unknown]	143	[2.3]	77	[6.6]						
Hormone receptor										
positive	5674	(90.2)	986	(88.0)	0.038	83	(9.2)	83	(9.2)	n.s.
negative	613	(9.8)	135	(12.0)		818	(90.8)	818	(90.8)	
[unknown]	125	[1.9]	32	[2.7]						
Chemotherapy					n.s.					n.s.
no	4581	(71.4)	855	(74.2)		660	(73.3)	660	(73.3)	
yes	1831	(28.6)	298	(25.8)		241	(26.7)	241	(26.7)	
Endocrine therapy					<0.001					n.s.
no	3076	(48.0)	651	(56.5)		485	(53.8)	485	(53.8)	
yes	3336	(52.0)	502	(43.5)		416	(46.2)	416	(46.2)	

* Percentages of the presented subcategories are related to the sum of each item with available data; missing values are not taken into account. Hormone receptor positive: estrogen and/or progesterone positive (>1%). BCS: breast conserving surgery, RT: radiotherapy, n.s.: not significant.

2.2. Outcome

The median follow-up for the entire cohort was 95.2 months (95%CI: 92.5–97.9) and 109.4 months (95% CI: 104.3–114.5) for the matched cohort. Of the 7565 BC patients, 521 (6.9%) developed local recurrences, 160 (2.1%) lymph node recurrences, and 607 (8.0%) distant metastases.

The cumulative incidence of local recurrence (LR) for the BCT group was 3.2% after 5 years and 8.2% after 10 years. In contrast, the mastectomy group had significantly higher local failure rates with 5.0% 5-year LR and 12.6% 10-year LR rates, respectively ($p < 0.001$, Table 2).

Table 2. Cumulative incidence of local recurrences (LR) and lymph node recurrences (LNR) and Kaplan-Meier estimates of distant recurrence-free survival (DRFS) and overall survival (OS) for patients of the different cohorts. BCS + RT: breast-conserving surgery with postoperative radiotherapy; Mastectomy: mastectomy without radiotherapy; y: years.

Outcome	Treatment Modality	Entire Cohort Diagnosis 1998–2014 7565 Patients			Case Control Cohort Diagnosis 1998–2014 1802 Patients		
		5 y (%)	10 y (%)	*p*	5 y (%)	10 y (%)	*p*
LR				<0.001			0.025
	BCS + RT	3.2	8.2		4.6	9.4	
	Mastectomy	5.0	12.6		4.8	12.9	
LNR				<0.001			<0.001
	BCS + RT	0.9	2.2		0.7	2.0	
	Mastectomy	2.6	5.7		2.5	5.8	
DRFS				<0.001			0.013
	BCS + RT	94.5	90.2		93.8	89.4	
	Mastectomy	92.0	84.8		93.1	85.5	
OS				<0.001			<0.001
	BCS + RT	95.2	86.7		93.8	85.3	
	Mastectomy	90.5	77.6		92.2	79.3	

Multivariable Cox analysis for local recurrence-free survival identified mastectomy (hazard ratio [HR], 1.476; 95% confidence interval [CI], 1.164–1.872, $p < 0.001$) as a significant predictor for local failure. Table 3 summarizes other classic prognostic risk factors that had a significant impact on LR risk at multivariable analysis, including young age <40 years ($p < 0.001$), higher tumor stage ($p < 0.001$), high tumor grade ($p < 0.001$) and negative hormone receptor status ($p = 0.012$). In the matched cohort, type of local treatment, age at diagnosis, and tumors stage confirmed their significant impact on LR risk estimates.

Table 3. Multivariable Cox regression analysis for local recurrence free survival.

Variable	Entire Cohort (n = 7565) Local Recurrence Free Survival			Case Control Cohort (n = 1802) Local Recurrence Free Survival		
	Hazard Ratio HR	95% CI	*p*-Value	Hazard Ratio HR	95% CI	*p*-Value
Local therapy			<0.001			0.013
BCS + RT	1			1		
Mastectomy	1.476	1.164-1.872		1.517	1.092–2.108	
Age at diagnosis			<0.001			<0.001
<40 years	1			1		
40–49 years	0.931	0.671–1.291		0.802	0.475–1.353	
50–59 years	0.521	0.370–0.732		0.309	0.172–0.554	
60–69 years	0.393	0.274–0.565		0.360	0.199–0.651	
≥70 years	0.357	0.228–0.561		0.168	0.075–0.379	
Tumour stage			<0.001			0.020
T1N0	1			1		
T2N0	1.177	0.899–1.541		0.916	0.584–1.434	
T1N1	1.147	0.855–1.538		1.014	0.601–1.712	
T2N1	2.091	1.565–2.795		1.969	1.204–3.220	
Resection status			0.604			0.330
R0	1			1		
R1/R2	0.808	0.360–1.812		1.773	0.560–5.618	
Grade			<0.001			0.320
G1	1			1		
G2	2.063	1.438–2.959		1.719	0.821–3.599	
G3/4	2.415	1.619–3.601		1.526	0.676–3.444	

Table 3. *Cont.*

Variable	Entire Cohort (n = 7565) Local Recurrence Free Survival			Case Control Cohort (n = 1802) Local Recurrence Free Survival		
	Hazard Ratio HR	95% CI	p-Value	Hazard Ratio HR	95% CI	p-Value
Hormone receptor			0.012			0.104
positive	1			1		
negative	1.466	1.087–1.975		1.575	0.911–2.721	
Chemotherapy			0.402			0.462
yes	1			1		
no	1.110	0.870–1.417		1.172	0.768–1.789	
Endocrine therapy			0.382			0.955
yes	1			1		
no	0.808	0.360–1.812		1.010	0.706–1.447	

Similarly, lymph node recurrences (LNR) were more frequent in patients undergoing mastectomy only. The cumulative incidence of LNR at 5 and 10 years in the BCT group were 0.9% and 2.2%, respectively, compared to 2.6% and 5.7% in patients receiving mastectomy ($p < 0.001$). This observation was still significant on multivariable analysis. Type of local therapy (mastectomy HR 2.442; 95% CI, 1.675–3.560, $p < 0.001$), higher tumor stage ($p = 0.006$) and high tumor grade ($p < 0.001$) did significantly affect the risk of LNR. Focusing on the impact of the type of local treatment in the matched cohort, mastectomy was also correlated with an increased rate of LNR (HR 1.517; 95% CI, 1.092–2.108, $p = 0.013$, Table 4).

Table 4. Multivariable Cox regression analysis for lymph node recurrence-free survival (LNRFS).

Variable	Entire Cohort (n = 7565) Lymph Node Recurrence-Free Survival (LNRFS)			Case Control Cohort (n = 1802) Lymph Node Recurrence-Free Survival (LNRFS)		
	Hazard Ratio HR	95% CI	p-Value	Hazard Ratio HR	95% CI	p-Value
Local therapy			<0.001			0.013
BCS + RT	1			1		
Mastectomy	2.442	1.675–3.560		1.517	1.092–2.108	
Age at diagnosis			0.025			0.030
<40 years	1			1		
40–49 years	1.795	0.857–3.762		1.758	0.576–5.361	
50–59 years	1.143	0.539–2.423		0.715	0.215–2.376	
60–69 years	1.399	0.661–2.960		0.871	0.262–2.890	
≥70 years	0.603	0.238–1.526		0.286	0.058–1.411	
Tumor stage			0.006			0.331
T1N0	1			1		
T2N0	1.754	1.130–2.724		1.175	0.535–2.584	
T1N1	1.274	0.749–2.168		1.433	0.593–3.463	
T2N1	2.300	1.383–3.825		2.186	0.931–5.134	
Resection status			0.366			
R0	1			1		
R1/R2	0.403	0.056–2.888		NA *		
Grade			<0.001			0.082
G1	1			1		
G2	1.451	0.755–2.787		1.121	0.327–3.840	
G3	3.651	1.841–7.242		2.284	0.623–8.371	
Hormone receptor			0.120			0.973
positive	1			1		
negative	1.523	0.897–2.586		0.982	0.342–2.819	
Chemotherapy			0.221			0.593
yes	1			1		
no	1.303	0.853–1.990		1.223	0.585–2.557	
Endocrine therapy			0.193			0.702
yes	1			1		
no	0.770	0.520–1.141		0.885	0.475–1.652	

* NA: not applicable, HR not estimable because no event in the R1/2 group.

Ten-year distant metastasis-free survival (DMFS) in the entire cohort was statistically different in the univariate analysis—with 90.2% DMFS in the BCT group, compared to 84.8% in the mastectomy group ($p < 0.001$). This was also seen in a comparable magnitude in the matched cohort ($p = 0.013$). Overall, patients treated with postoperative radiotherapy after BCS showed improved distant control, independent from other covariates in multivariable Cox regression analysis (mastectomy HR 1.257; 95% CI, 1.006–1.570, $p = 0.044$). Other factors correlated with poor DMFS in this cohort were advanced tumor stage ($p < 0.001$), high tumor grade ($p < 0.001$) and negative hormone receptor status ($p = 0.050$). Also in the matched cohort, the positive effect of BCT on DMFS was observed ($p = 0.008$, Table 5).

Table 5. Multivariable Cox regression analysis for distant metastasis free survival.

Variable	Entire Cohort (*n* = 7565) Distant Metastasis Free Survival (DMFS)			Case Control Cohort (*n* = 1802) Distant Metastasis Free Survival (DMFS)		
	Hazard Ratio HR	**95% CI**	***p*-Value**	**Hazard Ratio HR**	**95% CI**	***p*-Value**
Local therapy			0.044			0.008
BCS + RT	1			1		
Mastectomy	1.257	1.006–1.570		1.537	1.121–2.107	
Age at diagnosis			0.677			0.053
<40 years	1			1		
40–49 years	0.860	0.608–1.216		0.600	0.351–1.027	
50–59 years	0.826	0.592–1.153		0.497	0.292–0.845	
60–69 years	0.785	0.556–1.106		0.437	0.246–0.777	
≥70 years	0.891	0.601–1.321		0.592	0.314–1.118	
Tumor stage			<0.001			0.001
T1N0	1			1		
T2N0	1.895	1.489–2.411		1.258	0.820–1.932	
T1N1	1.577	1.196–2.080		1.520	0.933–2.477	
T2N1	3.755	2.930–4.812		2.516	1.608–3.936	
Resection status			0.209			0.587
R0	1			1		
R1/R2	1.445	0.813–2.568		1.377	0.435–4.364	
Grade			<0.001			
G1	0.215	0.141–0.327		NA *		
G2	0.514	0.421–0.629		NA		
G3	1			1		
Hormone receptor			0.050			0.706
positive	1			1		
negative	1.327	1.000–2.586		1.110	0.646–1.907	
Chemotherapy			0.656			0.517
yes	1			1		
no	0.951	0.762–1.186		0.874	0.583–1.312	
Endocrine therapy			0.013			0.174
yes	1			1		
no	0.770	0.627–0.946		0.782	0.549–1.114	

* NA: not applicable, HR not estimable because no event in the R1/2 group.

Among patients treated with BCS plus RT, 10-year OS estimates were 86.7%, and for those treated with mastectomy 77.6% ($p < 0.001$). In multivariable Cox regression analysis, the use of mastectomy was again independently associated with less favorable outcome, with an HR of 1.268 (95% CI, 1.055–1.525, $p = 0.011$). Further risk factors correlated with poor OS in this cohort were older age ($p < 0.001$), advanced tumor stage ($p < 0.001$), and high tumor grade ($p < 0.001$). This effect could be confirmed in multivariable analysis for the matched cohort, where type of local treatment (mastectomy HR 1.452; 95% CI, 1.124–1.875, $p = 0.004$, Table 6), older age ($p < 0.001$), advanced tumor stage ($p < 0.001$), and high tumor grade ($p = 0.033$) were independent risk factors.

Table 6. Multivariable Cox regression analysis for overall survival.

Variable	Entire Cohort (n = 7565) Overall Survival (OS)			Case Control Cohort (n = 1802) Overall Survival (OS)		
	Hazard Ratio HR	95% CI	p-Value	Hazard Ratio HR	95% CI	p-Value
Local therapy			0.011			0.004
BCS + RT	1			1		
Mastectomy	1.268	1.055–1.525		1.452	1.124–1.875	
Age at diagnosis			<0.001			<0.001
<40 years	1			1		
40–49 years	1.011	0.674–1.517		0.439	0.240–0.804	
50–59 years	1.273	0.870–1.861		0.599	0.346–1.038	
60–69 years	1.757	1.203–2.565		0.854	0.494–1.476	
≥70 years	4.552	3.089–6.710		2.335	1.342–4.065	
Tumor stage			<0.001			<0.001
T1N0	1			1		
T2N0	1.763	1.446–2.150		1.633	1.175–2.270	
T1N1	1.529	1.214–1.925		1.375	0.887–2.130	
T2N1	2.892	2.337–3.580		2.589	1.786–3.753	
Resection status			0.608			0.712
R0	1			1		
R1/R2	1.144	0.685–1.911		1.184	0.484–2.896	
Grade			<0.001			0.033
G1	1			1		
G2	1.406	1.100–1.798		1.968	1.028–3.768	
G3	2.165	1.645–2.848		2.432	1.227–4.820	
Hormone receptor			0.076			0.606
positive	1			1		
negative	1.254	0.986–1.612		1.135	0.702–1.834	
Chemotherapy			0.481			0.708
yes	1			1		
no	1.075	0.880–1.313		1.075	0.736–1.570	
Endocrine therapy			0.662			0.709
yes	1			1		
no	1.039	0.876–1.232		0.946	0.708–1.26	

3. Discussion

The present study showed that patients treated with BCS followed by radiotherapy (RT) in a population reflecting "real life" in this clinical setting, had an improved outcome regarding local control, distant control, and overall survival compared to those who underwent a mastectomy. These findings were also confirmed in the matched cohort after adjusting for confounders.

The results presented here are in line with those of other studies investigating the same clinical setting. A population-based analysis of van Maaren et al. [4] of 37,207 breast cancer patients treated in the Netherlands between 01/2000 and 12/2004 obtained similar results. BCS was associated with a significantly improved 10-year overall survival (HR 0.81, 95% CI: 0.78–0.85, $p < 0.0001$). Furthermore, in a representative cohort of patients diagnosed in 2003, BCT had a significant impact on relative survival (HR 0.76, 95% CI: 0.64–0.91, $p = 0.003$). In contrast to the present analysis, distant metastasis-free survival (HR 0.88, 95% CI: 0.77–1.01, $p = 0.070$) was not significantly different in the Dutch cohort, with exception of the T1N0 subgroup (HR 0.60, 95% CI: 0.42–0.85, $p = 0.004$). Yet, in the present analysis, the occurrence of lymph node metastases and distant metastases were both decreased in patients treated with breast-conserving surgery and radiotherapy compared to mastectomy.

Although locoregional and distant control rates are lacking in most of the published experiences [16–19], two studies addressed these issues in a similar BC cohort as in the present study [20,21]. An analysis of the prospective Swedish Multicenter Cohort Study including 2767 patients compared BCS with postoperative RT and mastectomy without RT. Similar to the present analysis, the axillary recurrence-free survival rate at 13 years was significantly reduced after mastectomy without irradiation as compared to BCS (98.3% versus 96.2%, $p < 0.001$) [21]. Moreover, locoregional recurrence was a strong independent predictor of breast cancer death, (HR: 4.28, 95% CI: 2.55–7.17) and overall survival (HR: 2.64, 95% CI: 1.66–4.19).

The axillary recurrence rates decrease after BCS with RT in comparison to mastectomy, which may have different explanations. Of note, in the present study, 23.5% of patients treated in the BCT group had a positive nodal status with 1–3 involved lymph nodes. While after the AMAROS trial [22], the debate about the role of regional nodal irradiation continues, results from the ACOSOG Z0011 trial [23] and the IBCSG 23-01 trial [24] demonstrated that patients with low-volume nodal disease who are treated with BCS and whole breast RT, can safely avoid axillary lymph node dissection without affecting locoregional control or survival rates [25]. The potential rationale behind this observation is that radiation originating from whole-breast tangential field RT after BCS could exert some protective effect on axillary recurrence rates by controlling the minimal residual disease [21]. It is noteworthy, that the dose to axillary lymph node levels I and II usually is significantly lower than the prescribed dose and can range from 5% to 80% of the prescribed dose (mean value 48.7%). Even in patients receiving regional nodal irradiation of 50 Gray (Gy) to the supra-/infraclavicular lymph node levels (corresponding to levels IV, III and interpectoral lymph nodes), level I receives a reduced dose coverage of mean 41.3 Gy [26,27]. The potential influence of whole breast irradiation, especially in cases of pN+, needs further evaluation in randomized studies.

Regarding distant control, in a single center experience of 6137 cases, Wang et al. [20] observed that patients undergoing BCS plus RT showed a significantly increased 5-year metastasis-free survival ($p < 0.003$) and overall survival ($p < 0.036$) compared with mastectomy. But how could these results be interpreted? Is RT able to add something more than just improved locoregional control? The EBCTCG meta-analysis [28] proved a concrete direct relationship between improved local control and favorable breast cancer specific survival outcome. Nevertheless, the underlying biological mechanisms remain unclear. The oncological community has generated various hypotheses regarding the heterogeneous biology of BC and the impact of available treatment options. A commonly accepted hypothesis is that the addition of RT represents an effective curative treatment for a selected subset of patients who would otherwise have relapsed locally and subsequently would have developed metastases. The fact that the survival benefit only occurs in the framework of successful local control, indicates that RT is involved in events occurring within the treated radiotherapy fields. RT prevents local recurrences through the successful eradication of residual tumor clones or tumor cell clusters within the breast, which are not detected at primary diagnosis. Regarding the beneficial effect on distant tumor control, this interpretation assumes that the metastatic process consists of different waves of cell migration and metastases with differing invasive properties [29]. Hence, RT appears to have unique biological effects to prevent early distant dissemination of cancer cells to distant organs. Furthermore, several potential interactions with the immune system are advocated, including radiation-induced tumor-specific immunity capable of rejecting the colonizing clonogenic cells [29]. Nevertheless, it remains challenging to assess the relative contribution of the interactions between systemic and locoregional treatments on the outcome, as well as that of the individual drugs and RT volumes [15].

The present results of patients treated in a "real life" clinical setting are different from those reported from historical randomized trials of the 1980s, which described similar survival for BCT and mastectomy [30,31]. A key to interpreting these different findings could be that the management of breast cancer has changed considerably over time. Fisher et al. [31] documented a 5-year local recurrence rate of 7.7% for the BCT group and 14.3% in the twenty-year follow-up of the NSABP trial B-06. The 5-year and 10-year cumulative incidence of local recurrences in the present analysis were 3.2% and 8.2%, respectively, suggesting improved local control rates with modern breast cancer therapy, even in the setting outside of randomized trials. The modern multimodal treatment approach, including diagnostics, surgery, systemic therapy, and RT procedures, has improved significantly over the last decades and might explain the survival difference in patients treated with breast-conserving surgery plus radiotherapy as compared to patients treated with mastectomy. [15] The 10-year overall survival was significantly improved for patients receiving BCS plus radiotherapy: 86.7% with BCT and 77.6% with mastectomy alone ($p < 0.001$). This difference was also observed in the matched cohort ($p < 0.001$). Improved breast cancer specific and overall survival have been found in several population-based cohorts studies [3,5,32–37]. Regarding early-stage breast cancer, Hwang et al. [32] analyzed patients diagnosed with stage I or II breast cancer between 1990 and 2004 and reported improved OS and DSS compared to patients with mastectomy (adjusted hazard ratio for OS entire cohort = 0.81, 95% CI: 0.80–0.83). A registry-based study in Norway also showed comparable results to the present analysis [5]. In multivariate analysis, patients who underwent mastectomy for T1-2/N0-1 BC had an adjusted hazard ratio of 1.65 (95% CI: 1.50–1.82) for OS compared to those who underwent BCT. Similarly, in the present matched cohort, the outcome in terms of OS for patients receiving BCS plus RT was improved (HR: 1.452, 95%CI: 1.124–1.875). Onitilo et al. [35] also compared BCS $\pm$ RT versus mastectomy. While overall survival was similar for BCS alone and mastectomy, BCS plus radiation was superior compared to mastectomy alone. The authors concluded, that the survival benefit was not only related to the surgical approach itself but that the addition of adjuvant RT results in a prognostic advantage of BCS plus radiation over mastectomy [35].

We controlled for all variables available in the registry. Unfortunately, we could not account for host-related factors like comorbidities, performance status, or clinician- and patient-related preferences, which may have influenced the clinical treatment decision-making process. It is known that older patients or patients with comorbidities often receive non-standard treatments. A recent analysis of 7581 early stage BC patients diagnosed in 9 European countries analyzed the influence of comorbidities on receiving standard treatments and found that mastectomy was mainly given to elderly women and women with comorbidities [38]. There are several other limitations to effectiveness research due to unpredictable confounding factors and consequently, misinterpretations of treatment and mortality effects should be avoided [39]. In fact, the present observational study may suffer from a "confounding by severity" [40], considering that the severity of the disease (e.g., high-risk factors, tumor biology) could be a potential confounder influencing the indication for mastectomy. Furthermore, survival estimates might be affected by non-tumor-related factors such as age or comorbidities, which could lead to more non-breast cancer deaths. However, we conducted a matched cohort analysis to directly address these concerns and control for these imbalances. Finally, we want to underline that patients of the present study were treated at two specialized breast cancer centers, which in general could have improved outcomes as compared to other settings.

Many previous studies have performed similar analyses with comparable results [4,20,21]. However, a specific characterizing element of the present study is the additional matched case control analysis. This methodology was not used in previously published experiences, which further strengthens the evidence that breast-conserving therapy should be the preferred treatment for patients with early-stage breast cancer when it is medically feasible and appropriate. More specifically, in the present study, we could show that breast-conserving therapy had improved outcome regarding local control, distant control and overall survival as compared to mastectomy alone–even in the matched cohort. Patients were matched regarding a number of variables in order to reduce confounding: 1:1 match for tumor lateralization, tumor size, lymph node status, tumor grade, hormone receptor status, administration of chemotherapy/endocrine therapy and age match with a tolerance of ± 2 years for age at diagnosis. This resulted in a cohort, where for each mastectomy patient an exactly matched BET patient with exactly the same tumor formula and treatment history was present. Even in this matched cohort analysis, the effect of the choice of surgical treatment on oncologic outcome remained statistically significant.

Since many people still believe that mastectomy may be a better choice, we recommend generating more external validity, such as this retrospective study, in order to gain wide public attention. It is well known that there are a number of barriers to compliance with treatment recommendations, including lack of outcome expectancy. If a physician believes that a treatment will not lead to an improved outcome, he is less likely to follow the treatment recommendations. Another explanation for the widespread underuse of treatments that were beneficial in controlled trials could be the lack of consideration of external validity [14]. In general, we hope that the present study contributes to the existing evidence regarding the effectiveness of BCS and radiotherapy in this setting.

4. Materials and Methods

For the present analysis, all female patients with a first primary unilateral invasive breast cancer diagnosed between 1998 and 2014 and treated at two Breast Cancer Centers (Red Cross Hospital or LMU Munich, München, Germany) were identified. All data were retrieved from the Munich Cancer Registry. The cancer registry routinely collects data on patient's demographics, primary tumor site, the extent of disease (TNM), histology, treatment, and follow-up. Survival information was obtained systematically through death certificates of health offices. Patients were considered eligible after receiving mastectomy without postoperative radiotherapy (RT) or breast-conserving surgery followed by RT. Patients were excluded if they received neoadjuvant chemotherapy, or in case of histology of ductal carcinoma in situ ($n = 1.412$), lymphoma ($n = 10$) or sarcoma ($n = 57$), or in case of unknown date of initial diagnosis (e.g., tumors from death certificate information only [DCO], $n = 58$). Patients were also excluded if surgery information or pathologic tumor stage was incomplete or missing.

For the present study, women with tumor stages pT1pN0, pT2pN0, pT1pN1 and pT2pN1 (all M0) were selected. For comparison of the standard BCT and mastectomy approaches, we excluded patients with tumor stage ≥pT3 or more than 3 positive lymph nodes (pN2), as postmastectomy RT (PMRT) would have been routinely recommended in these high-risk patients.

Over the last decades, the use of PMRT was under debate for most intermediate risk patients with small tumor size and limited nodal disease (1–3 positive lymph nodes). Although previous studies provided evidence for a possible survival benefit in intermediate-risk patients [41], PMRT was not uniformly recommended at that time. The standard RT regimen at the Department of Radiation Oncology of the LMU Munich during the observation period was whole-breast irradiation following BCS (50.4 Gy in 28 fractions) using a 3-dimensional conformal tangential field technique with a photon or electron boost of 10–16 Gy to the tumor bed [42].

In order to reduce selection bias and confounding, a subgroup analysis of a matched cohort was performed. To compare treatment outcomes within a set of similar patients, 1:1 case-control matching on the following variables was performed: age at diagnosis, tumor lateralization, tumor size, lymph node status, tumor grade, hormone receptor status, administration of chemotherapy and endocrine therapy. The Hormone receptor was defined positive if estrogen and/or progesterone were positive (>1%).

Statistical analyses were conducted using IBM SPSS Statistics version 24.0 (IBM, Amonk, NY, USA). Frequency data were analyzed using the Chi-Square test. Tolerances values of the case-control matching were set to 2 years for age at diagnosis and 0 (exact matches) for all other above-mentioned variables. Cumulative incidence analysis (CI) was used to calculate the time to LR and LNR and the differences were assessed using the Gray's test for equality of cumulative incidence functions and was performed using R environment for statistical computing and visualization (version. 3.4.0). Distant metastasis-free survival (DMFS) and overall survival (OS) were estimated by the Kaplan-Meier method and tested using the log-rank test. The observation period began after diagnosis of the invasive tumor and ended at the date of distant metastasis occurrence or date of death or the last follow-up for cases without events. In addition, Cox proportional hazards models were used to identify independent prognostic factors related to local recurrence-free survival (LRFS), lymph node recurrence-free survival (LNRFS), DMFS and OS for the different cohorts. The significance level in all analyses was set at 5%.

5. Conclusions

In contrast to the highly selected and homogeneous study populations of randomized trials, this observational analysis included a large patient cohort reflecting "real-life" clinical practice involving a more diverse population, including elderly patients. A fundamental finding of the present study was that patients treated with BCS followed by RT had improved outcome in clinical practice regarding local control, distant control and overall survival as compared to mastectomy alone. Even if randomized trials provide the least biased estimates to compare treatments and remain the gold standard of efficacy research in oncology, observational data should be appreciated when weighing treatment options for breast cancer surgery. As a result of the present study, it seems advisable to continue to encourage future patients to receive BCS with RT rather than mastectomy when it is medically feasible and appropriate.

Author Contributions: Conceptualization, S.C., C.M., E.B., U.G., F.A. and C.B.; Data curation, S.C.; Formal analysis, S.C. and D.R.; Methodology, S.C., D.R., F.A. and M.N.; Project administration, C.B.; Resources, M.B. and N.H.; Supervision, C.B.; Validation, S.C., D.R., S.S. and M.N.; Visualization, S.C. and M.P.; Writing—original draft, S.C., D.R., M.P. and S.S.; Writing—review & editing, S.C., D.R., M.P., S.S., M.B., N.H., C.M., E.B., U.G., F.A., M.N. and C.B.

References

1. Fisher, B.; Bauer, M.; Margolese, R.; Poisson, R.; Pilch, Y.; Redmond, C.; Fisher, E.; Wolmark, N.; Deutsch, M.; Montague, E.; et al. 5-year results of a randomized clinical-trial comparing total mastectomy and segmental mastectomy with or without radiation in the treatment of breast-cancer. *N. Engl. J. Med.* **1985**, *312*, 665–673. [CrossRef] [PubMed]
2. Veronesi, U.; Zucali, R.; Luini, A. Local-control and survival in early breast-cancer—The Milan Trial. *Int. J. Radiat. Oncol. Biol. Phys.* **1986**, *12*, 717–720. [CrossRef]
3. Agarwal, S.; Pappas, L.; Neumayer, L.; Kokeny, K.; Agarwal, J. Effect of breast conservation therapy vs mastectomy on disease-specific survival for early-stage breast cancer. *JAMA Surg.* **2014**, *149*, 267–274. [CrossRef] [PubMed]
4. Van Maaren, M.C.; de Munck, L.; de Bock, G.H.; Jobsen, J.J.; van Dalen, T.; Linn, S.C.; Poortmans, P.; Strobbe, L.J.A.; Siesling, S. 10 year survival after breast-conserving surgery plus radiotherapy compared with mastectomy in early breast cancer in the Netherlands: A population-based study. *Lancet Oncol.* **2016**, *17*, 1158–1170. [CrossRef]
5. Hartmann-Johnsen, O.J.; Kåresen, R.; Schlichting, E.; Nygård, J.F. Survival is Better After Breast Conserving Therapy than Mastectomy for Early Stage Breast Cancer: A Registry-Based Follow-up Study of Norwegian Women Primary Operated Between 1998 and 2008. *Ann. Surg. Oncol.* **2015**, *22*, 3836–3845. [CrossRef] [PubMed]
6. Corradini, S.; Bauerfeind, I.; Belka, C.; Braun, M.; Combs, S.E.; Eckel, R.; Harbeck, N.; Hölzel, D.; Kiechle, M.; Niyazi, M.; et al. Trends in use and outcome of postoperative radiotherapy following mastectomy: A population-based study. *Radiother. Oncol.* **2017**, *122*, 2–10. [CrossRef]
7. Gu, J.; Groot, G.; Holtslander, L.; Engler-Stringer, R. Understanding women's choice of mastectomy versus breast conserving therapy in early-stage breast cancer. *Clin. Med. Insights Oncol.* **2017**, *11*, 1–7. [CrossRef]
8. Lee, W.Q.; Tan, V.K.M.; Choo, H.M.C.; Ong, J.; Krishnapriya, R.; Khong, S.; Tan, M.; Sim, Y.R.; Tan, B.K.; Madhukumar, P.; et al. Factors influencing patient decision-making between simple mastectomy and surgical alternatives. *BJS Open* **2018**. [CrossRef]
9. Shaverdian, N.; Wang, X.; Hegde, J.V.; Aledia, C.; Weidhaas, J.B.; Steinberg, M.L.; McCloskey, S.A. The patient's perspective on breast radiotherapy: Initial fears and expectations versus reality. *Cancer* **2018**, *124*, 1673–1681. [CrossRef]
10. Agarwal, S.; Agarwal, S.; Neumayer, L.; Agarwal, J.P. Therapeutic nipple-sparing mastectomy: Trends based on a national cancer database. *Am. J. Surg.* **2014**, *208*, 93–98. [CrossRef]
11. Sisco, M.; Kyrillos, A.M.; Lapin, B.R.; Wang, C.E.; Yao, K.A. Trends and variation in the use of nipple-sparing mastectomy for breast cancer in the United States. *Breast Cancer Res. Treat.* **2016**, *160*, 111–120. [CrossRef] [PubMed]
12. Li, M.; Chen, K.; Liu, F.; Su, F.; Li, S.; Zhu, L. Nipple sparing mastectomy in breast cancer patients and long-term survival outcomes: An analysis of the SEER database. *PLoS ONE* **2017**, *12*, e0183448. [CrossRef] [PubMed]

13. Troiano, G.; Nante, N.; Cozzolino, M. The Angelina Jolie effect—Impact on breast and ovarian cancer prevention A systematic review of effects after the public announcement in May 2013. *Health Educ. J.* **2017**, *76*, 707–715. [CrossRef]
14. Corradini, S.; Niyazi, M.; Niemoeller, O.M.; Li, M.; Roeder, F.; Eckel, R.; Schubert-Fritschle, G.; Scheithauer, H.R.; Harbeck, N.; Engel, J.; et al. Adjuvant radiotherapy after breast conserving surgery—A comparative effectiveness research study. *Radiother Oncol* **2014**, *114*, 28–34. [CrossRef]
15. Poortmans, P.M.P.; Arenas, M.; Livi, L. Over-irradiation. *Breast* **2017**, *31*, 295–302. [CrossRef] [PubMed]
16. Abdulkarim, B.S.; Cuartero, J.; Hanson, J.; Deschênes, J.; Lesniak, D.; Sabri, S. Increased risk of locoregional recurrence for women with T1-2N0 triple-negative breast cancer treated with modified radical mastectomy without adjuvant radiation therapy compared with breast-conserving therapy. *J. Clin. Oncol.* **2011**, *29*, 2852–2858. [CrossRef] [PubMed]
17. Zumsteg, Z.S.; Morrow, M.; Arnold, B.; Zheng, J.; Zhang, Z.; Robson, M.; Traina, T.; McCormick, B.; Powell, S.; Ho, A.Y. Breast-conserving therapy achieves locoregional outcomes comparable to mastectomy in women with T1-2N0 triple-negative breast cancer. *Ann. Surg. Oncol.* **2013**, *20*, 3469–3476. [CrossRef] [PubMed]
18. Adkins, F.C.; Gonzalez-Angulo, A.M.; Lei, X.; Hernandez-Aya, L.F.; Mittendorf, E.A.; Litton, J.K.; Wagner, J.; Hunt, K.K.; Woodward, W.A.; Meric-Bernstam, F. Triple-negative breast cancer is not a contraindication for breast conservation. *Ann. Surg. Oncol.* **2011**, *18*, 3164–3173. [CrossRef]
19. Kim, K.; Park, H.J.; Shin, K.H.; Kim, J.H.; Choi, D.H.; Park, W.; Do Ahn, S.; Kim, S.S.; Kim, D.Y.; Kim, T.H.; et al. Breast Conservation Therapy Versus Mastectomy in Patients with T1-2N1 Triple-Negative Breast Cancer: Pooled Analysis of KROG 14-18 and 14-23. *Cancer Res. Treat.* **2018**, *50*, 1316–1323. [CrossRef]
20. Wang, J.; Wang, S.; Tang, Y.; Jing, H.; Sun, G.; Jin, J.; Liu, Y.; Song, Y.; Wang, W.; Fang, H.; et al. Comparison of Treatment Outcomes With Breast-conserving Surgery Plus Radiotherapy Versus Mastectomy for Patients With Stage I Breast Cancer: A Propensity Score-matched Analysis. *Clin. Breast Cancer* **2018**, *18*, e975–e984. [CrossRef]
21. De Boniface, J.; Frisell, J.; Bergkvist, L.; Andersson, Y. Breast-conserving surgery followed by whole-breast irradiation offers survival benefits over mastectomy without irradiation. *Br. J. Surg.* **2018**, 1607–1614. [CrossRef]
22. Donker, M.; Van Tienhoven, G.; Straver, M.E.; Meijnen, P.; Van De Velde, C.J.; Mansel, P.R.E.; Cataliotti, P.L.; Westenberg, A.H.; Klinkenbijl, J.H.; Orzalesi, L.; et al. Radiotherapy or surgery of the axilla after a positive sentinel node in breast cancer (EORTC 10981-22023 AMAROS): A randomised, multicentre, open-label, phase 3 non-inferiority trial. *Lancet Oncol.* **2014**, *15*, 1303–1310. [CrossRef]
23. Giuliano, A.; Huntm, K.; Ballman, K.; Beitsch, P.D.; Whitworth, P.W.; Blumencranz, P.W.; Leitch, A.M.; Saha, S.; McCall, L.M.; Morrow, M. Axillary dissection vs no axillary dissection in women with invasive breast cancer and sentinel node metastasis: A randomized clinical trial. *JAMA* **2011**, *305*, 569–575. [CrossRef]
24. Galimberti, V.; Cole, B.F.; Zurrida, S.; Viale, G.; Luini, A.; Veronesi, P.; Baratella, P.; Chifu, C.; Sargenti, M.; Intra, M.; et al. Axillary dissection versus no axillary dissection in patients with sentinel-node micrometastases (IBCSG 23-01): A phase 3 randomised controlled trial. *Lancet. Oncol.* **2013**, *14*, 297–305. [CrossRef]
25. Pazos, M.; Schönecker, S.; Reitz, D.; Rogowski, P.; Niyazi, M.; Alongi, F.; Matuschek, C.; Braun, M.; Harbeck, N.; Belka, C.; et al. Recent Developments in Radiation Oncology: An Overview of Individualised Treatment Strategies in Breast Cancer. *Breast Care* **2018**, *13*, 285–291. [CrossRef]
26. Pazos, M.; Fiorentino, A.; Gaasch, A.; Schönecker, S.; Reitz, D.; Heinz, C.; Niyazi, M.; Duma, M.N.; Alongi, F.; Belka, C.; et al. Dose variability in different lymph node levels during locoregional breast cancer irradiation: The impact of deep-inspiration breath hold. *Strahlenther. Onkol.* **2019**, *195*, 13–20. [CrossRef]
27. Nguyen, M.H.; Lavilla, M.; Kim, J.N.; Fang, L.C. Cardiac sparing characteristics of internal mammary chain radiotherapy using deep inspiration breath hold for left-sided breast cancer. *Radiat. Oncol.* **2018**, *13*, 103. [CrossRef]
28. Early Breast Canc Trialists, C.; Darby, S.; McGale, P.; Correa, C.; Taylor, C.; Arriagada, R.; Clarke, M.; Cutter, D.; Davies, C.; Ewertz, M.; et al. Effect of radiotherapy after breast-conserving surgery on 10-year recurrence and 15-year breast cancer death: Meta-analysis of individual patient data for 10,801 women in 17 randomised trials. *Lancet* **2011**, *378*, 1707–1716.

29. Formenti, S.C.; Demaria, S. Local control by radiotherapy: Is that all there is? *Breast Cancer Res.* **2008**, *10*, 215. [CrossRef]
30. Veronesi, U.; Cascinelli, N.; Mariani, L.; Greco, M.; Saccozzi, R.; Luini, A.; Aguilar, M.; Marubini, E. Twenty-year follow-up of a randomized study comparing breast-conserving surgery with radical mastectomy for early breast cancer. *N. Engl. J. Med.* **2002**, *347*, 1227–1232. [CrossRef]
31. Fisher, B.; Anderson, S.; Bryant, J.; Margolese, R.G.; Deutsch, M.; Fisher, E.R.; Jeong, J.; Wolmark, N. Twenty-year follow-up of a randomized trial comparing total mastectomy, lumpectomy, and lumpectomy plus irradiation for the treatment of invasive breast cancer. *N. Engl. J. Med.* **2002**, *347*, 1233–1241. [CrossRef]
32. Hwang, S.; Lichtensztajn, D.; Gomez, S.; Fowble, B.; Clarke, C. Survival After Lumpectomy and Mastectomy for Early Stage Invasive Breast Cancer. *Cancer* **2013**, *119*, 1402–1411. [CrossRef]
33. Fisher, S.; Gao, H.; Yasui, Y.; Dabbs, K.; Winget, M. Survival in stage I-III breast cancer patients by surgical treatment in a publicly funded health care system. *Ann. Oncol.* **2015**, *26*, 1161–1169. [CrossRef] [PubMed]
34. Hofvind, S.; Holen, Å.; Aas, T.; Roman, M.; Sebuødegård, S.; Akslen, L.A. Women treated with breast conserving surgery do better than those with mastectomy independent of detection mode, prognostic and predictive tumor characteristics. *Eur. J. Surg. Oncol.* **2015**, *41*, 1417–1422. [CrossRef]
35. Onitilo, A.A.; Engel, J.M.; Stankowski, R.V.; Doi, S.A.R. Survival Comparisons for Breast Conserving Surgery and Mastectomy Revisited: Community Experience and the Role of Radiation Therapy. *Clin. Med. Res.* **2015**, *13*, 65–73. [CrossRef] [PubMed]
36. Chen, K.; Liu, J.; Zhu, L.; Su, F.; Song, E.; Jacobs, L.K. Comparative effectiveness study of breast-conserving surgery and mastectomy in the general population: A NCDB analysis. *Oncotarget* **2015**, *6*, 40127–40140. [CrossRef]
37. Chen, Q.-X.; Wang, X.-X.; Lin, P.-Y.; Zhang, J.; Li, J.-J.; Song, C.-G.; Shao, Z.-M. The different outcomes between breast-conserving surgery and mastectomy in triple-negative breast cancer: A population-based study from the SEER 18 database. *Oncotarget* **2017**, *8*, 4773–4780. [CrossRef]
38. Minicozzi, P.; Van Eycken, L.; Molinie, F.; Innos, K.; Guevara, M.; Marcos-Gragera, R.; Castro, C.; Rapiti, E.; Katalinic, A.; Torrella, A.; et al. Comorbidities, age and period of diagnosis influence treatment and outcomes in early breast cancer. *Int. J. Cancer* **2018**. [CrossRef]
39. Giordano, S.H.; Kuo, Y.-F.; Duan, Z.; Hortobagyi, G.N.; Freeman, J.; Goodwin, J.S.; Foley, N.H.; Bray, I.; Watters, K.M.; Das, S.; et al. Limits of observational data in determining outcomes from cancer therapy. *Cancer* **2008**, *112*, 2456–2466. [CrossRef]
40. Salas, M.; Hofman, A.; Stricker, B.H. Confounding by indication: An example of variation in the use of epidemiologic terminology. *Am. J. Epidemiol.* **1999**, *149*, 981–983. [CrossRef]
41. Overgaard, M.; Nielsen, H.M.; Overgaard, J. Is the benefit of postmastectomy irradiation limited to patients with four or more positive nodes, as recommended in international consensus reports? A subgroup analysis of the DBCG 82 b&c randomized trials. *Radiother. Oncol.* **2007**, *82*, 247–253. [PubMed]
42. Corradini, S.; Pazos, M.; Schönecker, S.; Reitz, D.; Niyazi, M.; Ganswindt, U.; Schrodi, S.; Braun, M.; Pölcher, M.; Mahner, S.; et al. Role of postoperative radiotherapy in reducing ipsilateral recurrence in DCIS: An observational study of 1048 cases. *Radiat. Oncol.* **2018**, *13*, 25. [CrossRef] [PubMed]

9

Liver Kinase B1—A Potential Therapeutic Target in Hormone-Sensitive Breast Cancer in Older Women

Binafsha Manzoor Syed [1,2], Andrew R Green [1], David A L Morgan [3], Ian O Ellis [1] and Kwok-Leung Cheung [1,*]

1 Nottingham Breast Cancer Research Centre, School of Medicine, University of Nottingham, Nottingham DE22 3DT, UK; drbinafsha@hotmail.com (B.M.S.); andrew.green@nottingham.ac.uk (A.R.G.); ian.ellis@nottingham.ac.uk (I.O.E.)

2 Medical Research Centre, Liaquat University of Medical & Health Sciences, Jamshoro 71000, Pakistan

3 Department of Oncology, Nottingham University Hospitals, Nottingham NG5 1PB, UK; dalmorgan@me.com

* Correspondence: kl.cheung@nottingham.ac.uk

Abstract: *Background*: The role of liver kinase B1 (LKB1), a serine/threonine kinase, has been described in the development of PeutzJagher's syndrome, where a proportion (~45%) of patients have developed breast cancer in their lifetime. Cell line studies have linked LKB1 with oestrogen receptors (ER) and with the Adenosine monophosphate-activated protein kinase (AMPK) pathway for energy metabolism. However, limited studies have investigated protein expression of LKB1 in tumour tissues and its intracellular relationships. This study aimed to investigate the intracellular molecular relationships of LKB1 in older women with early operable primary breast cancer and its correlation with long-term clinical outcome. *Methods*: Between 1973 and 2010, a consecutive series of 1758 older ($\geq$70 years) women with T0-2N0-1M0 breast carcinoma were managed in a dedicated facility. Of these, 813 patients underwent primary surgery, and 575 had good quality tumour samples available for tissue microarray construction. LKB1 was assessed in 407 cases by indirect immunohistochemistry (IHC). Tumours with 30% or more of cells with cytoplasmic LKB1 expression were considered positive. LKB1 expression was compared with tumour size, histological grade, axillary lymph node stage, ER, PgR, EGFR, HER2, HER3, HER4, BRCA1&2, p53, Ki67, Bcl2, Muc1, E-Cadherin, CD44, basal (CK5, CK5/6, CK14 and CK17) and luminal (CK7/8, CK18 and CK19) cytokeratins, MDM2 and MDM4, and correlated with long-term clinical outcome. *Results*: Positive LKB1 expression was seen in 318 (78.1%) patients, and was significantly associated with high tumour grade, high Ki67, over-expression of HER2, VEGF, HER4, BRCA2, MDM2 and negative expression of CD44 ($p < 0.05$). There was no significant correlation with tumour size, axillary lymph node status, ER, PgR, p53, basal or luminal cytokeratins, Bcl2, Muc1, EGFR, HER3, MDM4, E-cadherin and BRCA1. LKB1 did not show any significant influence on survival in the overall population; however, in those patients receiving adjuvant endocrine therapy for ER positive tumours, those with positive LKB1 had significantly better 5-year breast cancer specific survival when compared to those without such expression (93% versus 74%, $p = 0.03$). *Conclusion*: LKB1 expression has shown association with poor prognostic factors in older women with breast cancer. However, LKB1 expression appears to be associated with better survival outcome among those patients receiving adjuvant endocrine therapy. Further research is required to explore its potential role as a therapeutic target.

Keywords: LKB1; Breast Cancer; Older women; Metformin; Endocrine therapy

---

1. Introduction

Liver kinase B1 (LKB1) or serine/threonine kinase-11, a 436-amino acid chain protein with a molecular weight of 49 kDa, is associated with the development of Peutz-Jeghers syndrome (PJS) [1,2].

In addition, approximately 45% of PJS patients have been reported to develop breast cancer in their lifetime [3]. LKB1 is known to work as a tumour suppressor gene as well as an upstream kinase which is linked to the cellular functions during normal state and in metabolic stress response [4,5]. LKB1 is normally located in the nucleus, however, upon activation, it is relocated to the cytoplasm, where it acts as a co-activator of the oestrogen receptor (ER), controls the citric acid cycle (KREB's cycle) and cell energy metabolism via the adenosine mono-phosphate activated protein kinase (AMPK) pathway, and inhibits the production of the aromatase enzyme [6–11]. It has also been reported to control the cell cycle at the G0–G1 check point via the p53 pathway, to be associated with angiogenesis through the control of Vascular Endothelial Growth Factor (VEGF) and with cell polarity [8,11,12]. A proposed mechanism of LKB1 function in breast cancer cells is presented in Figure 1. Previously, reported data linked LKB1 with poor prognostic factors [11]. A cell line study on MDA-MB-231 cells showed an association of LKB1 with gemcitabine resistance [13]. Additionally, cell line studies suggested that LKB1 is involved in DNA repair, thus deficient cells demonstrate delayed repair and respond well to DNA-based therapy, such as PARP inhibitors [14]. Cell-based studies showed that LKB1-null cells possess invasion and breast cancer stem cell like properties. However, LKB1 enhancing therapy (i.e., Honokoil, a bioactive molecule) showed improving outcome by reducing cellular invasiveness and stemness [15], thus suggesting a therapeutic significance.

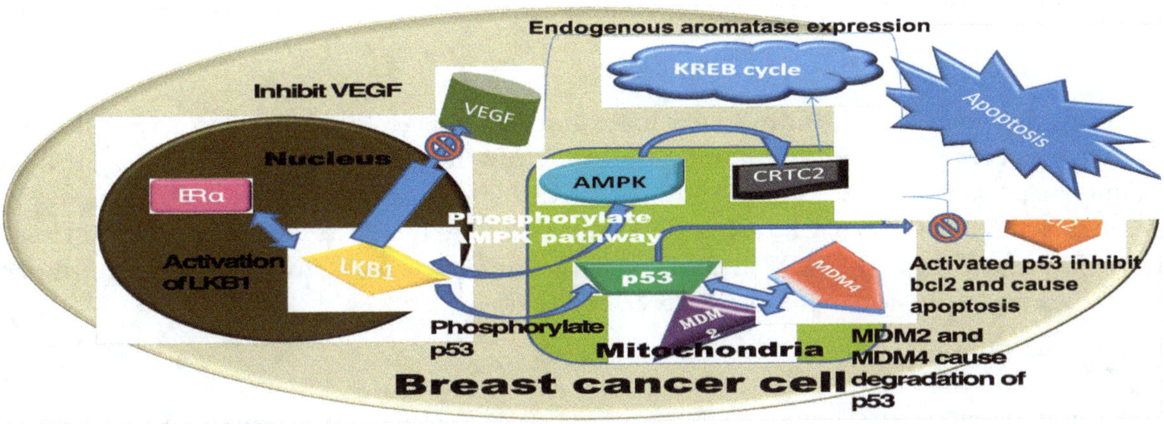

Figure 1. Proposed intracellular mechanism of action of LKB1 as suggested in the cell line studies [7–9,12,16]. VEGF: Vascular Endothelial Growth factor, KREB: Citric acid cycle, ER: Oestrogen receptor, CRTC2: Creb-regulated transcription co-activator 2, MDM2/4: Mouse double minute 2/4.

Currently available literature is based on in vitro or in vivo model studies, or gene technologies, such as Western blot. However, there is limited information available on the subject of using immunohistochemistry (IHC), which is currently a widely used technique for analysis of therapeutic targets in clinical practice. This study was designed to analyse the association of LKB1 with other biological markers of known significance in breast cancer and to correlate its expression with long-term clinical outcome in older women with primary breast cancer.

2. Materials and Methods

2.1. Patients

Over 37 years (1973–2010), 1758 older (≥70 years) women with early operable primary breast cancer (T0-2, N0-1, M0) were managed in a dedicated facility in a single institution with clinical information available from diagnosis till death/last follow-up. Eight hundred and thirteen patients underwent primary surgery (with optimal adjuvant therapy as per unit policy at the time [17]) and among them, good quality formalin-fixed paraffin-embedded surgical specimens were available from 575 patients for tissue microarray (TMA) construction. The management pattern over this period of time was evolving, a detailed description of which was reported earlier [17]. Briefly during the

1970s and 1980s, ER status was not available and there was no consensus on recommendations for adjuvant systemic therapy. During the 1990s, adjuvant endocrine therapy was advised based on the clinical judgement of the treating physician and/or the patient's choice. In the recent decade, there have been structured recommendations for the use of adjuvant endocrine therapy. Those patients with ER positive tumours and Nottingham Prognostic Index (NPI) <3 (excellent prognostic group) were not given any adjuvant systemic therapy, those with an NPI of 3–3.4 (good prognostic group) were offered endocrine therapy and given the choice of tamoxifen or a non-steroidal aromatase inhibitor, and those with an NPI of >3.4 (moderate to poor prognostic group) were given a non-steroidal aromatase inhibitor. Adjuvant chemotherapy was considered in fit, relatively younger patients with moderate to poor prognostic tumours, in particular those with ER negative tumours. Trastuzumab was considered in relatively fit patients with HER2 positive tumours having moderate to poor prognosis.

2.2. *Tissue Microarray Construction*

Tissue microarrays (TMAs) of formalin-fixed paraffin-embedded tumour sections were constructed as described [18]. Briefly, 0.6 mm-diameter cores of the representative part of the tumour blocks were implanted in the TMA blocks using Beecher's manual tissue microarrayer (MP06 Beecher Instruments Inc, Sun Prairie, WI, USA).

2.3. *Immunohistochemistry*

LKB1 and 24 other biological markers including ER, progesterone receptor (PgR), Epidermal Growth Factor Receptor (EGFR), Human Epidermal Growth Factor Receptor (HER)-2, HER3, HER4, Breast Cancer Associated gene (BRCA)1&2, p53, Ki67, B-Cell Lymphoma (Bcl)2, Mucin (MUC)1, E-Cadherin, basal (CK5, CK5/6, CK14 and CK17) and luminal (CK7/8, CK18 and CK19) cytokeratins, and Mouse Double Minute (MDM)2 and MDM4 were analysed using indirect IHC by StreptAvidin Biotin Complex and EnVision methods as described [19].

2.4. *Scoring*

Immunohistochemical staining of biological markers was assessed by the percentage of invasive tumour cells stained and by McCarty's immunohistochemical scoring (H-score) (range 0–300) [20]. The LKB1 expression of 30% or more positive cells was considered positive (Figure 2a–d). Previously, studies have shown that the active form of LKB1 is found in the cytoplasm and is associated with other markers and outcome of breast cancer; thus, cytoplasmic expression of LKB1 was considered in our study [21].

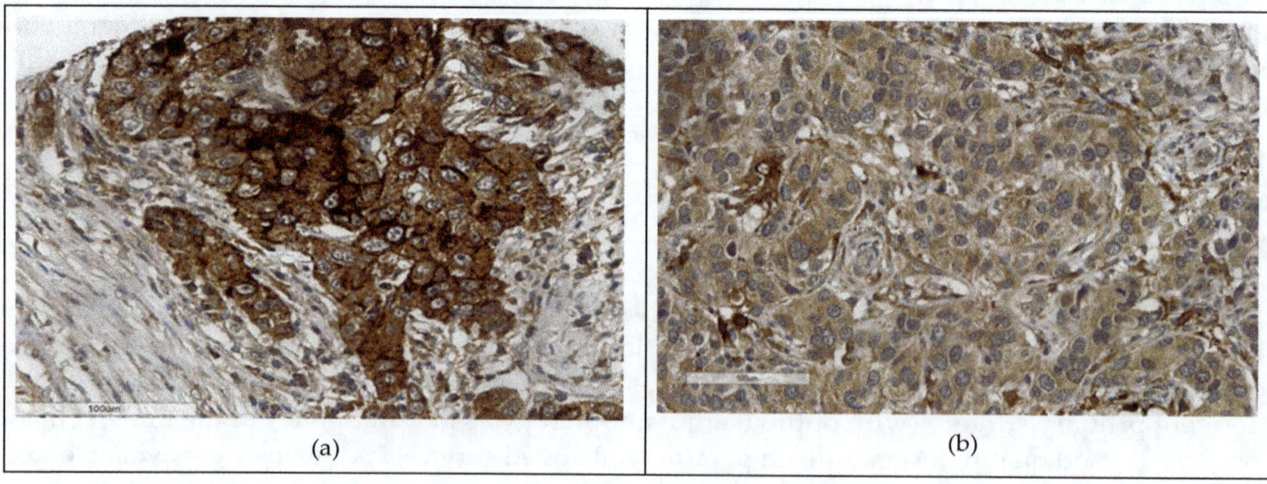

(a) (b)

Figure 2. *Cont.*

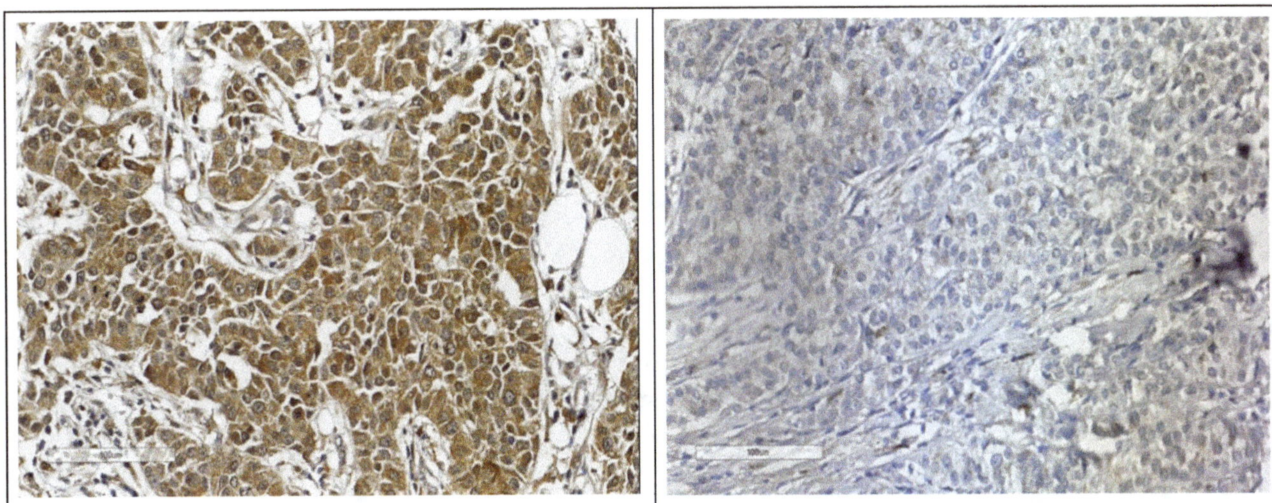

(c) (d)

Figure 2. Immunohistochemichemical expression of LKB1 in Breast cancer cells. (**a**–**c**) Positive cytoplasmic expression, (**d**) LKB1 negative.

2.5. *Statistical Analysis*

X-tile bio-informatics software (Yale University, New Haven, CT, USA) was used to define cut-offs for positivity of the expression of the biological markers based on breast cancer specific survival (BCSS) [22]. The cut-offs for all the biological markers were determined by using the same metric in X-tile. The cut-off values to define positive expression are the same as reported earlier [23]. The Statistical Package for Social Sciences (SPSS, version 16.0, Chicago, IL, USA) was used for data collection and analysis. A Chi-squared test was used for the analysis of the association of the LKB1 with other biomarkers in terms of expression. The clinical outcome was evaluated in terms of BCSS, metastases free survival, local recurrence free survival and regional recurrence free survival, breast cancer specific survival was defined as survival from the date of diagnosis till death from breast cancer; metastases free, local recurrence free and regional recurrence free survivals were calculated from the date of diagnosis till the appearance of the respective recurrences. Survival was analysed by using Kaplan-Meier methods with application of log-rank and generalised Wilcoxon tests, as appropriate. A p-value of <0.05 was considered significant.

2.6. *Ethical Consideration*

The study was approved by the Nottingham Research Ethics Committee 2 under ethical approval number C2020313.

3. Results

3.1. *Patients*

Of the 575 patients who had TMAs constructed from surgical specimens, 168 cores were lost during the IHC process and 407 cases had LKB1 measured. The median age of the patients was 76 (range 70–91) years, with the majority having had no axillary lymph node involvement (54.2%). Most of the patients (n = 296 (72.7%)) underwent a mastectomy and 46.6% of patients (n = 189) received adjuvant endocrine therapy. None of these patients received chemotherapy. The median follow-up was 60 months (longest = 261 months).

3.2. Pattern of LKB1 Expression and Association with Other Clinico-Pathological Parameters and Biological Markers

Overall, 78.1% (n = 318) of patients showed positive cytoplasmic expression of LKB1 in their tumours.

3.2.1. Pathological Parameters

The expression of LKB1 was significantly associated with high histological grade (among LKB1 positive, grade 1&2 = 44.5%, grade 3 = 55.5%; among LKB1 negative, grade 1&2 = 59.2% and grade 3 = 40.8%, p = 0.01).However there was no statistically significant correlation with tumour size(among LKB1 positive, <3 cm = 81.7% and among LKB1 negative, <3 cm = 75.6%, p = 0.15) and axillary lymph node status (among LKB1 positive:, stage 1&2 = 87.1%, stage 3 = 12.9%, among LKB1 negative, stage 1&2 = 89.5%, stage 3 = 10.5%, p = 0.41).

3.2.2. Biological Markers

The positive expression of LKB1 was significantly associated with positive expression of HER2 (p = 0.003), Ki67 (p = 0.01), VEGF (p = 0.002), HER4 (p = 0.001), BRCA2 (p = 0.01) and MDM2 (p < 0.001), and negative expression of CD44 (p = 0.03). However, there was no statistically significant correlation with, ER, PgR, p53, basal or luminal cytokeratins, Bcl2, Muc1, EGFR, HER3, MDM4, E-cadherin, and BRCA1.A, as summarised in Table 1.

Table 1. Intracellular relationships between LKB1 with biological markers in older women with early operable primary breast cancer.

Biomarker	LKB1 Positive N (%)	LKB1 Negative N (%)	p-Value
ER + ve	211 (69.0)	61 (72.6)	0.30
PgR + ve	168 (55.1)	52 (61.9)	0.16
HER2 + ve	30 (9.6)	2 (2.4)	0.01
Ki67 + ve	114 (35.8)	20 (22.5)	0.01
MUC1 + ve	274 (89.0)	73 (86.9)	0.36
Bcl2 + ve	250 (83.1)	69 (83.1)	0.56
P53 + ve	123 (41.1)	31 (39.7)	0.46
CK5 + ve	104 (33.7)	21 (24.7)	0.07
CK5/6 + ve	128 (45.2)	33 (42.3)	0.37
CK7/8 + ve	301 (97.4)	84 (98.8)	0.38
CK14 + ve	73 (25.8)	15 (18.5)	0.11
CK17 + ve	70 (23.4)	14 (16.7)	0.11
CK18 + ve	286 (97.3)	81 (96.4)	0.45
CK19 + ve	291 (95.4)	79 (96.3)	0.49
EGFR + ve	65 (23.0)	12 (14.8)	0.07
BRCA2 + ve	160 (56.7)	35 (42.7)	0.01
VEGF + ve	234 (88.6)	56 (73.7)	0.002
CD44 + ve	61 (19.7)	25 (29.8)	0.03
MDM2 + ve	296 (96.7)	60 (74.1)	<0.001
E-Cadherin + ve	191 (63.2)	48 (57.1)	0.18
Expression of LKB1 in molecular classes of breast cancer			
Luminal A	79 (76.0)	25 (24.0)	0.09
Luminal B	56 (75.7)	18 (24.3)	
Low ER Luminal	36 (81.8)	8 (18.2)	
All low expression/normal like	13 (76.5)	4 (23.5)	
Basal Like	19 (73.1)	7 (26.9)	
HER2 positive	25 (96.2)	1 (3.8)	

ER: Oestrogen receptor, HER2: Human Epidermal Receptor 2.

3.3. Correlation with Molecular Classes of Breast Cancer

The expression of LKB1 was correlated with molecular classes (subtypes) of breast cancer found in older women (published previously [23]). The results showed no significant difference in the expression across them (Table 1).

3.4. Association of LKB1 with Clinical Outcome

Breast Cancer Specific Survival (BCSS)

At a median follow-up of 60 months (longest 261 months), LKB1 did not show any significant association with BCSS (Figure 3a. However, among those who received adjuvant endocrine therapy (n = 267), patients with ER positive disease and positive LKB1 expression (ER+/LKB1+) showed significantly better BCSS (5-year: 93%versus 74%, $p = 0.03$) (Figure 3b). However, in the absence of adjuvant endocrine therapy, LKB1 did not produce any significant impact on survival ($p = 0.85$). For patients with positive LKB1, positive expression of ER ($p < 0.001$, Figure 4a), PgR ($p = 0.001$, Figure 4b), MUC1 ($p = 0.003$, Figure 4c) and Bcl2 ($p < 0.001$, Figure 4d) was associated with significantly better BCSS but poorer BCSS in cases of positive expression of HER2 ($p < 0.001$, Figure 4e), Ki67 ($p = 0.01$, Figure 4f), CK17 ($p = 0.02$, Figure 4g) and EGFR ($p = 0.03$, Figure 4h).

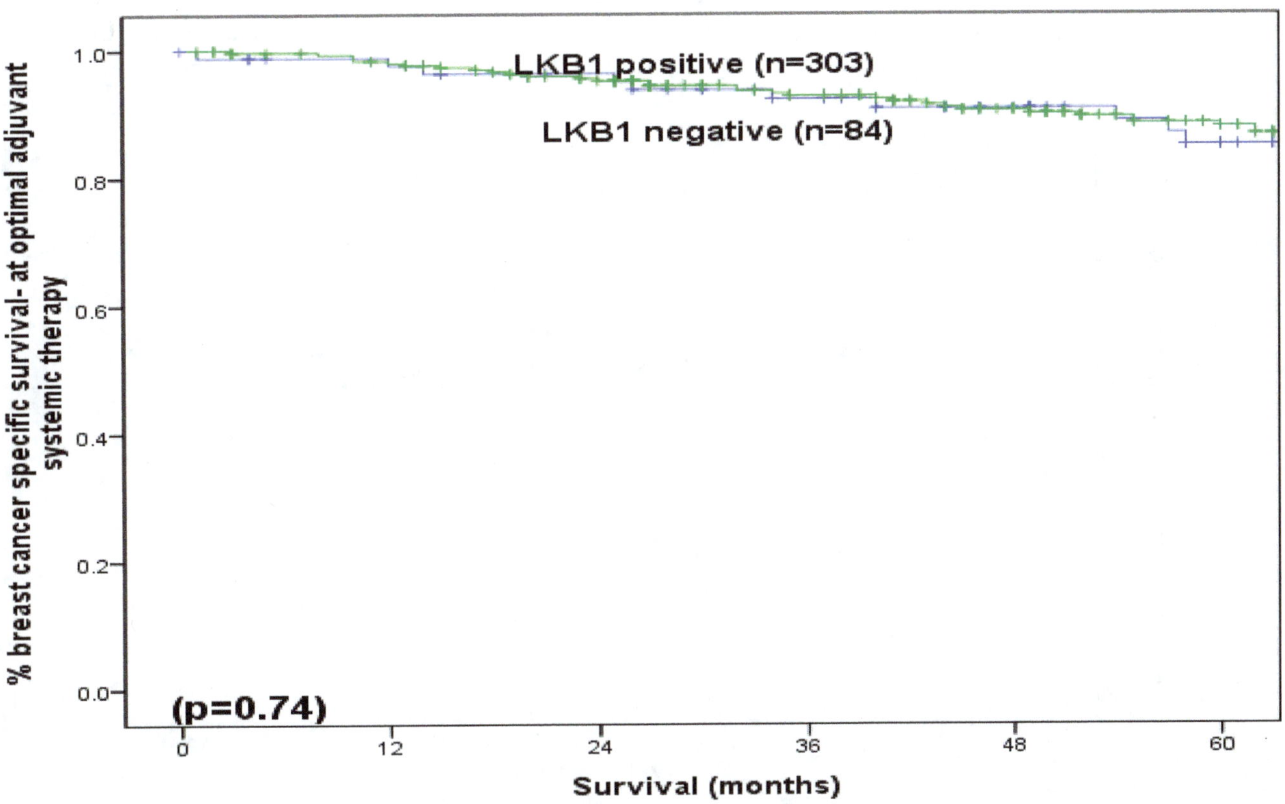

(a)

Figure 3. *Cont.*

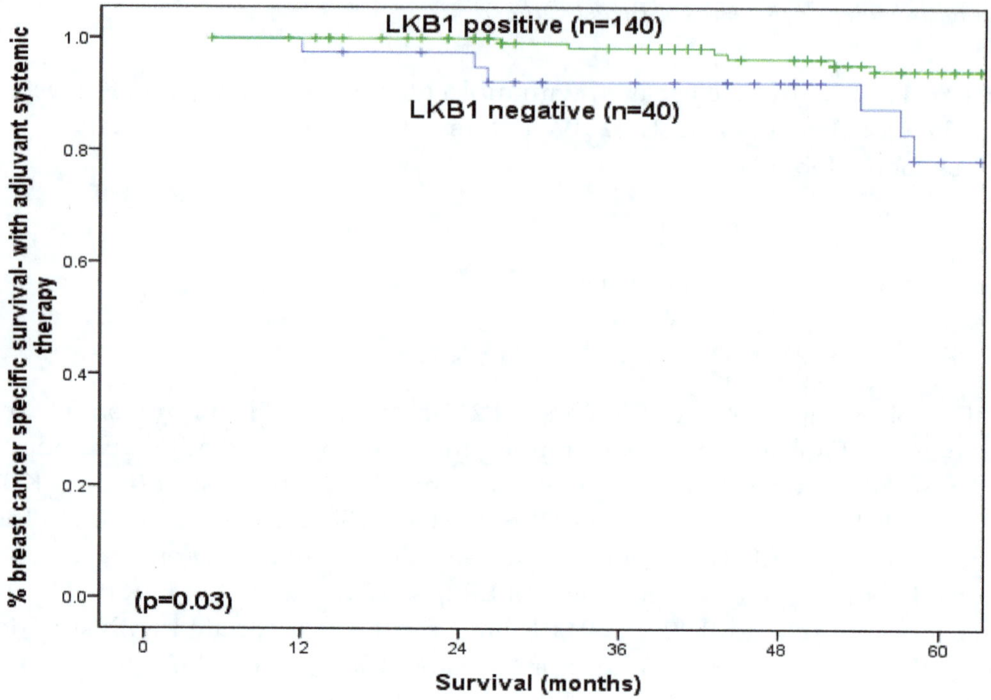

(b)

Figure 3. (a) Breast cancer specific survival according to the expression of LKB1 in older women with early operable primary breast cancer (all patients). (b) Breast cancer specific survival according to the expression of LKB1 in older women with early operable primary breast cancer who received adjuvant endocrine therapy.

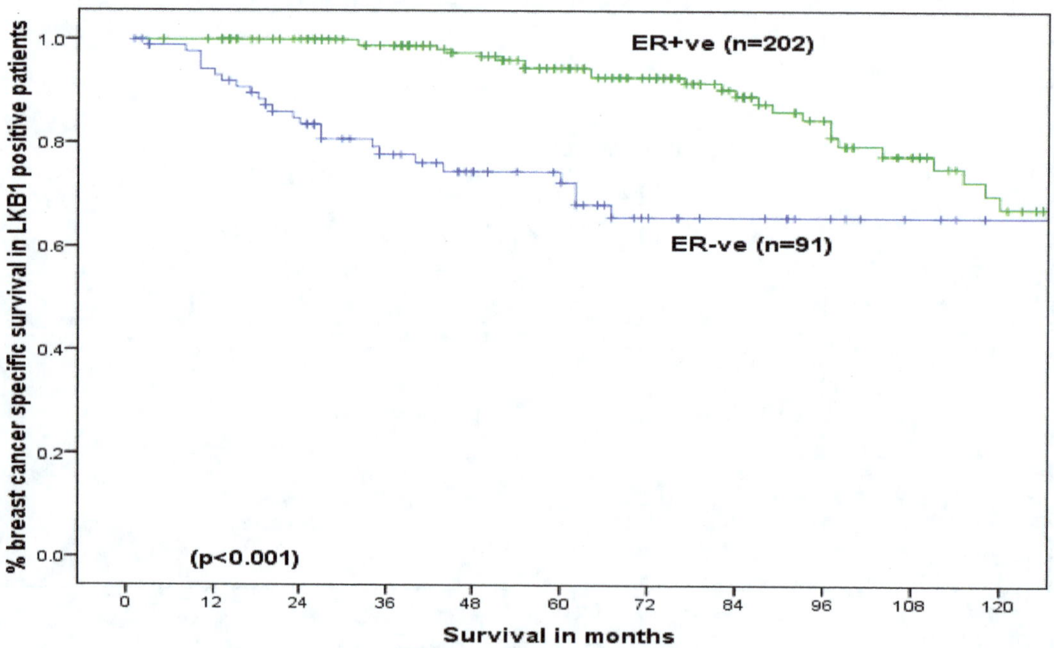

(a)

Figure 4. *Cont.*

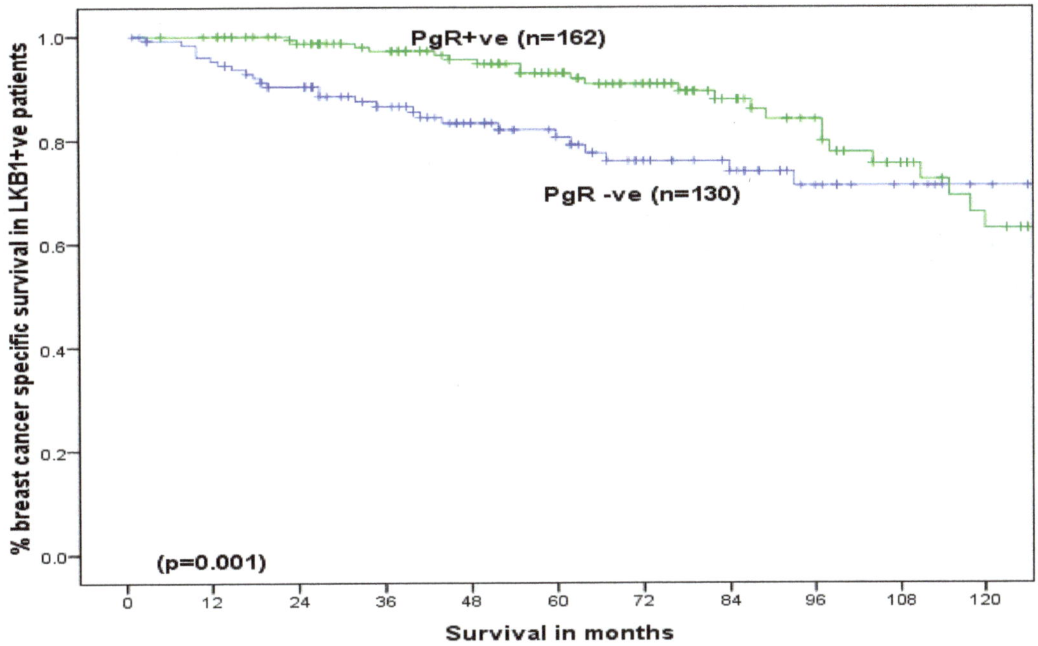

(b)

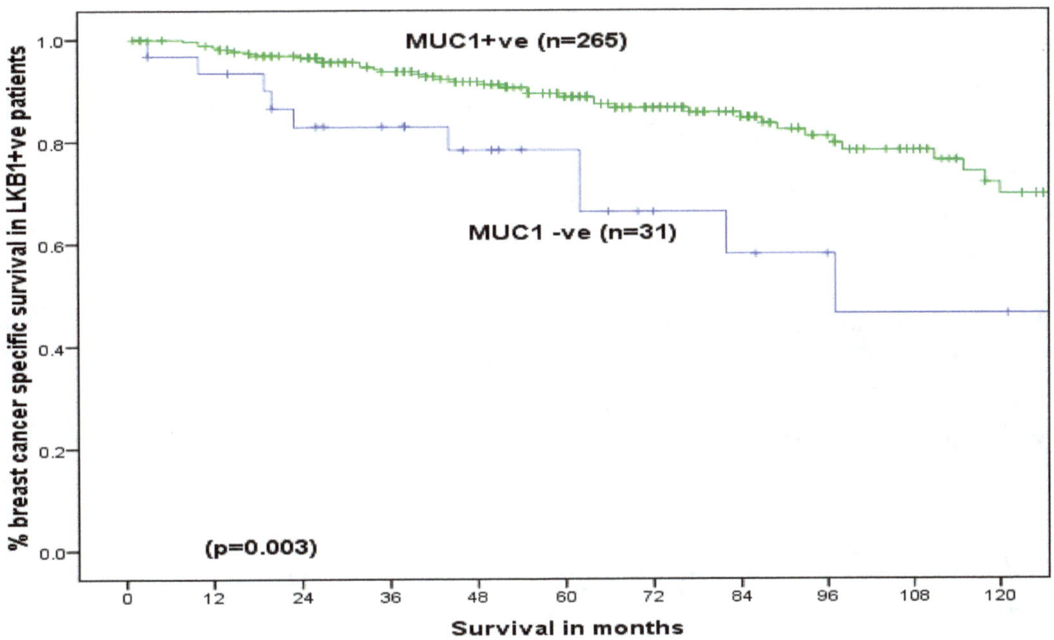

(c)

Figure 4. *Cont.*

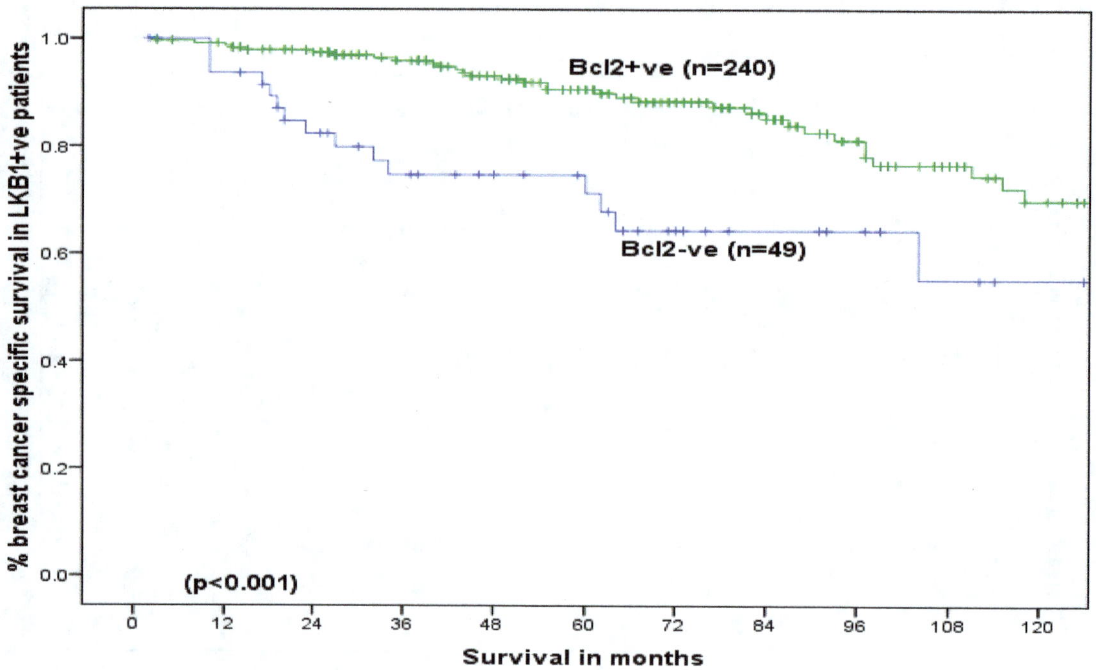

(**d**)

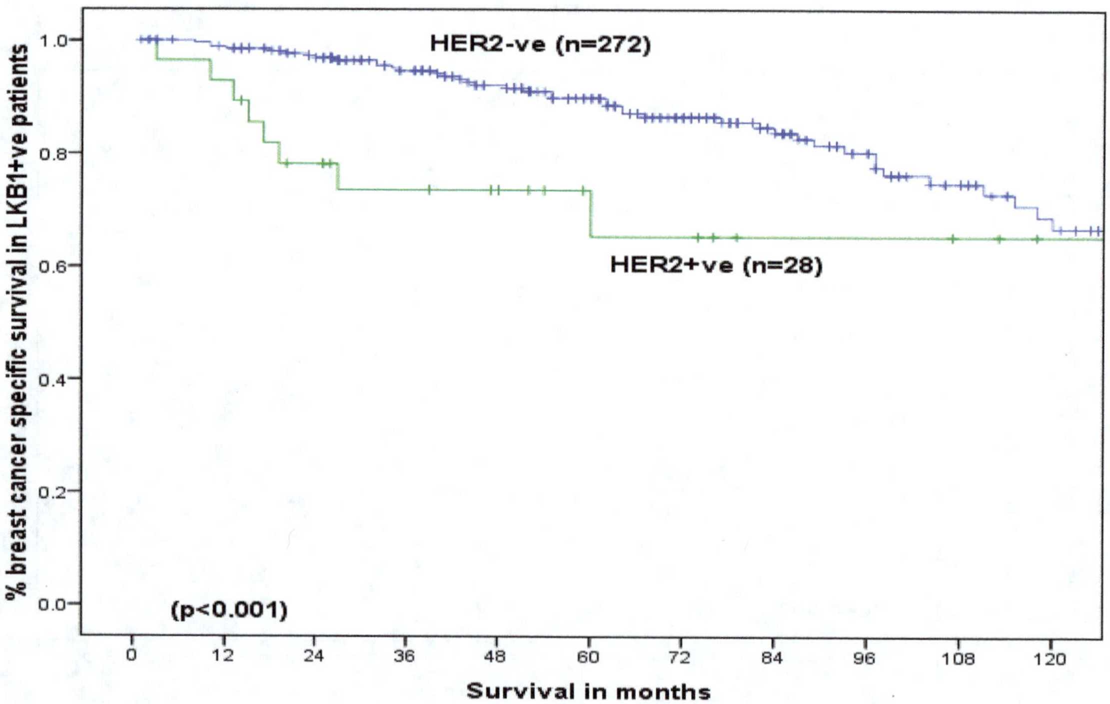

(**e**)

Figure 4. *Cont.*

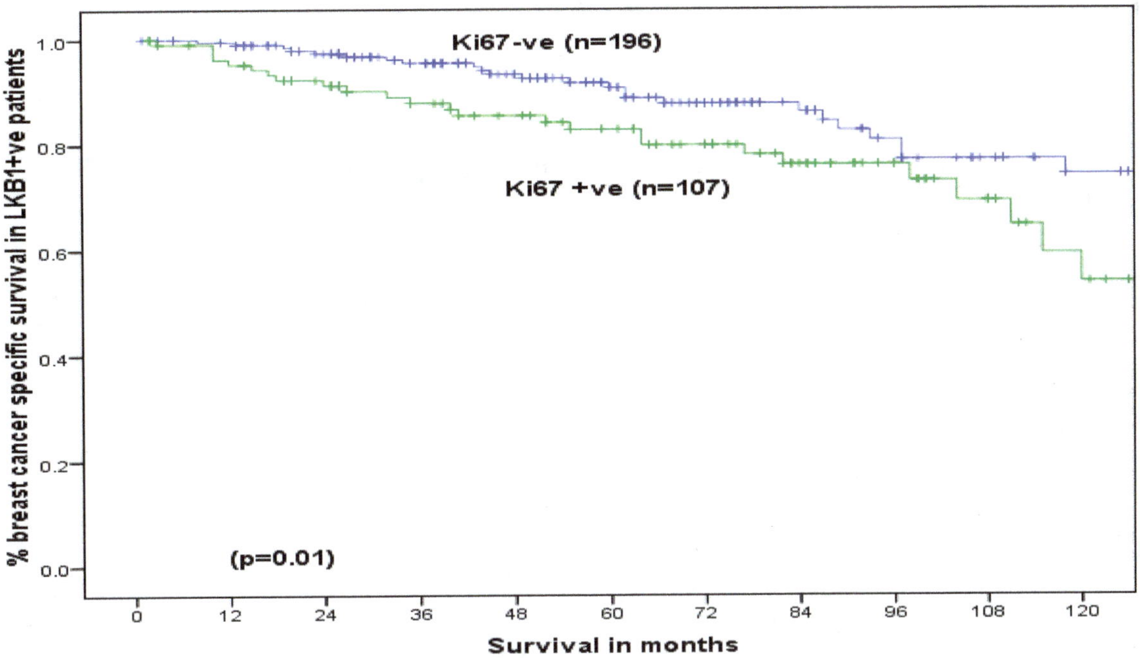

(f)

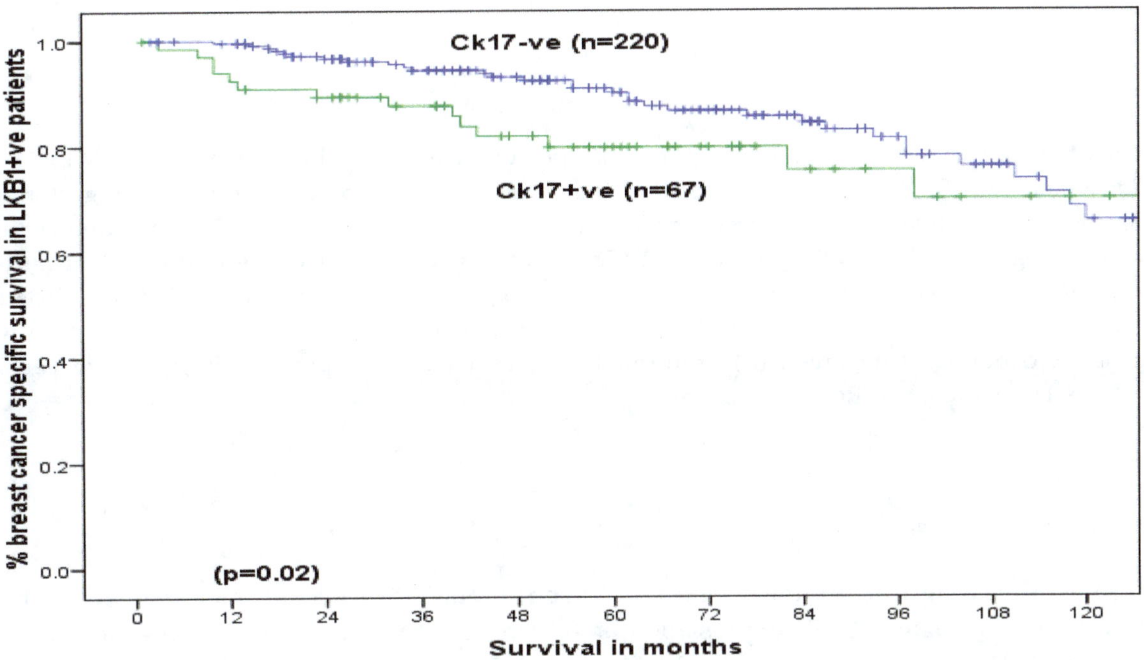

(g)

Figure 4. *Cont.*

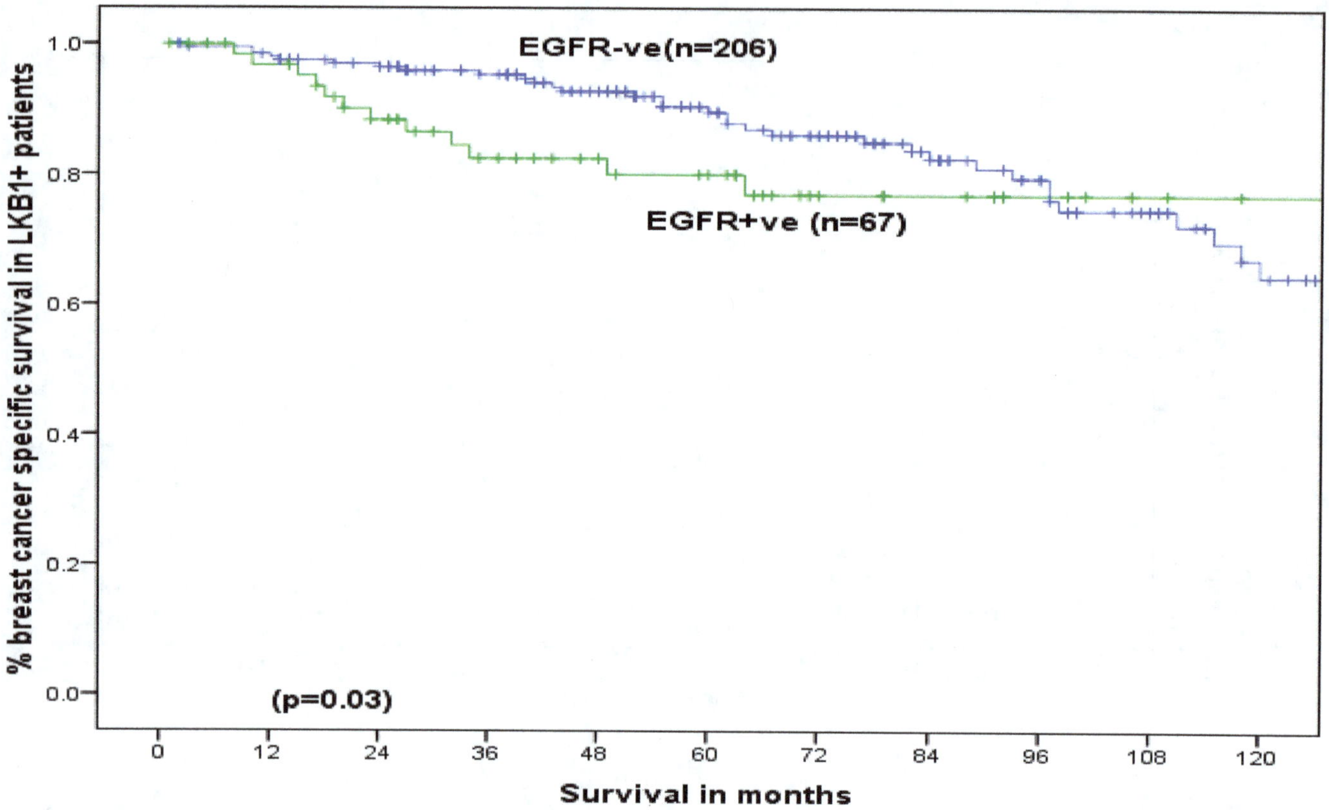

(**h**)

Figure 4. Breast cancer specific survival in LKB1 positive early operable primary breast cancer in older women: (**a**) Oestrogen receptor positive versus oestrogen receptor negative. (**b**) Progesterone receptor(PgR) positive versus Progesterone Receptor negative, (**c**) Mucin (MUC)-1 positive versus Mucin 1 negative, (**d**) B-Cell Lymphoma-2 (Bcl2) positive versus B-Cell Lymphoma 2 negative, (**e**) Human Epidermal Growth Factor Receptor-2(HER2) positive versus Human Epidermal Growth Factor Receptor-2 negative, (**f**) Ki67 positive versus Ki67 negative, (**g**) Cytokeratin 17(CK17) positive versus Cytokeratin 17 negative, (**h**) Epidermal Growth Factor Receptor (EGFR) positive versus Epidermal Growth Factor Receptor negative.

3.5. Recurrence Free Survival

There was no significant correlation between metastases-, local recurrence- or regional recurrence-free survival and LKB1 expression ($p > 0.05$). Figure S1a–e). Nevertheless, among patients with positive LKB1, positive expression of ER ($p < 0.001$, Figure 5a), PgR ($p = 0.001$, Figure 5b), MUC1 ($p = 0.002$, Figure 5c), Bcl2 ($p = 0.004$, Figure 5d) and negative expression of HER2 were associated with better metastases-free survival ($p = 0.01$, Figure 5e). While Ki67 (Figure S2a), CK17 (Figure S2b) and EGFR (Figure S2c) did not show any significant influence on metastases free survival.

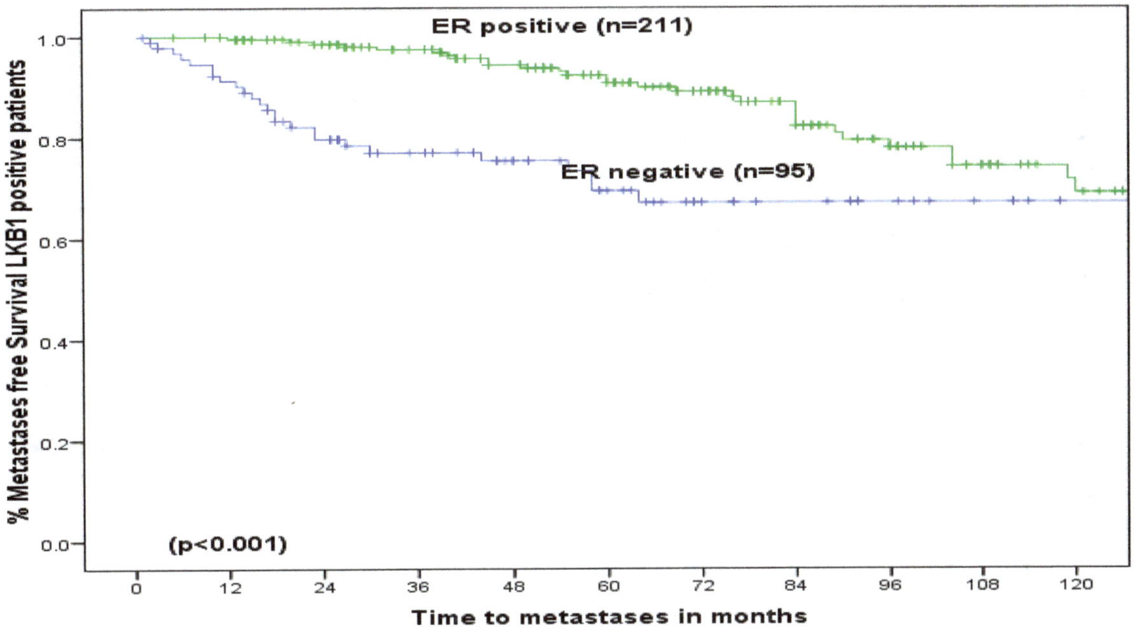

(a)

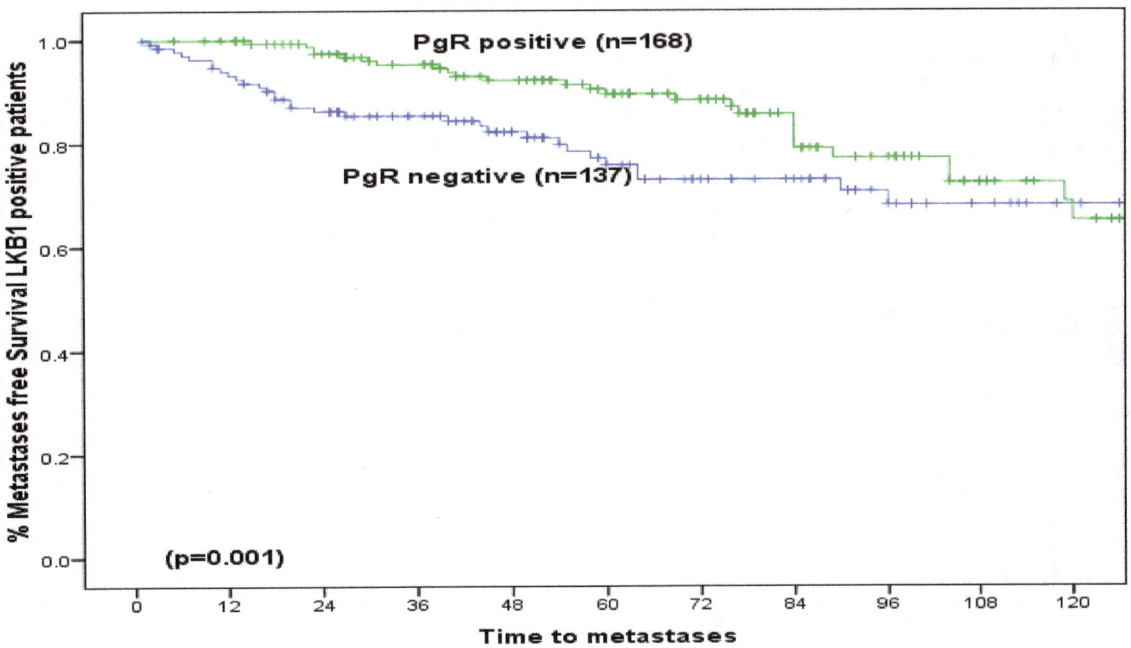

(b)

Figure 5. *Cont.*

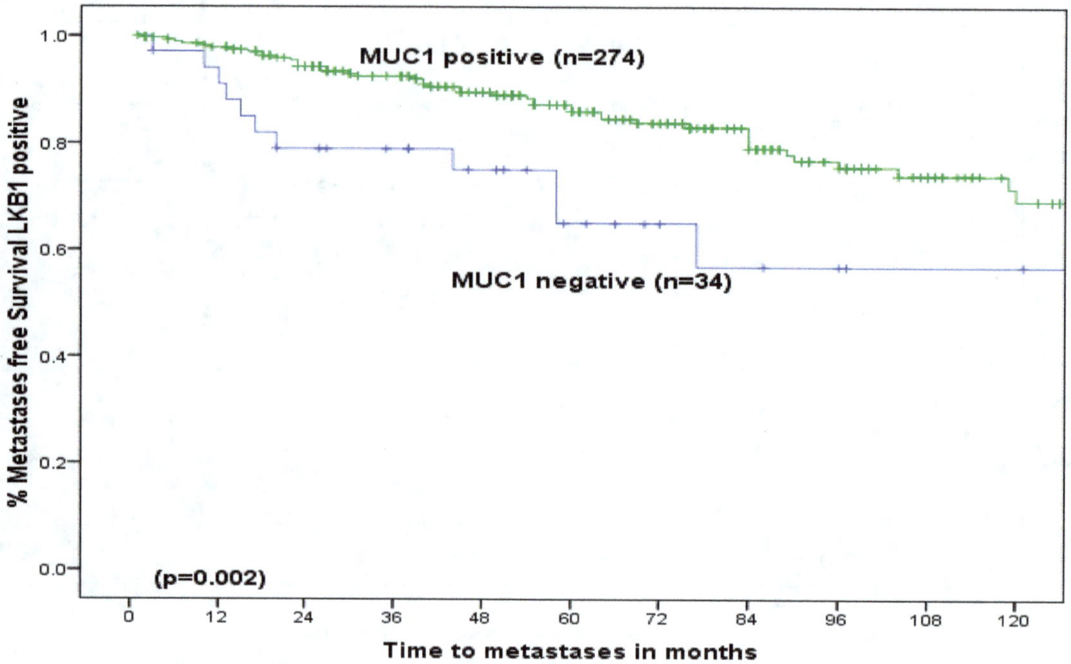

(c)

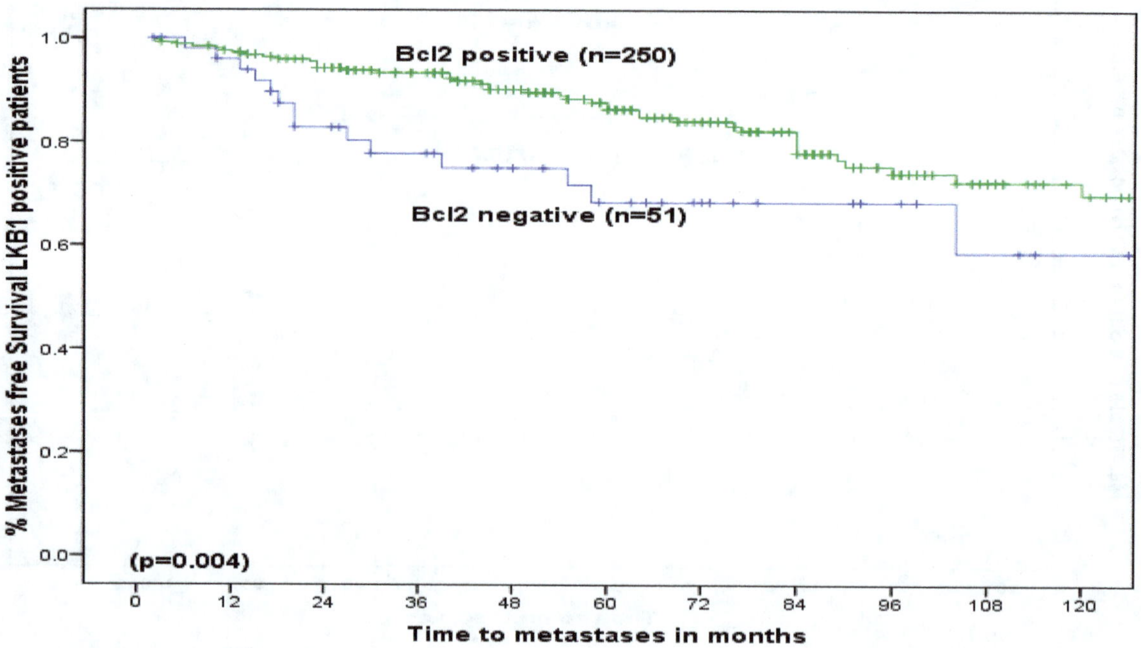

(d)

Figure 5. *Cont.*

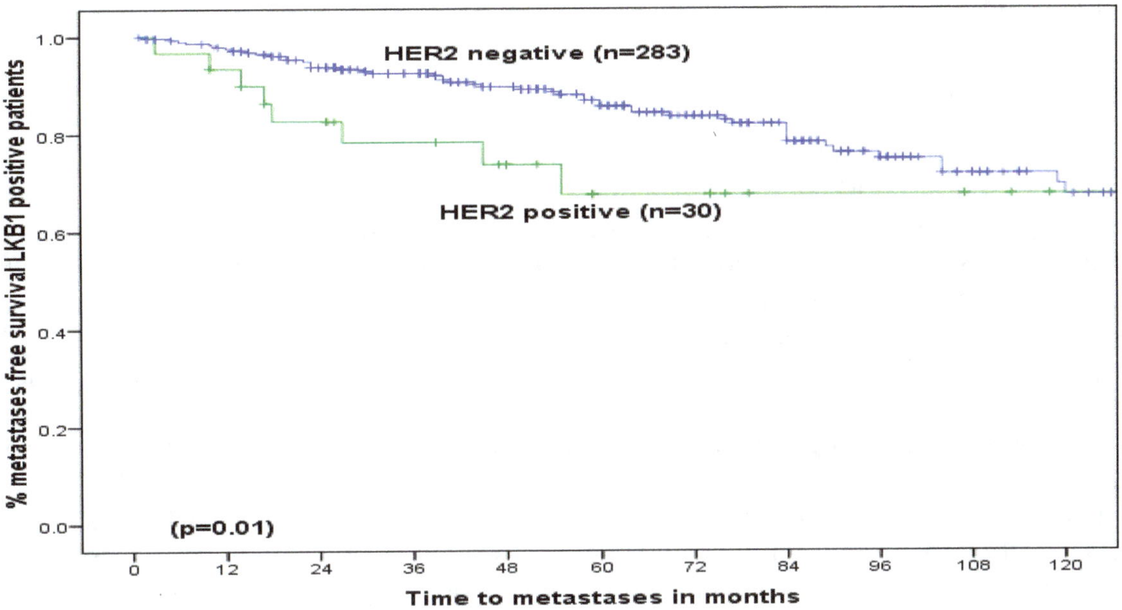

(e)

Figure 5. (**a**) Metastasis-free survival in LKB1 positive early operable primary breast cancer in older women: ER positive versus ER negative. (**b**) Metastasis-free survival in LKB1 positive early operable primary breast cancer in older women: PgR positive versus PgR negative. (**c**) Metastasis-free survival in LKB1 positive early operable primary breast cancer in older women: MUC1 positive versus MUC1 negative. (**d**) Metastasis-free survival in LKB1 positive early operable primary breast cancer in older women: Bcl2 positive versus Bcl2 negative. (**e**) Metastasis-free survival in LKB1 positive early operable primary breast cancer in older women: HER2 positive versus HER2 negative.

4. Discussion

Results of the analysis showed that cytosolic expression of LKB1 was associated with high-grade tumours and positive expression of HER2, Ki67 and VEGF. Within the population with LKB1 positive tumours, BCSS was significantly better in patients who received adjuvant endocrine therapy.

The expression of LKB1 in tumours cells was previously reported as 71%, which is slightly lower than the expression reported in our population (78%) [24]. This could be explained by the age of the population, as our study included patients 70 years or older, while the previously reported data included four groups with median ages of 48, 54, 61 and 62 years [24]. In our study, the association between LKB1 positivity and the factors mentioned above suggests its role as a possible poor prognostic indicator. The association of LKB1 expression with high histological grade suggests a poor prognostic indication as reported previously, where IHC was used for the detection of LKB1 protein expression [24]. While in vitro studies reported a negative correlation between both LKB1 mutation and grade and VEGF and a positive correlation with hormone receptor expression [1,3,12,25], these studies analysed LKB1 using Western blot and RT-PCR [1,3,11]. A recently presented study suggested that the nuclear location of LKB1 was associated with better survival while cytosolic expression is an indicator of poor prognosis [25]. Another study analysed both nuclear and cytoplasmic expression ($n = 32$) on IHC in early operable primary breast cancer with ER and PgR positive expression [26]. High cytoplasmic expression was seen in 62.5% of cases, which was not associated with age, ER, PgR and HER2, but was shown to be significantly associated with smaller tumour size [26]. In this study, the nuclear expression was also associated with smaller tumours and better survival. A high LKB1 gene expression has been reported to be linked to a high ER expression [24]. The expression of LKB1 has shown its association with CD44, which is a marker of stemness in breast cancer stem cells. Previously, the available literature showed LKB1 as a factor for maintenance of stem cells in haemopoetic cells in a mouse model study, where animals with LKB1 deletion had progressive pancytopenia and reduction in haemopoetic cell proliferation [27–29]. In this study, LKB1 has also shown its significant association with VEGF, probably linked to tumour growth and invasion. A recent study has demonstrated the influence of LKB1 on tumour invasion and metastases in colorectal cancer and suggested it to be a potential therapeutic marker [30].

The expression of LKB1 among molecular classes or subtypes has not been reported in the literature. Though it did not show any remarkable findings in our data analyses, its relatively high expression in the HER2 over-expressing class may be linked to some relationship with growth factor pathways. As it was previously reported, it may be a potential predictor of overall survival among HER2 positive breast cancer patients [24].

The prognostic significance of LKB1 was clinically demonstrated in the group of patients who received adjuvant endocrine therapy. This is an interesting finding, which is in line with the data previously reported, which suggested that within the stress environment, 17β oestradiol stimulatesthe AMPK pathway. The same study has also suggested that LKB1 is required for the ER mediated activation of AMPK [31,32]. The tumour analysis of the patients included in the TAMRAD randomized GINECO trial (the trial compared tamoxifen versus tamoxifen plus everolimus in ER+ metastatic breast cancers). It reported that the patients with a low cytoplasmic expression of LKB1 demonstrated a 67% reduction in the risk of disease progression with everolimus (a mammalian target of rapamycin (mTOR) inhibitor) plus tamoxifen, when compared to the tamoxifen only arm [33]. On the other hand, high cytoplasmic expression was associated with less benefit with everolimus therapy, consistent with our results, suggesting the predictive role of LKB1 in patients with ER positive tumours.

In addition, LKB1 has been previously reported to inhibit the aromatase enzyme via the AMP-activated protein kinase, thus supporting its potential role in the prediction of the response to primary endocrine therapy in older women [7,10,26].

The study has limitation of not including the comparison with the younger women and not studying the gene expression and mutations in older women. Precisely defining an expression cut-off based on IHC remains a challenge as this could vary between laboratories.

5. Conclusions

The available literature reported on LKB1 are primarily based on in vitro and in vivo studies using Western blot or PCR techniques. Our work describes a novel study which analysed the relationship between LKB1 and other biomarkers and clinical outcome in a large series of older patients with breast cancer by using IHC. Given the availability of IHC in clinical practice, this study possesses translational significance. The study has demonstrated significant correlations between LKB1 and biological markers of established significance. It has also shown its significant influence on the clinical outcome (notably BCSS) in older women receiving adjuvant endocrine therapy. Further studies are required to investigate and compare the expression of LKB1 in and with the younger patients and to delineate the precise role of LKB1 as a potential therapeutic target in breast cancer management. Studies are also required to understand the detailed genetics of LKB1.

Supplementary Materials:
Figure S1: (a) Metastasis-free survival according to the expression of LKB1 in older women with early operable primary breast cancer (all patients). (b) Local recurrence-free survival according to the expression of LKB1 in older women with early operable primary breast cancer (all patients). (c) Regional recurrence free survival according to the expression of LKB1 in older women with early operable primary breast cancer (all patients). (d) Metastasis-free survival according to the expression of LKB1 in older women with early operable primary breast cancer who received adjuvant endocrine therapy, Figure S2. (a) Metastases free survival in LKB1 positive early operable primary breast cancer in older women: Ki67 positive versus Ki67 negative. (b) Metastasis-free survival in LKB1 positive early operable primary breast cancer in older women: CK17 positive versus CK17 negative. (c) Metastasis-free survival in LKB1 positive early operable primary breast cancer in older women: EGFR positive versus EGFR negative.

Author Contributions: B.M.S. designed study, collected data, analysed data and wrote manuscript; A.R.G. supervised study, analysed data, written manuscript; D.A.L.M. supervised study, analysed data and wrote manuscript; I.O.E.: supervised study, analysed data and wrote manuscript; K.L.C. conceived idea, designed study, collected data, analysed data and wrote manuscript.

References

1. Collins, S.P.; Reoma, J.L.; Gamm, D.M.; Uhler, M.D. LKB1, a novel serine/threonine protein kinase and potential tumour suppressor, is phosphorylated by cAMP-dependent protein kinase (PKA) and prenylated in vivo. *Biochem. J.* **2000**, *345*, 673–680. [CrossRef] [PubMed]
2. Marignani, P.A.; Negishi, Y.; Ui, N.; Nakajima, M.; Kawashima, K.; Maruyama, K.; Takizawa, T.; Endo, H.; Kanai, F.; Carpenter, C.L. LKB1 Associates with Brg1 and Is Necessary for Brg1-induced Growth Arrest. *J. Biol. Chem.* **2001**, *276*, 32415–32418. [CrossRef] [PubMed]
3. McCarthy, A.; Lord, C.J.; Savage, K.; Grigoriadis, A.; Smith, D.P.; Weigelt, B.; Reis-Filho, J.S.; Ashworth, A.; Reis-Filho, J.S. Conditional deletion of the Lkb1 gene in the mouse mammary gland induces tumour formation. *J. Pathol.* **2009**, *219*, 306–316. [CrossRef] [PubMed]
4. Liu, X.; Xiao, Z.-D.; Han, L.; Zhang, J.; Lee, S.-W.; Wang, W.; Lee, H.; Zhuang, L.; Chen, J.; Lin, H.-K.; et al. LncRNA NBR2 engages a metabolic checkpoint by regulating AMPK under energy stress. *Nature* **2016**, *18*, 431–442. [CrossRef] [PubMed]
5. Trapp, E.K.; Majunke, L.; Zill, B.; Sommer, H.; Andergassen, U.; Koch, J.; Harbeck, N.; Mahner, S.; Friedl, T.W.P.; Janni, W.; et al. LKB1 pro-oncogenic activity triggers cell survival in circulating tumor cells. *Mol. Oncol.* **2017**, *11*, 1508–1526. [CrossRef] [PubMed]
6. Boudeau, J.; Sapkota, G.; Alessi, D.R. LKB1, a protein kinase regulating cell proliferation and polarity. *FEBS Lett.* **2003**, *546*, 159–165. [CrossRef]
7. Brown, K.; McInnes, K.; Simpson, E. The regulation of LKB1 by hormones and its implications for post-menopausal breast cancer. *Breast Cancer Res. Treat.* **2007**, S125.
8. Cheng, H.; Liu, P.; Wang, Z.C.; Zou, L.; Santiago, S.; Garbitt, V.; Gjoerup, O.V.; Iglehart, J.D.; Miron, A.; Richardson, A.L.; et al. SIK1 Couples LKB1 to p53-Dependent Anoikis and Suppresses Metastasis. *Sci. Signal.* **2009**, *2*, ra35. [CrossRef]
9. Nath-Sain, S.; Marignani, P.A. LKB1 Catalytic Activity Contributes to Estrogen Receptor α Signaling. *Mol. Biol. Cell* **2009**, *20*, 2785–2795. [CrossRef]
10. Hunger, N.I.; Docanto, M.; Simpson, E.R.; Brown, K.A. Metformin inhibits aromatase expression in human breast adipose stromal cells via stimulation of AMP-activated protein kinase. *Breast Cancer Res. Treat.* **2010**, *123*, 591–596.
11. Li, J.; Liu, J.; Li, P.; Mao, X.; Li, W.; Yang, J.; Liu, P. Loss of LKB1 disrupts breast epithelial cell polarity and promotes breast cancer metastasis and invasion. *J. Exp. Clin. Cancer Res.* **2014**, *33*, 70. [CrossRef] [PubMed]
12. Zhuang, Z.-G.; Di, G.-H.; Shen, Z.-Z.; Ding, J.; Shao, Z.-M. Enhanced Expression of LKB1 in Breast Cancer Cells Attenuates Angiogenesis, Invasion, and Metastatic Potential. *Mol. Cancer Res.* **2006**, *4*, 843–849. [CrossRef] [PubMed]
13. Xia, C.; Ye, F.; Hu, X.; Li, Z.; Jiang, B.; Fu, Y.; Cheng, X.; Shao, Z.; Zhuang, Z. Liver kinase B1 enhances chemoresistance to gemcitabine in breast cancer MDA-MB-231 cells. *Oncol. Lett.* **2014**, *8*, 2086–2092. [CrossRef] [PubMed]
14. Wang, Y.-S.; Chen, J.; Cui, F.; Wang, H.; Wang, S.; Hang, W.; Zeng, Q.; Quan, C.-S.; Zhai, Y.-X.; Wang, J.-W.; et al. LKB1 is a DNA damage response protein that regulates cellular sensitivity to PARP inhibitors. *Oncotarget* **2016**, *7*, 73389–73401. [CrossRef] [PubMed]
15. Sengupta, S.; Nagalingam, A.; Muniraj, N.; Bonner, M.Y.; Mistriotis, P.; Afthinos, A.; Kuppusamy, P.; LaNoue, D.; Korangath, P.; Shriver, M.; et al. Activation of tumor suppressor LKB1 by honokiol abrogates cancer stem-like phenotype in breast cancer via inhibition of oncogenic Stat3. *Oncogene* **2017**, *36*, 5709–5721. [CrossRef] [PubMed]
16. Simpson, E.; Brown, K. The link between the LKB1/AMPK pathway and aromatase in the breast provides a link between obesity and breast cancer. *Endocrine J.* **2010**, S198–S199.

17. Syed, B.M.; Johnston, S.J.; Wong, D.W.M.; Green, A.R.; Winterbottom, L.; Kennedy, H.; Simpson, N.; Morgan, D.A.L.; Ellis, I.O.; Cheung, K.L.; et al. Long-term (37 years) clinical outcome of older women with early operable primary breast cancer managed in a dedicated clinic. *Ann. Oncol.* **2011**, *23*, 1465–1471. [CrossRef]

18. Rakha, E.; Elsheikh, S.E.; Aleskandarany, M.A.; Habashi, H.O.; Green, A.R.; Powe, D.G.; El-Sayed, M.E.; Benhasouna, A.; Brunet, J.S.; Akslen, L.A.; et al. Triple-negative breast cancer: Distinguishing between basal and nonbasal subtypes. *Clin. Cancer Res.* **2009**, *15*, 2302–2310. [CrossRef]

19. Rao, V.S.; Garimella, V.; Hwang, M.; Drew, P.J. Management of early breast cancer in the elderly. *Int. J. Cancer* **2007**, *120*, 1155–1160. [CrossRef]

20. Weigelt, B.; Geyer, F.; Reis, J. Histological types of breast cancer: How special are they? *Mol. Oncol.* **2010**, *4*, 192–208. [CrossRef]

21. Avtanski, D.B.; Nagalingam, A.; Bonner, M.Y.; Arbiser, J.L.; Saxena, N.K.; Sharma, D. Honokiol activates LKB1-miR-34a axis and antagonizes the oncogenic actions of leptin in breast cancer. *Oncotarget* **2015**, *6*, 29947–29962. [CrossRef] [PubMed]

22. Tan, D.S.P.; Marchiò, C.; Jones, R.L.; Savage, K.; Smith, I.E.; Dowsett, M.; Reis-Filho, J.S. Triple negative breast cancer: Molecular profiling and prognostic impact in adjuvant anthracycline-treated patients. *Breast Cancer Res. Treat.* **2007**, *111*, 27–44. [CrossRef] [PubMed]

23. Syed, B.M.; Green, A.R.; Paish, E.C.; Soria, D.; Garibaldi, J.; Morgan, L.; Morgan, D.A.; Ellis, I.O.; Cheung, K.L. Biology of primary breast cancer in older women treated by surgery: With correlation with long-term clinical outcome and comparison with their younger counterparts. *Br. J. Cancer* **2013**, *108*, 1042–1051. [CrossRef] [PubMed]

24. Chen, I.-C.; Chang, Y.-C.; Lu, Y.-S.; Chung, K.-P.; Huang, C.-S.; Kuo, K.-T.; Wang, M.-Y.; Wu, P.-F.; Hsueh, T.-H.; Shen, C.-Y.; et al. Clinical Relevance of Liver Kinase B1(LKB1) Protein and Gene Expression in Breast Cancer. *Sci. Rep.* **2016**, *6*, 21374. [CrossRef] [PubMed]

25. Bouchekioua-Bouzaghou, K.; Poulard, C.; Rambaud, J.; Lavergne, E.; Hussein, N.; Billaud, M.; Bachelot, T.; Chabaud, S.; Mader, S.; Dayan, G.; et al. LKB1 when associated with methylatedERalpha is a marker of bad prognosis in breast cancer. *Int. J. Cancer* **2014**, *135*, 1307–1318. [PubMed]

26. Azim, H.A.; Kassem, L.; Treilleux, I.; Wang, Q.; Abu El Enein, M.; Anis, S.E.; Bachelot, T. Analysis of PI3K/mTOR Pathway Biomarkers and Their Prognostic Value in Women with Hormone Receptor–Positive, HER2-Negative Early Breast Cancer. *Transl. Oncol.* **2016**, *9*, 114–123. [CrossRef] [PubMed]

27. Gan, B.; Hu, J.; Jiang, S.; Liu, Y.; Sahin, E.; Zhuang, L.; Fletcher-Sananikone, E.; Colla, S.; Wang, Y.A.; Chin, L.; et al. Lkb1 regulates quiescence and metabolic homeostasis of haematopoietic stem cells. *Nature* **2010**, *468*, 701–704. [CrossRef]

28. Gurumurthy, S.; Xie, S.Z.; Alagesan, B.; Kim, J.; Yusuf, R.Z.; Saez, B.; Tzatsos, A.; Ozsolak, F.; Milos, P.; Ferrari, F.; et al. The Lkb1 metabolic sensor maintains haematopoietic stem cell survival. *Nature* **2010**, *468*, 659–663. [CrossRef]

29. Nakada, D.; Saunders, T.L.; Morrison, S.J. Lkb1 regulates cell cycle and energy metabolism in haematopoietic stem cells. *Nature* **2010**, *468*, 653–658. [CrossRef]

30. Chen, Y.; Liu, Y.; Zhou, Y.; You, H. Molecular mechanism of LKB1 in the invasion and metastasis of colorectal cancer. *Oncol. Rep.* **2018**, *41*, 1035–1044. [CrossRef]

31. Andrade-Vieira, R.; Xu, Z.; Colp, P.; Marignani, P.A. Loss of lkb1 Expression Reduces the Latency of ErbB2-Mediated Mammary Gland Tumorigenesis, Promoting Changes in Metabolic Pathways. *PLoS ONE* **2013**, *8*, e56567. [CrossRef]

32. Lipovka, Y.; Chen, H.; Vagner, J.; Price, T.J.; Tsao, T.S.; Konhilas, J.P. Oestrogen receptors interact with the alpha-catalytic subunit of AMP-activated protein kinase. *Biosci. Rep.* **2015**, *35*, e00264. [CrossRef] [PubMed]

33. Treilleux, I.; Arnedos, M.; Cropet, C.; Wang, Q.; Ferrero, J.-M.; Abadie-Lacourtoisie, S.; Levy, C.; Legouffe, E.; Lortholary, A.; Pujade-Lauraine, E.; et al. Translational studies within the TAMRAD randomized GINECO trial: Evidence for mTORC1 activation marker as a predictive factor for everolimus efficacy in advanced breast cancer. *Ann. Oncol.* **2014**, *26*, 120–125. [CrossRef] [PubMed]

10

Trends in Overall Survival and Treatment Patterns in Two Large Population-Based Cohorts of Patients with Breast and Colorectal Cancer

Doris van Abbema [1,2], Pauline Vissers [3], Judith de Vos-Geelen [1], Valery Lemmens [3,4], Maryska Janssen-Heijnen [5,6] and Vivianne Tjan-Heijnen [1,*]

1 Department of Internal Medicine, GROW-School for Oncology and Developmental Biology, Maastricht University Medical Center, Peter Debyelaan 25, 6229 HX Maastricht, The Netherlands
2 ACHIEVE Centre of Applied Research, Faculty of Health, Amsterdam University of Applied Sciences, Tafelbergweg 51, 1105 BD Amsterdam, The Netherlands
3 Department of Research, Netherlands Comprehensive Cancer Organisation (IKNL), Godebaldkwartier 419, 3511 DT Utrecht, The Netherlands
4 Department of Public Health, Erasmus Medical Center, Wytemaweg 80, 3015 CN Rotterdam, The Netherlands
5 Department of Clinical Epidemiology, VieCuri Medical Centre, Tegelseweg 210, 5912 BL Venlo, The Netherlands
6 Department of Epidemiology, GROW-School for Oncology and Developmental Biology, Maastricht University Medical Centre, Universiteitssingel 60, 6229 ER Maastricht, The Netherlands
* Correspondence: vcg.tjan.heijnen@mumc.nl

Abstract: Previous studies showed substantial improvement of survival rates in patients with cancer in the last two decades. However, lower survival rates have been reported for older patients compared to younger patients. In this population-based study, we analyzed treatment patterns and the survival of patients with breast cancer (BC) and colorectal cancer (CRC). Patients with stages I–III BC and CRC and diagnosed between 2003 and 2012 were selected from the Netherlands Cancer Registry (NCR). Trends in treatment modalities were evaluated with the Cochran-Armitage trend test. Trends in five-year overall survival were calculated with the Cox hazard regression model. The Ederer II method was used to calculate the five-year relative survival. The relative excess risk of death (RER) was estimated using a multivariate generalized linear model. During the study period, 98% of BC patients aged <75 years underwent surgery, whereas for patients ≥75 years, rates were 79.3% in 2003 and 66.7% in 2012 ($p < 0.001$). Most CRC patients underwent surgery irrespective of age or time period, although patients with rectal cancer aged ≥75 years received less surgery or radiotherapy over the entire study period than younger patients. The administration of adjuvant chemotherapy increased over time for CRC and BC patients, except for BC patients aged ≥75 years. The five-year relative survival improved only in younger BC patients (adjusted RER 0.95–0.96 per year), and was lower for older BC patients (adjusted RER 1.00, 95% Confidence Interval (CI) 0.98–1.02, and RER 1.00; 95% CI 0.98–1.01 per year for 65–74 years and ≥75 years, respectively). For CRC patients, the five-year relative survival improved over time for all ages (adjusted RER on average was 0.95 per year). In conclusion, the observed survival trends in BC and CRC patients suggest advances in cancer treatment, but with striking differences in survival between older and younger patients, particularly for BC patients.

Keywords: breast cancer; colorectal cancer; relative survival; older patients; geriatric oncology; cancer treatment

1. Introduction

Together with the aging of the population in Western countries, the number of older people with cancer has increased considerably in the last decade [1]. In the Netherlands, breast cancer (BC) is the most common cancer in women, with an estimated incidence rate of 66 new cases per 100,000 women [2]. The incidence of BC is highest in patients aged 70–74 years (212 per 100,000 women) [2]. One of the most common cancers in both men and women is colorectal cancer (CRC), with an estimated incidence of 65 new cases per 100,000 persons. Its incidence increases with age (415 per 100,000 per persons in those aged 75–79 years) [2].

Though the group of older patients has increased considerably, evidence to guide treatment of these patients remains limited [3]. Many clinical trials exclude older patients from participating [4], and older patients who do participate in clinical trials may not be representative of the general older population, as clinical trials often exclude older patients with comorbidities or poor overall health [5].

Several population-based studies showed that the survival rate of BC patients has improved substantially in the last two decades [1,6–8]. This has been attributed particularly to mammographic screening programs [9] and advances in treatment (e.g., improved radiotherapy techniques and new systemic therapeutic agents such as third-generation chemotherapy, aromatase inhibitors, and HER2-targeted therapies). Clinical guidelines, as well as international position papers, state that surgery is recommended for early-stage BC patients [3,10]. Adjuvant chemotherapy is recommended for node-positive or high-risk node-negative disease, and endocrine therapy is recommended for high-risk receptor-positive disease [3,10]. However, population-based studies showed that older BC patients are less likely to receive standard care, which has been linked to lower survival rates in older patients [6,8,11].

Surgery is recommended in early-stage CRC patients. To reduce the risk of recurrence after surgery, clinical guidelines recommend that all lymph node-positive patients should be considered for adjuvant treatment, e.g., radiotherapy, or chemotherapy [12,13]. Several population-based studies showed that the administration of adjuvant chemotherapy has increased considerably in recent years, and that this is associated with improved survival [14,15]. However, the administration of adjuvant chemotherapy is considerably less common in older patients [14].

Several studies state that age should not be a contraindication for surgery or adjuvant chemotherapy [16]. Trends in survival and treatment have been published before, but this has not clarified the differences in survival rates between cancers. The aim of this study was to investigate trends in survival rates and treatment patterns over time for older versus younger patients with BC and CRC in the Netherlands.

2. Results

Between 2003 and 2012, 127,146 patients were diagnosed with stages I–III BC in the Netherlands, while 85,629 patients were diagnosed with stages I–III CRC (Table 1). The median age of patients with BC was 60 years (range 18 to 103), and the median age of patients with CRC was 71 years (range 18 to 102).

Table 1. Clinical characteristics of 127,146 breast cancer (BC) and 85,629 colorectal cancer (CRC) patients, diagnosed in 2003–2012.

Characteristics	BC		CRC	
	n	%	*n*	%
Gender				
Male	-		45,783	53.5
Female	127,146	100	39,846	46.5
Age (years)				
15–44	15,206	12	2077	2.4
45–54	30,539	24	6457	7.5
55–64	31,830	25	17,969	21
65–74	27,095	21.3	26,839	31.3
≥75	22,476	17.7	32,287	37.7
Year of diagnosis				
2003	11,669	9.2	7367	8.6
2004	11,848	9.3	7813	9.1
2005	11,845	9.3	7877	9.2
2006	12,264	9.6	8190	9.6
2007	12,725	10	8510	9.9
2008	12,836	10.1	8713	10.2
2009	12,999	10.2	8877	10.4
2010	13,102	10.3	9135	10.7
2011	13,838	10.9	9486	11.1
2012	14,020	11	9661	11.3
Stage				
I	56,579	44.5	19,453	22.7
II	52,049	40.9	33,363	39
III	18,518	14.6	32,813	38.3

2.1. *Stage at Diagnosis*

The stages at diagnosis according to age are presented in Figure 1. BC patients aged ≤45 or ≥75 years were more often diagnosed with stage II or III cancer compared to those aged 45–75 years ($p < 0.001$). Stage II was diagnosed in 51.7% and stage III in 17.9% of the BC patients aged ≥75 years. The percentage of CRC patients with stage II disease steadily increased with age (32.5% in CRC patients aged 45–54 years, and 44.3% in CRC patients aged ≥75 years), while stage III decreased with age (46.7% in CRC patients aged 45–54 years, and 33.3% in CRC patients aged ≥75 years, $p < 0.001$).

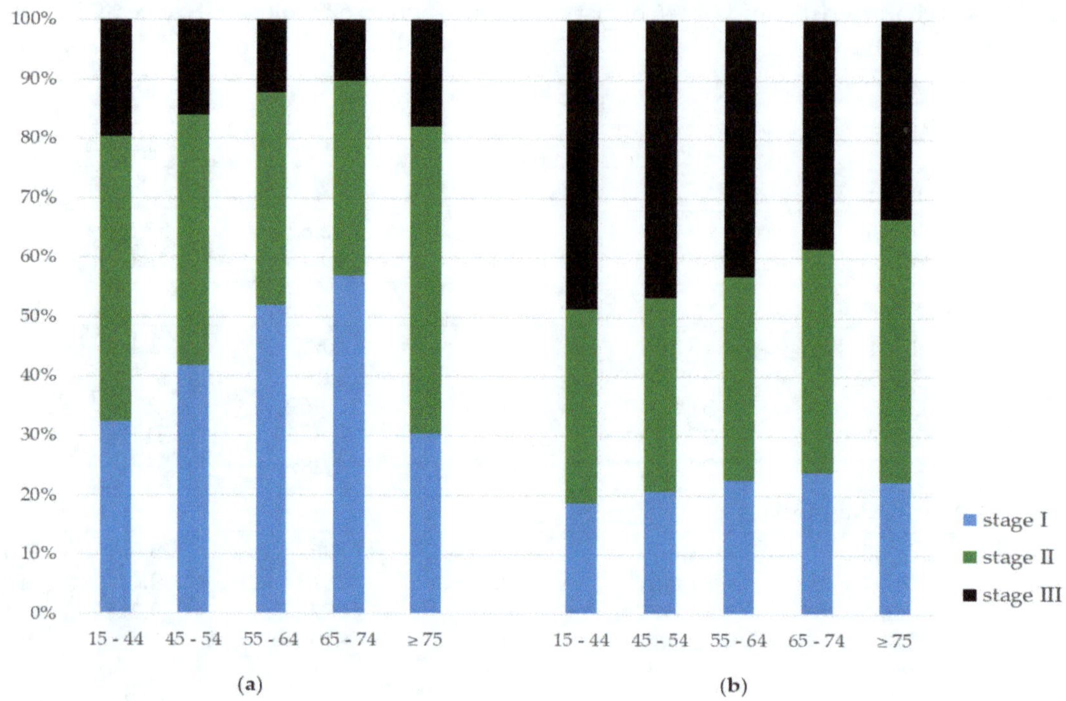

Figure 1. Tumor stage by age at diagnosis: (**a**) breast cancer, and (**b**) colorectal cancer.

2.2. Trends in Treatment

The time trends for all treatments for BC patients between 2003 and 2012 are presented in Figure 2. Over the entire study period, 98.0% of patients with stages I–III BC who were younger than 75 years underwent surgery, whereas for those aged 75 years or over, surgery rates declined from 79.3% in 2003 to 66.7% in 2012 ($p < 0.001$, Figure 2a). The proportion of BC patients undergoing lymph node dissection for node-positive disease decreased over time for all age groups (Figure 2b). The use of radiotherapy after breast-conserving surgery increased significantly for all age groups but was lowest among patients aged 75 years and older (73.6% in 2003 vs. 84.1% in 2012, $p < 0.001$) and highest among patients aged 45–54 years (84.4% in 2003 vs. 96.2% in 2012, $p < 0.001$, Figure 2c). Primary endocrine therapy as a monotherapy in BC patients was almost exclusively used for patients aged 75 years or over, and increased significantly over time (16.5% in 2003 and 28.7% in 2012, $p < 0.001$, Figure 2d). The use of adjuvant chemotherapy in stages II and I BC patients increased significantly over time for all age groups, except for patients aged 75 years or older. Its use was associated with age, with more than 90% of patients younger than 55 years and less than 9% of patients aged 65 years or older in 2012 receiving it, and hardly any patients aged 75 years or older (Figure 2e,f).

As CRC patients are treated according to tumor location, i.e., colon cancer (CC) or rectal cancer (RC), we report the treatments received for CC and RC separately (Figure 3). In CC, the number of patients aged 75 years or older who underwent surgery declined significantly over time (98.1% in 2003 vs. 94.2% in 2012, $p < 0.001$, Figure 3a). The percentage of chemotherapy treatment in stage III CC patients aged 55 years or older increased significantly over time (Figure 3b), although the percentage of those aged 75 years or older who received chemotherapy remained considerably lower (16.3% in 2003 vs. 23.5% in 2012, $p < 0.001$). The percentage of RC patients aged 45 years or older who underwent surgery declined significantly over time, the greatest decrease being observed in RC patients aged 75 years or older (from 91.8% in 2003 to 81.1% in 2012, $p < 0.001$) (Figure 3c). The use of radiotherapy in stage III RC increased significantly over time for all age groups but became less frequent with increasing age (91.8% of patients aged 55–64 years compared to 80.2% of patients aged 75 years or older in 2012, Figure 3d). The number of RC patients aged 75 years or older undergoing surgery was lower than that of younger patients. The percentage of I-III RC patients aged 75 years or older who received primary radiotherapy as a single treatment modality increased significantly, from 3.8% in 2003 to 9.4% in 2013 ($p < 0.001$, Figure 3e). The use of chemoradiation in stage II RC patients increased significantly in all age groups, ranging from 19.8% to 71.6% in 2012, but again this was highly dependent on age, with the lowest use in the age group of 75 years and older (Figure 3f).

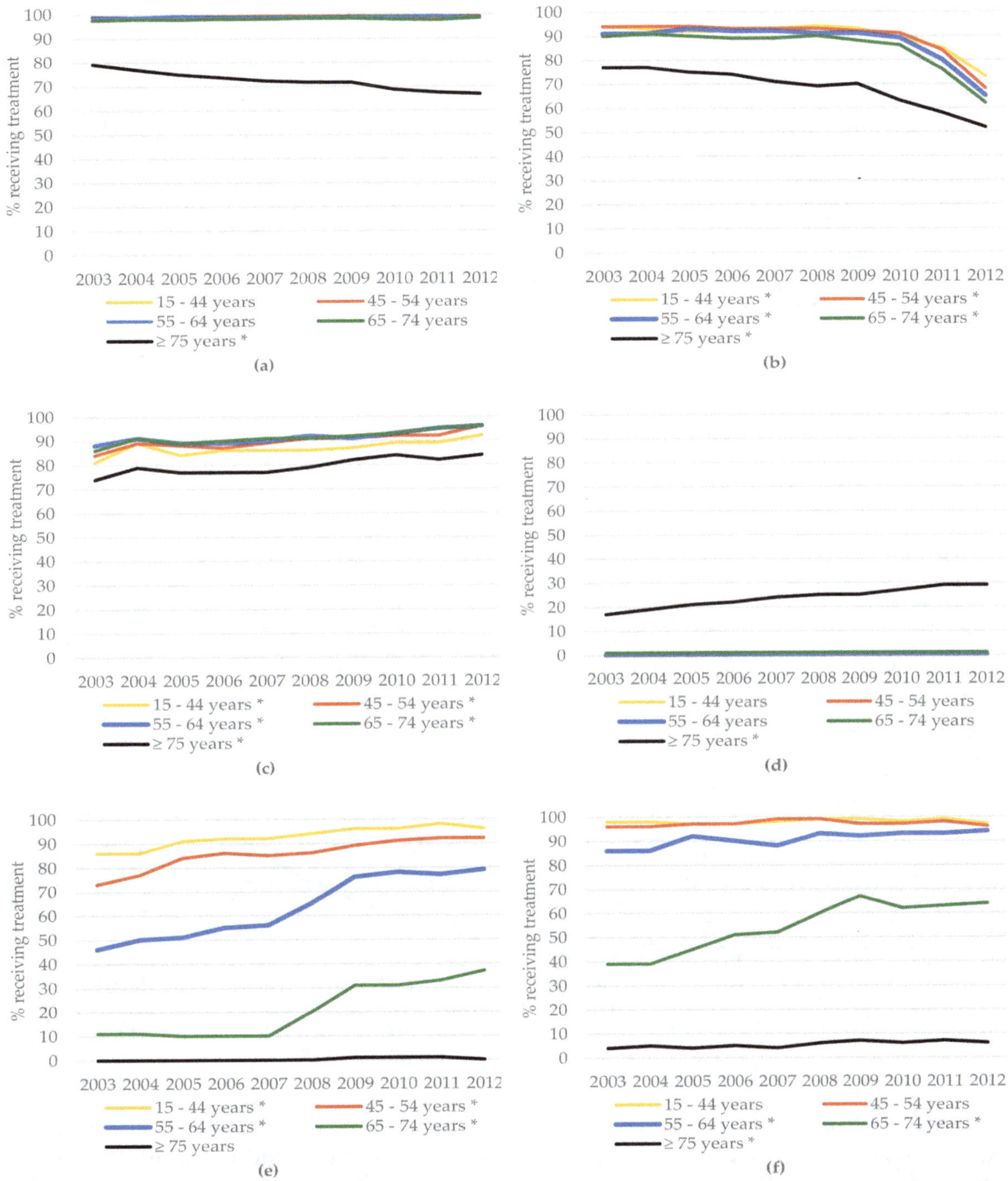

Figure 2. Time trends in the treatment of breast cancer (BC) patients according to age group: (**a**) surgery in BC patients stages I–III, (**b**) lymph node dissection in BC patients stages I–III with node-positive disease, (**c**) radiotherapy after breast-conserving surgery in BC patients stages I–III, (**d**) primary endocrine therapy in BC patients stages I–III, (**e**) chemotherapy in BC patients stage II, and (**f**) chemotherapy in BC patients stage III. * Significant ($p < 0.05$) difference in treatment over time using the Cochran–Armitage trend test.

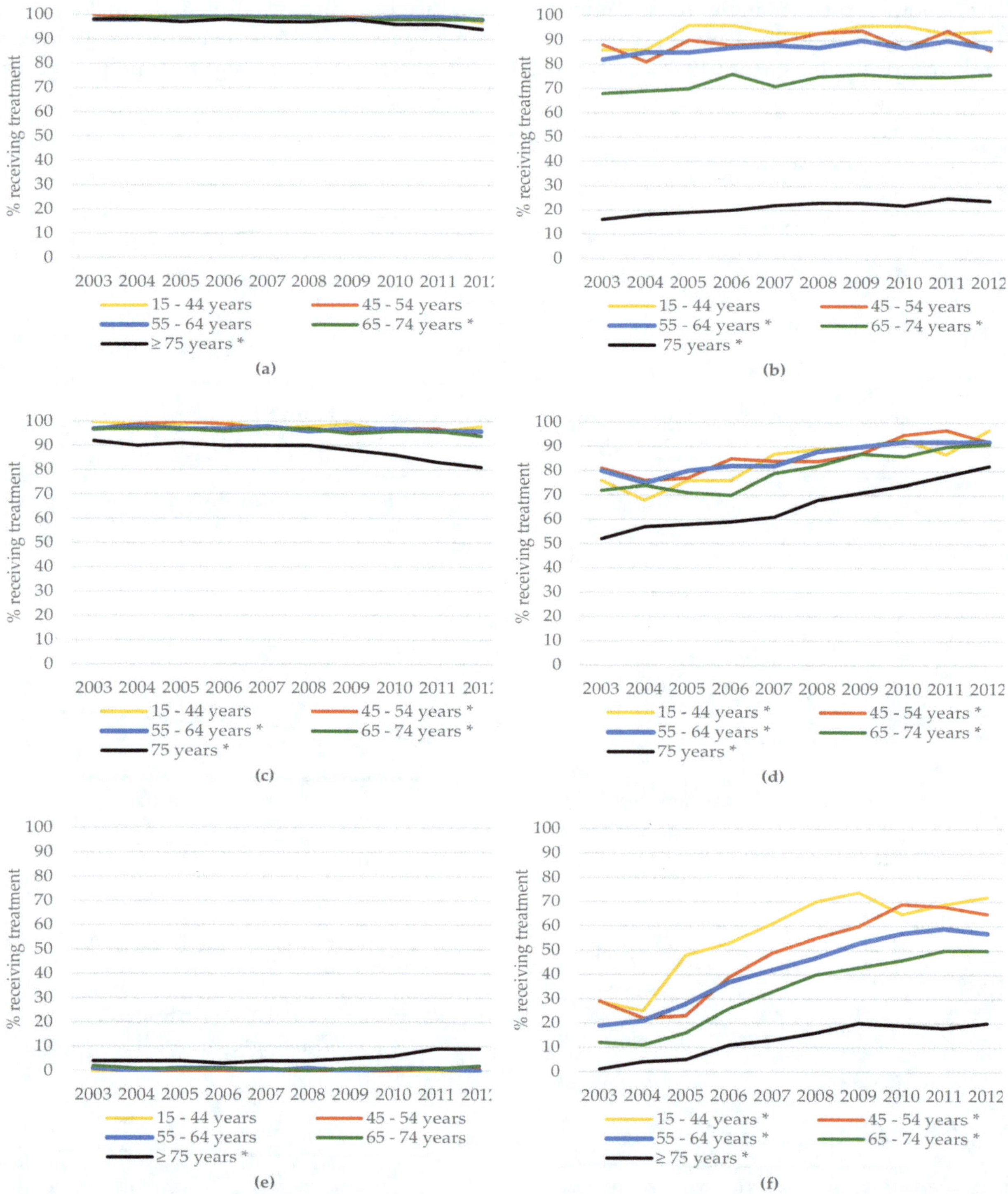

Figure 3. Time trends of treatment in colon cancer (CC) and rectal cancer (RC) patients according to age group: (**a**) surgery in CC patients stages I–III, (**b**) chemotherapy in CC patients stage III, (**c**) surgery in RC patients stages I–III, (**d**) radiotherapy in RC patients stage III, (**e**) primary radiotherapy as a single treatment modality in RC patients stage III, and (**f**) chemoradiation in RC patients stages II–III. * Significant ($p < 0.05$) difference in treatment over time using the Cochran–Armitage trend test.

2.3. *Trends in Survival*

The 5-year overall survival of BC patients is presented in Figure 4. The 5-year overall survival improved in BC patients (adjusted hazard ratio (HR) 0.78, 95% CI 0.73–0.83) in the period 2003–2012. The 5-year overall survival improved slightly in patients aged 75 years or older (adjusted HR 0.99, 95%

CI 0.98–0.99) and did not significantly improve in patients aged 65–74 years (adjusted HR 0.99, 95% CI 0.98–1.01). In the multivariable Cox regression analysis, the overall survival improved in the period 2003–2012 and was influenced significantly by age (Table 2). The 5-year relative survival improved in BC patients, from 89.7% in 2003 to 93.1% in 2012 (adjusted relative excess risk (RER) 0.97, 95% CI 0.97–0.98 per year) (Figure 5). The 5-year relative survival rate improved significantly for BC patients aged 65 years or younger over the period between 2003 and 2012. In contrast, the relative survival for BC patients aged 75 years or older did not increase significantly over the same period (crude RER 0.99, 95% CI 0.97–1.02). After adjustment for age, stage, and treatment, the RER for BC patients aged 65–74 years was no longer significant (adjusted RER 1.00, 95% CI 0.98–1.01), and the RER for patients aged 75 years or older remained non-significant (adjusted RER 1.00, 95% CI 0.98–1.01).

Table 2. Multivariate Cox hazard analysis of five-year overall survival.

Variable	BC		CRC	
	HR (95% CI) [a]	p	HR (95% CI) [a]	p
Year of diagnosis (per year)	0.98 (0.97–0.98)	<0.001	0.96 (0.96–0.97)	<0.001
Age		<0.001		<0.001
15–44 years	1.04 (0.97–1.11)		**0.87 (0.76–0.98)**	
45–54 years	1.00 (ref)		1.00 (ref)	
55–64 years	**1.35 (1.28–1.43)**		**1.25 (1.17–1.34)**	
65–74 years	**2.06 (1.95–2.18)**		**1.81 (1.70–1.93)**	
≥75 years	**4.89 (4.60–5.18)**		**3.43 (3.22–3.65)**	
Gender	-			<0.001
Male	-		1.00 (ref)	
Female			**0.82 (0.80–0.84)**	
Stage		<0.001		<0.001
I	1.00 (ref)		1.00 (ref)	
II	**1.79 (1.72–1.87)**		**1.50 (1.44–1.55)**	
III	**4.14 (3.96–4.32)**		**2.74 (2.64–2.84)**	
Grade		<0.001		<0.001
Well differentiated	1.00 (ref)		1.00 (ref)	
Moderately differentiated	**1.29 (1.22–1.35)**		1.02 (0.97–1.07)	
Poorly differentiated and undifferentiated	**2.14 (2.03–2.25)**		**1.46 (1.38–1.55)**	
Unknown	**1.67 (1.57–1.77)**		**1.12 (1.06–1.19)**	
Surgery		<0.001		<0.001
No	1.00 (ref)		1.00 (ref)	
Yes	**0.30 (0.28–0.32)**		**0.14 (0.14–0.15)**	
Radiotherapy		<0.001		<0.001
No	1.00 (ref)		1.00 (ref)	
Yes	**0.63 (0.61–0.65)**		**0.76 (0.74–0.78)**	
Chemotherapy		<0.05		<0.001
No	1.00 (ref)		1.00 (ref)	
Yes	**0.95 (0.90–0.99)**		**0.64 (0.62–0.66)**	
Hormone therapy		<0.001		
No	1.00 (ref)		-	
Yes	**0.55 (0.53–0.57)**			

[a] Adjusted for all variables included in the model. HR, hazard ratio. Significant ($p < 0.05$) HR values are indicated in bold. ref, reference 95% CI, 95% Confidence Interval.

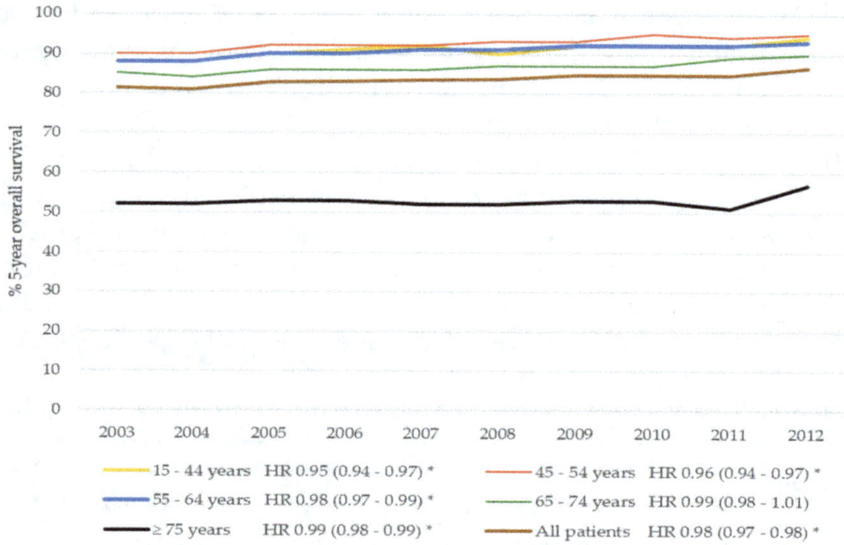

Figure 4. Five-year overall survival in BC patients over time per age group. HR indicates hazard ratio per year, adjusted for grade, stage, and treatment. * Significant ($p < 0.05$).

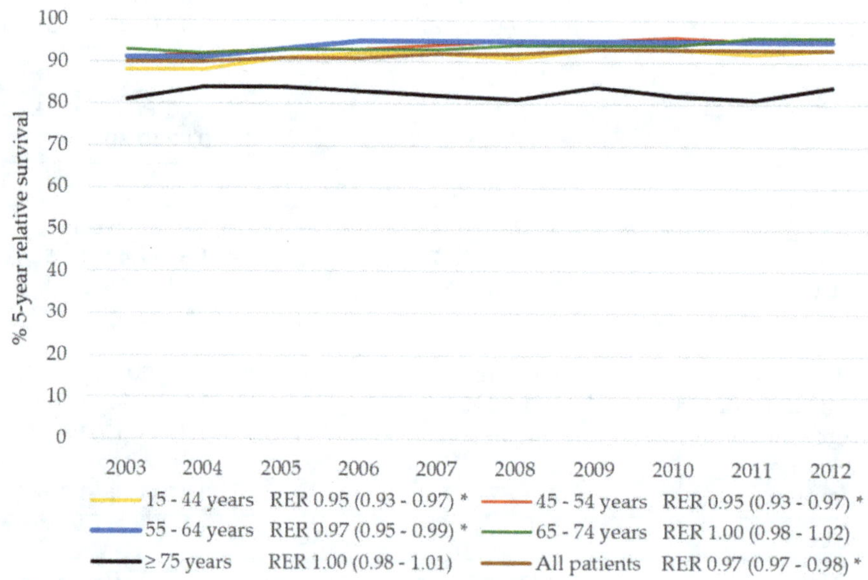

Figure 5. Five-year relative survival in BC patients over time per age group. RER indicates relative excess risk per year, adjusted for grade, stage, and treatment. * Significant ($p < 0.05$).

Similarly, the 5-year overall survival improved for all CRC patients (Figure 6). Overall survival in CRC patients was influenced by the year of diagnoses and age. Other factors affecting 5-year overall survival were, stage, grade, gender, and treatment. The relative survival for CRC patients improved from 76.0% in 2003 to 80.3% in 2012 (adjusted RER 0.95, 95% CI 0.94–0.95 per year, Figure 7). Most overall improvement was observed in the CRC patients aged 65–74 years. In this group, the 5-year relative survival increased by 7.9% between 2003 and 2012 (adjusted RER 0.94, 95% CI 0.93–0.95). In contrast to the BC cohort, the RERs for patients with CRC in all age groups had improved significantly after adjustment for grade, sex, stage, and treatment (adjusted RERs varying between 0.94 and 0.96 per year).

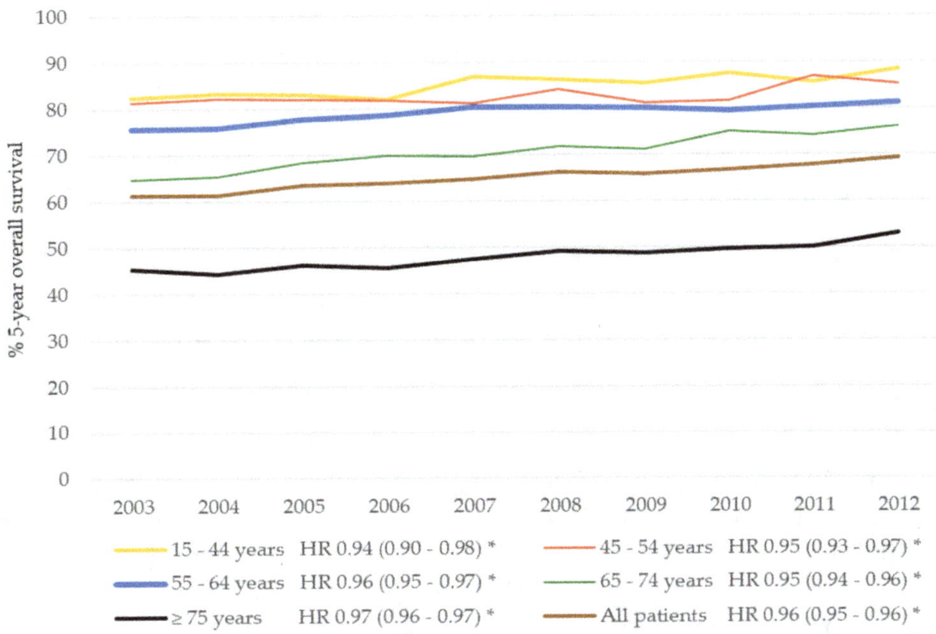

Figure 6. Five-year overall survival in CRC patients over time per age group. HR indicates the hazard ratio per year, adjusted for grade, stage, gender, and treatment. * Significant ($p < 0.05$).

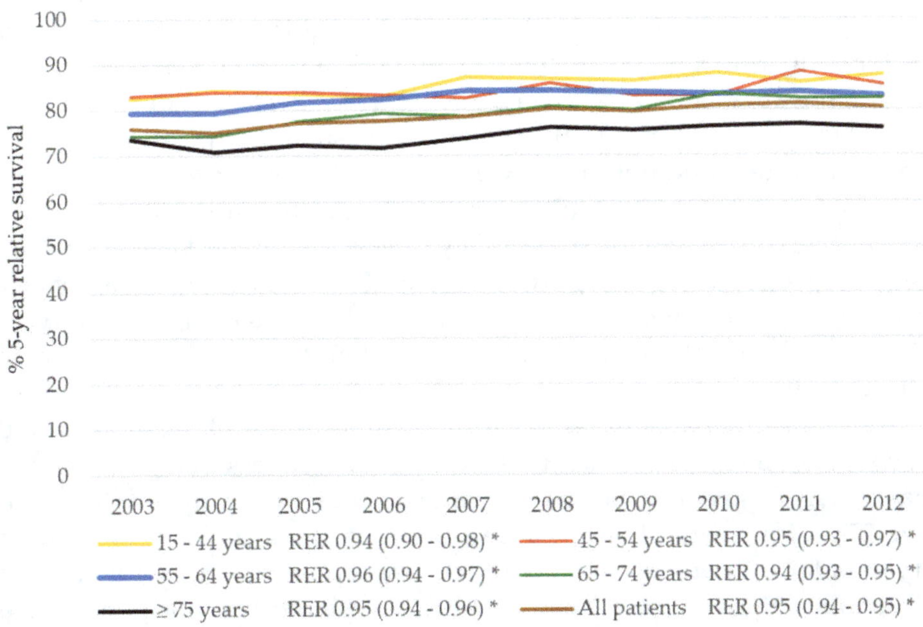

Figure 7. Five-year relative survival in CRC patients over time per age group. RER indicates the relative excess risk per year, adjusted for grade, stage, gender, and treatment. * Significant ($p < 0.05$).

3. Discussion

The findings of our population-based study show that 5-year overall and relative survival improved for BC patients and for CRC patients in the Netherlands between 2003 and 2012. The difference in 5-year survival between older and younger CRC patients decreased during the study period, and the greatest improvement in overall and relative survival was observed for older CRC patients. Among BC patients, substantial improvement of 5-year relative survival was seen only for younger BC patients. The overall and relative survival and its improvement over time were lower for older BC patients.

Previous population-based studies found that overall and relative survival among older BC patients did not change in the last decade [17,18]. This lack of improvement has been attributed to differences in the delivery of cancer care between older and younger BC patients, e.g., the influence of comorbid conditions on the selection of cancer treatments [19,20]; the lower likelihood of receiving breast surgery, radiotherapy, or adjuvant chemotherapy for older BC patients compared to younger BC patients [6]; and mammographic screening being offered only to younger women [9]. The survival and treatment differences observed in our study suggest possible limitations of cancer treatment, as well as reticence about cancer treatment, for older BC patients.

The most notable finding was the decreasing proportion of older BC patients receiving surgery, and the increasing proportion receiving primary endocrine therapy. Previous population-based studies in the Netherlands confirm this finding [6,17,21]. Van de Glas et al. showed that the proportion of older BC patients that did not receive breast surgery increased substantially from 9.2% in 1995 to 30.1% in 2011 [17]. Moreover, previous population-based studies showed that the proportion of older BC patients receiving primary endocrine therapy is higher in the Netherlands than in other European countries [22–24]. The EUROCARE breast cancer group found lower survival rates in European countries, like England and Ireland, where older BC patients are treated more often with primary endocrine therapy omitted [22]. This increased use of primary endocrine therapy may have been influenced by a meta-analysis, in which seven randomized controlled trials were included [25]. This meta-analysis showed that, compared to those treated with primary endocrine therapy, surgery alone seemed to have no beneficial impact on the overall survival rate (HR 0.98, 95% CI 0.74–1.30). However, BC patients who underwent surgery with adjuvant endocrine therapy had a borderline significantly improved overall survival rate (HR 0.86, 95% CI 0.73–1.00) and a significantly better disease-free survival. The HR for endocrine therapy alone was 0.65 (95% CI 0.53–0.81) [25].

Recent reports have advocated that primary endocrine therapy should only be considered in frail older BC patients [26]. Guidelines in the Netherlands state that patients with operable tumors should be treated with surgery and not primary endocrine therapy, irrespective of age [10]; also, the International Society of Geriatric Oncology (SIOG) recommends that primary endocrine therapy should only be offered to BC patients with a life expectancy of less than three years, or who are unfit for or refuse surgery [3]. However, as a large proportion of older BC patients are currently being treated with primary endocrine therapy, it is not clear if this recommendation is being followed consistently. In a small retrospective study in the Netherlands, Hamakers et al. found that the reason for not carrying out surgery was not always clearly stated in medical charts. When documented, reasons were often higher age, poor overall health, patient preference, and comorbidities [21]. Additionally, Sierink et al. found in a small cohort in the Netherlands that BC patients are less likely to receive surgery when they are older, have been diagnosed with more comorbidities, or have been diagnosed with a more advanced disease [27]. However, other studies found that age was the most important reason for foregoing surgery in older BC patients, even when adjustments were made for comorbidities [28–30].

Several studies found that the main factor for surgical morbidity in BC patients are comorbidities and not age [31]. Breast surgery can be considered a low morbidity surgery [32]. Approximately one third of BC patients develop breast and/or axillar wound infections, seromas, and hematomas after surgery, depending on the type of surgery. These surgical morbidities are often minor and treated in an outpatient setting [32]. Moreover, van de Glas et al. demonstrated that relative mortality was not influenced by postoperative complications in older BC patients [33].

Our study showed that the proportion of surgery in older CRC patients remains high. Many studies have shown that age should not prohibit surgery in CRC patients [16]. In RC, however, the proportion of patients aged ≥75 years that received primary chemoradiation increased from 0% in 2003 to almost 20% in 2012. Recently, foregoing surgery after chemoradiation has been shown to be safe for RC patients in whom a complete clinical response is seen [34].

In the present study, the proportion of older BC patients receiving adjuvant chemotherapy was lower than that of younger BC patients. In Europe, different rates of adjuvant chemotherapy in BC patients have been reported, with lower rates in the Netherlands [22]. There has been conflicting evidence regarding the benefits of this treatment for older BC patients. Data from the Early Breast Cancer Trial demonstrated a decreasing benefit from adjuvant chemotherapy with age [35,36], although relatively few BC patients aged 70 years or older have been included in clinical trials [5]. Nevertheless, the results of this meta-analysis may have contributed to the lower use of adjuvant chemotherapy in older BC patients [35]. Other recent studies suggest a possible benefit from adjuvant chemotherapy in older BC patients, especially in those with HER2-positive disease [37,38]. Recently, Du et al. compared the effectiveness of adjuvant chemotherapy between older BC and CRC patients, and found that chemotherapy might be effective in BC patients up to the age of 79 years [39].

Possible explanations why older BC patients receive adjuvant chemotherapy less often are frailty, poor functional status, or comorbidities. In addition, older patients are less willing to accept possible side effects associated with adjuvant chemotherapy compared with younger patients, and are concerned about negative influences of adjuvant chemotherapy. Most older BC patients receive adjuvant endocrine therapy because they are more likely to have a receptor positive disease, which tends to grow more slowly, are usually well differentiated, and respond better to endocrine therapy. However, there are side effects associated with endocrine therapy, like deep vein thrombosis or pulmonary emboli [40].

The 5-year overall and relative survival improved in older CRC patients in our study. In a population-based study, Van den Broek et al. showed that 5-year relative survival had increased significantly in CC patients aged <65 years and ≥75 years over the period from 1991 to 2005, but not in patients aged 65–74 years [41]. In our study the greatest overall improvement of relative survival was seen in CRC patients aged 65–74 years (74.4% in 2003 vs. 82.3% in 2012). In the ≥75 years age group, relative survival improved significantly, but still lagged behind the survival of younger age groups. However, the difference in survival between younger and older CRC patients reported by the EUROCARE working group [1,7] diminished over time in our study. This improved survival could be partly attributed to the increased use of adjuvant chemotherapy in older patients [14], but also to other factors, such as improved preoperative staging and improved surgery [42].

This study had some limitations. Information on patient characteristics, such as comorbidities, was not available. Furthermore, we can draw no conclusions about aspects such as quality of life, maintaining functional status, risk of recurrence, or complications, as we had no data for these outcomes. Although we adjusted the analyses for potential confounders, there may still have been some confounding by other factors. Finally, we did not have data on the causes of mortality. On the other hand, the use of data for two different tumor types means that our study does provide important insights into the differential treatment and survival trends by age. Another strength of our study is the large number of patients with BC and CRC included from the Netherlands Cancer Registry, with at least 5 years of follow-up.

4. Materials and Methods

4.1. Patients

For this population-based study, we selected all patients with primary BC and CRC stages I–II diagnosed between 2003 and 2012 from the Netherlands Cancer Registry (NCR). We only selected patients with stages I–III, as this group could potentially be treated with curative intent. Furthermore, only female BC patients were selected. The NCR records all newly diagnosed malignancies in the Netherlands after notification from the nationwide automated pathological archive (PALGA). This data is supplemented with data from the National Registry of Hospital Discharge Diagnosis. Trained registrars from the NCR routinely collect data from medical records regarding patient, tumor, and treatment characteristics in all Dutch hospitals.

Cancer stage was based on the pathological TNM classification applicable at the time of cancer diagnosis. In case of a missing pathological TNM classification, the clinical TNM classification was used instead. Data regarding the vital status of all patients was available through linkage with the municipal personal records database, with complete follow-up until 31 December 2017. Patients were divided into five groups according to age: 15–44, 45–54, 55–64, 65–74, and 75 years or older. Primary cancer treatment retrieved from the NCR included surgery, radiotherapy, endocrine therapy, immunotherapy, and (neo-)adjuvant chemotherapy.

According to the Central Committee on Research involving Human Subjects (CCMO), this type of study does not require approval from an ethics committee in the Netherlands. The Privacy Review Board of the Netherlands Cancer Registry approved this study in January 2018 (K17.351).

4.2. Statistical Analyses

All analyses were performed in IBM SPSS statistics version 22.0 (SPSS, Chicago, IL, USA) or SAS statistics version 9.4 (SAS institute, Inc., Cary, NC, USA). Statistical significance was defined as $p \leq 0.05$.

The Cochran-Armitage trend test was used to test for differences in treatment over time. Treatments are presented as percentages per age group and period.

The Cox hazard analysis was used to calculate the overall survival. The hazard ratio (HR) was calculated according to age group and cancer stage, and adjusted for cancer stage, grade, gender, and treatment.

As cause of death is not available in the NCR, relative survival was used as an estimation of the disease-specific survival, and was calculated using the Ederer II method, i.e., as the observed overall survival of patients in the study divided by the expected overall survival in a matched group of the general population by age, sex, and year [11]. The expected survival was obtained from national life tables. The relative excess risk of death (RER) was estimated using a multivariate generalized linear model with a Poisson distribution. The RER was calculated according to age and cancer type, and adjusted for cancer stage, grade, gender, and treatment. The treatment variables were added to investigate the effect of treatment on the RER.

5. Conclusions

In this population-based study analyzing oncological treatment patterns and relative survival of BC and CRC patients, we observed substantial differences between younger and older patients. Although the observed survival trends in BC and CRC patients suggest advances in cancer treatment, we found that the survival of older BC patients in particular was strikingly lower. Moreover, the differences in relative survival between younger and older BC patients revealed in previous studies were found to have continued to increase in recent years. Inequalities in the provision of cancer care to older BC patients need to be investigated in future cancer research. Selection criteria for specific treatments could eventually lead to individualized and optimized treatment for older cancer patients.

Author Contributions: Conceptualization, D.v.A., P.V., V.L., M.J.-H., and V.T.-H.; methodology, D.v.A., P.V., and V.T.-H.; formal analysis, D.v.A. and P.V.; investigation, D.v.A., P.V., and V.T.-H.; writing—original draft preparation, D.v.A.; writing—review and editing, P.V., J.d.V.-G., V.L., M.J.-H., and V.T.-H.

Acknowledgments: The authors would like to thank the Netherlands Cancer Registry for providing the data, and Jan Klerkx for proofreading the English text.

References

1. De Angelis, R.; Sant, M.; Coleman, M.P.; Francisci, S.; Baili, P.; Pierannunzio, D.; Trama, A.; Visser, O.; Brenner, H.; Ardanaz, E.; et al. Cancer survival in Europe 1999–2007 by country and age: Results of EUROCARE-5—A population-based study. *Lancet Oncol.* **2014**, *15*, 23–34. [CrossRef]
2. IKNL. Netherlands Comprehensive Cancer Organisation. Available online: http://www.cijfersoverkanker.nl/ (assessed on 1 March 2019).

3. Biganzoli, L.; Wildiers, H.; Oakman, C.; Marotti, L.; Loibl, S.; Kunkler, I.; Reed, M.; Ciatto, S.; Voogd, A.C.; Brain, E.; et al. Management of elderly patients with breast cancer: Updated recommendations of the International Society of Geriatric Oncology (SIOG) and European Society of Breast Cancer Specialists (EUSOMA). *Lancet Oncol.* **2012**, *13*, e148–e160. [CrossRef]
4. Hurria, A.; Levit, L.A.; Dale, W.; Mohile, S.G.; Muss, H.B.; Fehrenbacher, L.; Magnuson, A.; Lichtman, S.M.; Bruinooge, S.S.; Soto-Pérez-De-Celis, E.; et al. Improving the Evidence Base for Treating Older Adults With Cancer: American Society of Clinical Oncology Statement. *J. Clin. Oncol.* **2015**, *33*, 3826–3833. [CrossRef] [PubMed]
5. De Glas, N.A.; Hamaker, M.E.; Kiderlen, M.; De Craen, A.J.M.; Mooijaart, S.P.; Van De Velde, C.J.H.; Van Munster, B.C.; Portielje, J.E.A.; Liefers, G.J.; Bastiaannet, E. Choosing relevant endpoints for older breast cancer patients in clinical trials: An overview of all current clinical trials on breast cancer treatment. *Breast Cancer Res. Treat.* **2014**, *146*, 591–597. [CrossRef] [PubMed]
6. Bastiaannet, E.; Liefers, G.J.; De Craen, A.J.M.; Kuppen, P.J.K.; Van De Water, W.; Portielje, J.E.A.; Van Der Geest, L.G.M.; Janssen-Heijnen, M.L.G.; Dekkers, O.M.; Van De Velde, C.J.H.; et al. Breast cancer in elderly compared to younger patients in the Netherlands: Stage at diagnosis, treatment and survival in 127,805 unselected patients. *Breast Cancer Res. Treat.* **2010**, *124*, 801–807. [CrossRef]
7. Quaglia, A.; Tavilla, A.; Shack, L.; Brenner, H.; Janssen-Heijnen, M.; Allemani, C.; Colonna, M.; Grande, E.; Grosclaude, P.; Vercelli, M. The cancer survival gap between elderly and middle-aged patients in Europe is widening. *Eur. J. Cancer* **2009**, *45*, 1006–1016. [CrossRef] [PubMed]
8. Smith, B.D.; Jiang, J.; McLaughlin, S.S.; Hurria, A.; Smith, G.L.; Giordano, S.H.; Buchholz, T.A. Improvement in Breast Cancer Outcomes Over Time: Are Older Women Missing Out? *J. Clin. Oncol.* **2011**, *29*, 4647–4653. [CrossRef]
9. Bleyer, A.; Baines, C.; Miller, A.B. Impact of screening mammography on breast cancer mortality. International journal of cancer. *J. Int. Cancer* **2016**, *138*, 2003–2012. [CrossRef]
10. Richtlijn Mammacarcinoom. Available online: http://www.oncoline.nl/mammacarcinoom (assessed on 1 March 2019).
11. Hancke, K.; Denkinger, M.D.; Konig, J.; Kurzeder, C.; Wockel, A.; Herr, D.; Blettner, M.; Kreienberg, R. Standard treatment of female patients with breast cancer decreases substantially for women aged 70 years and older: A german clinical cohort study. *Ann. Oncol.* **2010**, *21*, 748–753. [CrossRef]
12. Richtlijn Rectumcarcinoom. Available online: http://www.oncoline.nl/rectumcarcinoom (assessed on 1 March 2019).
13. Richtlijn Coloncarcinoom. Available online: http://www.oncoline.nl/coloncarcinoom (assessed on 1 March 2019).
14. Van Steenbergen, L.N.; Lemmens, V.E.P.P.; Rutten, H.J.T.; Wymenga, A.N.M.; Nortier, J.W.R.; Janssen-Heijnen, M.L.G. Increased adjuvant treatment and improved survival in elderly stage III colon cancer patients in The Netherlands. *Ann. Oncol.* **2012**, *23*, 2805–2811. [CrossRef]
15. Van Steenbergen, L.N.; Elferink, M.A.G.; Krijnen, P.; Lemmens, V.E.P.P.; Siesling, S.; Rutten, H.J.T.; Richel, D.J.; Karim-Kos, H.E.; Coebergh, J.W.W.; Working Group Output of The Netherlands Cancer Registry; et al. Improved survival of colon cancer due to improved treatment and detection: A nationwide population-based study in The Netherlands 1989–2006. *Ann. Oncol.* **2010**, *21*, 2206–2212. [CrossRef]
16. Manceau, G.; Karoui, M.; Werner, A.; Mortensen, N.J.; Hannoun, L. Comparative outcomes of rectal cancer surgery between elderly and non-elderly patients: A systematic review. *Lancet Oncol.* **2012**, *13*, e525–e536. [CrossRef]
17. De Glas, N.A.; Jonker, J.M.; Bastiaannet, E.; De Craen, A.J.M.; Van De Velde, C.J.H.; Siesling, S.; Liefers, G.J.; Portielje, J.E.A.; Hamaker, M.E. Impact of omission of surgery on survival of older patients with breast cancer. *Br. J. Surg.* **2014**, *101*, 1397–1404. [CrossRef]
18. Bastiaannet, E.; Portielje, J.E.; Van De Velde, C.J.; De Craen, A.J.; Van Der Velde, S.; Kuppen, P.J.; Van Der Geest, L.G.; Janssen-Heijnen, M.L.; Dekkers, O.M.; Westendorp, R.G.; et al. Lack of Survival Gain for Elderly Women with Breast Cancer. *Oncologist* **2011**, *16*, 415–423. [CrossRef]
19. Janssen-Heijnen, M.L.; Houterman, S.; Lemmens, V.E.; Louwman, M.W.; Maas, H.A.; Coebergh, J.W.W. Prognostic impact of increasing age and co-morbidity in cancer patients: A population-based approach. *Crit. Rev. Oncol.* **2005**, *55*, 231–240. [CrossRef]
20. Louwman, W.; Janssen-Heijnen, M.; Houterman, S.; Voogd, A.; Van Der Sangen, M.; Nieuwenhuijzen, G.; Coebergh, J.; Van Der Sangen, M. Less extensive treatment and inferior prognosis for breast cancer patient with comorbidity: A population-based study. *Eur. J. Cancer* **2005**, *41*, 779–785. [CrossRef]

21. Hamaker, M.E.; Bastiaannet, E.; Evers, D.; Van De Water, W.; Smorenburg, C.H.; Maartense, E.; Zeilemaker, A.M.; Liefers, G.J.; Van Der Geest, L.; De Rooij, S.E.; et al. Omission of surgery in elderly patients with early stage breast cancer. *Eur. J. Cancer* **2013**, *49*, 545–552. [CrossRef] [PubMed]
22. Derks, M.G.M.; EURECCA Breast Cancer Group; Bastiaannet, E.; Kiderlen, M.; Hilling, D.E.; Boelens, P.G.; Walsh, P.M.; Van Eycken, E.; Siesling, S.; Broggio, J.; et al. Variation in treatment and survival of older patients with non-metastatic breast cancer in five European countries: A population-based cohort study from the EURECCA Breast Cancer Group. *Br. J. Cancer* **2018**, *119*, 121–129. [CrossRef]
23. Ojala, K.; Meretoja, T.J.; Mattson, J.; Leidenius, M.H.; Kaisu, O.; Johanna, M. Surgical treatment and prognosis of breast cancer in elderly—A population-based study. *Eur. J. Surg. Oncol. (EJSO)* **2019**, *45*, 956–962. [CrossRef]
24. Joerger, M.; Thürlimann, B.; Savidan, A.; Frick, H.; Rageth, C.; Lütolf, U.; Vlastos, G.; Bouchardy, C.; Konzelmann, I.; Bordoni, A.; et al. Treatment of breast cancer in the elderly: A prospective, population-based Swiss study. *J. Geriatr. Oncol.* **2013**, *4*, 39–47. [CrossRef]
25. Hind, D.; Wyld, L.; Reed, M.W. Surgery, with or without tamoxifen, vs tamoxifen alone for older women with operable breast cancer: Cochrane review. *Br. J. Cancer* **2007**, *96*, 1025–1029. [CrossRef]
26. Morgan, J.; Reed, M.; Wyld, L.; Reed, M.; Reed, M. Primary endocrine therapy as a treatment for older women with operable breast cancer—A comparison of randomised controlled trial and cohort study findings. *Eur. J. Surg. Oncol. (EJSO)* **2014**, *40*, 676–684. [CrossRef]
27. Sierink, J.; De Castro, S.; Russell, N.; Geenen, M.; Steller, E.; Vrouenraets, B. Treatment strategies in elderly breast cancer patients: Is there a need for surgery? *Breast* **2014**, *23*, 793–798. [CrossRef]
28. Lavelle, K.; Moran, A.; Howell, A.; Bundred, N.; Campbell, M.; Todd, C. Older women with operable breast cancer are less likely to have surgery. *Br. J. Surg.* **2007**, *94*, 1209–1215. [CrossRef]
29. Richards, P.; Ward, S.; Morgan, J.; Lagord, C.; Reed, M.; Collins, K.; Wyld, L. The use of surgery in the treatment of er+ early stage breast cancer in england: Variation by time, age and patient characteristics. *Eur. J. Surg. Oncol.* **2016**, *42*, 489–496. [CrossRef]
30. Morgan, J.L.; Richards, P.; Zaman, O.; Ward, S.; Collins, K.; Robinson, T.; Cheung, K.-L.; Audisio, R.A.; Reed, M.W.; Wyld, L. The decision-making process for senior cancer patients: Treatment allocation of older women with operable breast cancer in the UK. *Cancer Biol. Med.* **2015**, *12*, 308–315.
31. Houterman, S.; Janssen-Heijnen, M.L.G.; Verheij, C.D.G.W.; Louwman, W.J.; Vreugdenhil, G.; Van Der Sangen, M.J.C.; Coebergh, J.W.W. Comorbidity has negligible impact on treatment and complications but influences survival in breast cancer patients. *Br. J. Cancer* **2004**, *90*, 2332–2337. [CrossRef]
32. Vitug, A.F.; Newman, L.A. Complications in breast surgery. *Surg. Clin. N. Am.* **2007**, *87*, 431–451. [CrossRef]
33. De Glas, N.A.; Kiderlen, M.; Bastiaannet, E.; De Craen, A.J.M.; Van De Water, W.; Van De Velde, C.J.H.; Liefers, G.J. Postoperative complications and survival of elderly breast cancer patients: A FOCUS study analysis. *Breast Cancer Res. Treat.* **2013**, *138*, 561–569. [CrossRef]
34. Renehan, A.G.; Malcomson, L.; Emsley, R.; Gollins, S.; Maw, A.; Myint, A.S.; Rooney, P.S.; Susnerwala, S.; Blower, A.; Saunders, M.P.; et al. Watch-and-wait approach versus surgical resection after chemoradiotherapy for patients with rectal cancer (the oncore project): A propensity-score matched cohort analysis. *Lancet Oncol.* **2016**, *17*, 174–183. [CrossRef]
35. Effects of chemotherapy and hormonal therapy for early breast cancer on recurrence and 15-year survival: An overview of the randomised trials. *Lancet* **2005**, *365*, 1687–1717. [CrossRef]
36. Jakesz, R.; Jonat, W.; Gnant, M.; Mittlboeck, M.; Greil, R.; Tausch, C.; Hilfrich, J.; Kwasny, W.; Menzel, C.; Samonigg, H.; et al. Switching of postmenopausal women with endocrine-responsive early breast cancer to anastrozole after 2 years' adjuvant tamoxifen: Combined results of abcsg trial 8 and arno 95 trial. *Lancet* **2005**, *366*, 455–462. [CrossRef]
37. Cadoo, K.A.; Morris, P.G.; Cowell, E.P.; Patil, S.; Hudis, C.A.; McArthur, H.L. Adjuvant Chemotherapy and Trastuzumab Is Safe and Effective in Older Women With Small, Node-Negative, HER2-Positive Early-Stage Breast Cancer. *Clin. Breast Cancer* **2016**, *16*, 487–493. [CrossRef]
38. Muss, H.B. Adjuvant Chemotherapy in Older Women With Breast Cancer: Who and What? *J. Clin. Oncol.* **2014**, *32*, 1996–2000. [CrossRef]
39. Du, X.L.; Zhang, Y.; Parikh, R.C.; Lairson, D.R.; Cai, Y. Comparative Effectiveness of Chemotherapy Regimens in Prolonging Survival for Two Large Population-Based Cohorts of Elderly Adults with Breast and Colon Cancer in 1992–2009. *J. Am. Geriatr. Soc.* **2015**, *63*, 1570–1582. [CrossRef]

40. Crivellari, D.; Spazzapan, S.; Puglisi, F.; Fratino, L.; Scalone, S.; Veronesi, A. Hormone therapy in elderly breast cancer patients with comorbidities. *Crit. Rev. Oncol.* **2010**, *73*, 92–98. [CrossRef]
41. Van den Broek, C.B.; Dekker, J.W.; Bastiaannet, E.; Krijnen, P.; de Craen, A.J.; Tollenaar, R.A.; van de Velde, C.J.; Liefers, G.J. The survival gap between middle-aged and elderly colon cancer patients. Time trends in treatment and survival. *Eur. J. Surg. Oncol.* **2011**, *37*, 904–912. [CrossRef]
42. Hamaker, M.E.; Schiphorst, A.H.; Verweij, N.M.; Pronk, A. Improved survival for older patients undergoing surgery for colorectal cancer between 2008 and 2011. *Int. J. Color. Dis.* **2014**, *29*, 1231–1236. [CrossRef]

11

HDAC5 Inhibitors as a Potential Treatment in Breast Cancer Affecting Very Young Women

Sara S. Oltra [1], Juan Miguel Cejalvo [1], Eduardo Tormo [1,2], Marta Albanell [1], Ana Ferrer [1], Marta Nacher [1], Begoña Bermejo [1], Cristina Hernando [1], Isabel Chirivella [1], Elisa Alonso [2,3], Octavio Burgués [2,3], Maria Peña-Chilet [1], Pilar Eroles [1,2], Ana Lluch [1,2], Gloria Ribas [1,2,*] and María Teresa Martinez [1,*]

1 INCLIVA Biomedical Research Institute, Hospital Clínico Universitario Valencia, University of Valencia, 46010 Valencia, Spain; sara.oltra@uv.es (S.S.O.); juanmitch5@hotmail.com (J.M.C.); eduardo.tormo@uv.es (E.T.); marta.albanell.95@gmail.com (M.A.); ferrermartineza9@gmail.com (A.F.); martanacher13@gmail.com (M.N.); begobermejo@gmail.com (B.B.); c.hernandomelia@gmail.com (C.H.); chirivella_isa@gva.es (I.C.); mariapch84@gmail.com (M.P.-C.); pilar.eroles@uv.es (P.E.); lluch_ana@gva.es (A.L.)

2 Biomedical Research Centre Network in Cancer (CIBERONC), 46010 Valencia, Spain; elisa.alonso@uv.es (E.A.); octavioburgues@gmail.com (O.B.)

3 Pathology Department, Hospital Clínico Universitario Valencia, University of Valencia, 46010 Valencia, Spain

* Correspondence: gribasdespuig@gmail.com (G.R.); maitemartinez3@yahoo.es (M.T.M.)

Abstract: Background: Breast cancer in very young women (BCVY) defined as <35 years old, presents with different molecular biology than in older patients. High *HDAC5* expression has been associated with poor prognosis in breast cancer (BC) tissue. We aimed to analyze *HDAC5* expression in BCVY and older patients and their correlation with clinical features, also studying the potential of HDAC5 inhibition in BC cell lines. Methods: *HDAC5* expression in 60 BCVY and 47 older cases were analyzed by qRT-PCR and correlated with clinical data. The effect of the HDAC5 inhibitor, LMK-235, was analyzed in BC cell lines from older and young patients. We performed time and dose dependence viability, migration, proliferation, and apoptosis assays. Results: Our results correlate higher *HDAC5* expression with worse prognosis in BCVY. However, we observed no differences between *HDAC5* expression and pathological features. Our results showed greatly reduced progression in BCVY cell lines and also in all triple negative subtypes when cell lines were treated with LMK-235. Conclusions: In BCVY, we found higher expression of *HDAC5*. Overexpression of *HDAC5* in BCVY correlates with lower survival rates. LMK-235 could be a potential treatment in BCVY.

Keywords: breast cancer; young women; histone deacetylase; HDAC5 inhibitors; LMK-235

---

1. Introduction

Breast cancer is the most common cancer among women worldwide [1]. As a percentage of all cancers in young women, breast cancer rates increase during the third and fourth decades of life, from 2% at age 20 to more than 40% by age 40. This abrupt increase is attributable to routine screening mammography. Breast cancer incidence is similar among young women in both developed and developing countries [2], but in recent years, there has been an increase in breast cancer diagnoses in very young women [3]. The distribution of breast cancer subtypes and grades changes with age, with more aggressive phenotypes among young women compared with older counterparts [4]. Basal-like and Her2-enriched breast tumors are also more common in young than in older women [5]. Scientific evidence suggests that age at breast cancer diagnosis represents an independent prognostic survival factor [6]. Indeed, multiple studies conclude that early age at diagnosis of breast cancer is highly associated with an increased risk of recurrence and death [7].

Epigenetic modifications are reported to play an important role in the onset and progression of many diseases. Carcinogenesis can be explained by genetic alterations, but epigenetic processes such as DNA methylation, histone modifications, and non-coding RNA deregulation are also involved [8].

Histone deacetylases are essential for global acetylation patterns in the nucleus and the epigenetic regulation of gene expression [9]. Histone deacetylases (HDACs) have been stratified into classes I, IIA, IIB, III, and IV and increased expression of these isoenzymes has been observed in different tumors, also often associated with poor outcome [10–13]. It has been reported several times that their levels vary greatly in cancer cells and differ according to tumor type. Of the 18 human HDACs, HDAC5 (a class IIa HDAC) is involved in synoviocyte activation, neural regeneration and repair, differentiation of myoblasts, and recently, elevated expression of *HDAC5* has been correlated with worse prognosis in patients with breast cancer (BC) [14].

Histone deacetylase inhibitors (HDACi) are currently acquiring importance in cancer treatment, being the only approved epigenetic therapy in clinics altering histone proteins to date. HDACi have been classified into four groups depending on their structure: Hydroxamic acids, cyclic peptides, benzamides, and short chain fatty acids. The hydroxamic acids (vorinostat, belinostat, and panobinostat) have been approved by the FDA as anticancer treatments. However, they are limited by their nonspecificity, affecting all HDACs [15]. These are known as pan-HDAC inhibitors and may also cause numerous side effects due to their broader specificity. Therefore, in some cases, more selective inhibitors may be more effective in therapy [16–19].

A previous study based on evaluation of new HDAC inhibitors identified LMK235 (N-((6-(hydroxyamino)-6-oxohexyl)oxy)-3,5-dimethylbenzamide) as the most cytotoxic compound, displaying equipotent HDAC inhibition in pan-HDAC assay when compared to vorinostat. In contrast to vorinostat, LMK235 showed a novel HDAC isoform selectivity profile with a preference for HDAC4 and HDAC5 [20].

Previous group studies showed significant differences in miRNA expression [21] and methylation [22] profiles among breast cancer affecting very young women (<35 years) (BCVY) and breast cancer in older patients (>45 years) (BCO). Additionally, our group observed considerable hypomethylation of CpG regions that were regulating *HDAC5* expression in BCVY, and this methylation was related to significant *HDAC5* overexpression in BCVY patients [23]. In the present study, we analyse *HDAC5* expression in a large cohort of BC patients, to clarify the correlation between *HDAC5* overexpression and relapse and survival in BCVY and BCO and the inhibitory effect of LMK-235 in breast cancer cell lines from very young and older women with BC.

2. Results

2.1. Clinical-Pathologic Characteristics of Patients

A total of 107 patients were included, 60 were young women under 35 years (BCVY) and 47 samples from women over 45 years (BCO). The median age at breast cancer diagnosis in the young patient's group was 32 years (range, 20–35), and in the old patient's group was 69 years (range, 53–94). Hereditary cases with BRCA1 and BRCA2 mutations were excluded from the study. In BCVY cohort, the immunohistochemical analyses showed 39.9% (n = 24) of luminal patients, 11.6% (n = 7) HER2-positive, 21.6% (n = 13) luminal/HER2 and 23.3% (n = 14) triple negative. In BCO group, 59.5% (n = 28) of patients were luminal, 10.6% (n = 5) HER2-positive, 10.6% (n = 5) luminal/HER2 and 17% (n = 8) presented triple negative subtype. Median follow-up was 93.4 months (Table 1).

Table 1. Clinicopathological information of breast cancer (BC) samples and statistical results from the study of HDAC5 expression vs. clinicopathological features by age groups.

	BCVY	*p*-Value (HDAC5 ~ CP)	BCO	*p*-Value (HDAC5 ~ CP)
N	60		47	
Age mean (years ± SD)	32.1 ± 3.3		69.8 ± 9.3	
Histological subtypes (%)		0.46		0.40
Luminal A	16.6		27.6	
Luminal B	23.3		31.9	
TNBC	23.3		17.0	
Luminal/HER2	21.6		10.6	
HER2	11.6		10.6	
Unknown	3.6		2.3	
ER status (%)				
ER+	60.0	0.43	74.4	0.92
ER-	33.3		21.3	
Unknown	6.7		4.3	
PR status (%)				
PR+	50.0	0.44	57.4	0.44
PR-	43.3		38.3	
Unknown	6.7		4.3	
HER2 (%)				
HER2+	31.6	0.97	21.3	0.93
HER2-	61.6		74.5	
Unknown	6.8		4.2	
KI67 (%)		0.56		0.07
<15%	16.6		27.7	
15–30%	28.3		32.0	
>30%	38.3		27.7	
Unknown	16.8		12.6	
Grade (%)		0.16		2.8×10^{-3} **
I	13.2		23.3	
II	49.1		41.9	**
III	37.7		34.9	*
Unknown				
Tumour Size (%)		0.16		0.02 *
<2 cm	35.0		59.6	
2–5 cm	40.0		23.4	
>5 cm	20.0		8.5	
Unknown	5.0		8.5	
Axillary Affection (%)		0.98		0.17
POS	38.3		29.8	
NEG	56.6		63.8	
Unknown	5.1		6.4	
Exitus (%)	13.8	0.12	13.3	0.19
Relapse (%)	25.0	0.27	21.0	0.15

N: Sample size; SD: Standard deviation; TNBC: Triple negative subtype; ER: Estrogen receptor; PR: Progesterone receptor; BCVY: Breast cancer in very young women; BCO: Breast cancer in older women. P-values indicate statistics for the differences among HDAC5 expression and the different clinicopathological (CP) features included in the table by age groups. * p-value < 0.05, ** p-value < 0.01.

2.2. HDAC5 Overexpression in BCVY Patients Correlates with Poorer Prognosis

HDAC5 was significantly overexpressed in BCVY patients (p-value = 0.04) (Figure 1A). We found no appreciable differences among clinical features and *HDAC5* expression, apart from tumor grade in BCO patients (p-value = 2.8×10^{-3}) where the lower grades presented higher *HDAC5* expression (Figure S1A). Regarding molecular subtypes, we observed higher *HDAC5* expression in Luminal B and HER2 tumors from BCVY in comparison with BCO patients from the same subgroups. While BCO patients presented higher expression for Luminal A and Luminal/HER2 comparing to BCVY (Figure S1B). Despite no significant association, these results agree with higher expression of *HDAC5* for poor prognostic subtypes for each patient age groups in our cohort, that were HER2 for BCVY and Luminal/HER2 for BCO patients.

We observed similar percentages of cancer death between young and old patients, 13.8% (n = 9) and 13.3% (n = 6), respectively. However, *HDAC5* was significantly overexpressed in BCVY patients that died in comparison with BCO (p-value = 0.04) and a significant *HDAC5* overexpression was observed for BCO patients that survive when compare with BCO patients that died (p-value = 0.01) (Figure 1B). These results were in line with survival studies, where Kaplan–Meier curves showed a reduced survival trend for BCVY when *HDAC5* was overexpressed (Figure 2A) whereas BCO women presented poorer survival when *HDAC5* was repressed (Figure 2B). In terms of relapse, results were not as evident as survival (results not shown). For survival and relapse studies, samples were classified in high, medium or low, according to *HDAC5* expression. Despite no significant results observed for BCVY patients, survival studies indicated an important trend of worst survival for BCVY, contrary to the results observed for BCO. In this regard, *HDAC5* overexpression in BCVY could be related with the poorer outcome at this age group. It is worth to mention that the number of BC patients that experience relapse and/or death was reduced and further studies should be addressed in order to validate this tendency observed.

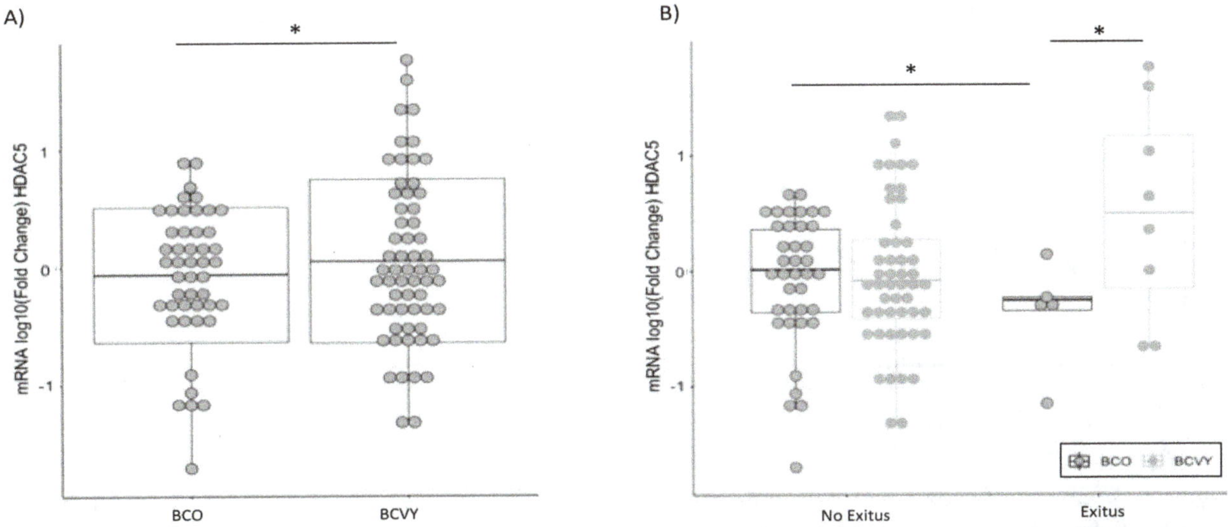

Figure 1. *HDAC5* expression in BCVY (n = 60) and BCO (n = 47) patients analyzed by qRT-PCR (**A**). *HDAC5* expression in BCVY and BCO patients regarding their status (exitus or no exitus) (**B**). BCVY: Breast cancer in very young women; BCO: Breast cancer in old women. * $p \leq 0.05$, ** $p \leq 0.01$.

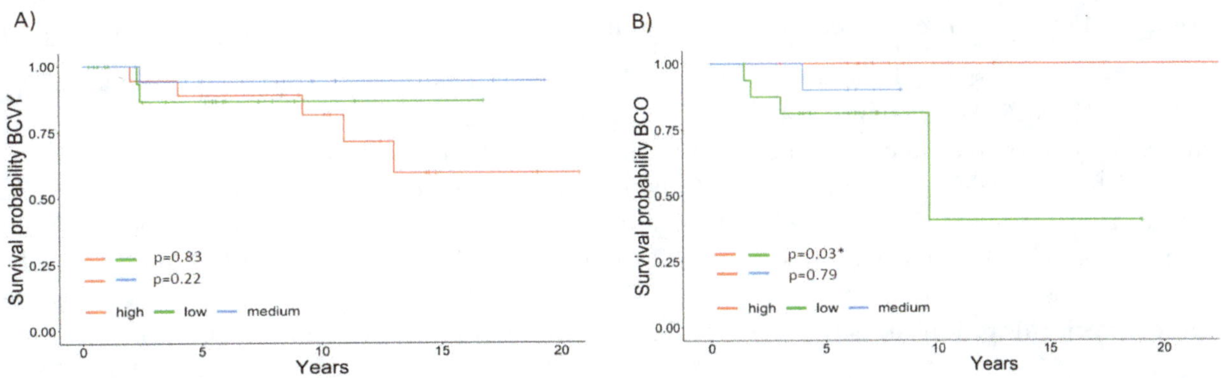

Figure 2. Association of *HDAC5* expression and survival in breast cancer patients. Survival curves for *HDAC5* expression in BCVY (n = 42) (**A**) and BCO patients (n = 28) (**B**). *HDAC5* expression was classified in high (red), medium (blue) or low (green). BCVY: Breast cancer in very young women; BCO: Breast cancer in old women. * $p \leq 0.05$.

2.3. *LMK-235 Inhibitor Reduces Proliferation in BC Cell Lines*

Breast cancer cell lines were exposed to increasing concentrations of HDAC5 inhibitor LMK-235 (0, 0.625, 1.25, 2.5, 5, 10, and 20 μM) for 24, 48, and 72 h. We observed that relative proliferation decreased in a dose- and time-dependent manner for some breast cancer cell lines (Figure 3). After 48 h treatment with low doses of LMK-235 (Figure 3A), cell viability of MDA-MB-231 and HCC1806 cell lines was severely compromised. Additionally, viability was notably diminished in the HCC1937 cell line after 72 h of treatment, showing similar results to MDA-MB-231 and HCC1806 cell lines (Figure 3B). Although no significant results were obtained for HCC1500 cell line after 48 h of treatment, the young cell line showed a 50% reduction in viability after 72 h of low dose LMK-235. Breast cancer cell lines that experienced significant viability reduction were triple negative subtype with the exception of HCC1500 luminal cell line established from young BC patients and showed higher reduction in comparison with the older luminal cell lines, MCF7 and BT474. Inhibitor studies reveal important response for triple negative BC cell lines to LMK-235 and for luminal cell lines from young women with BC not observed in older luminal cell lines.

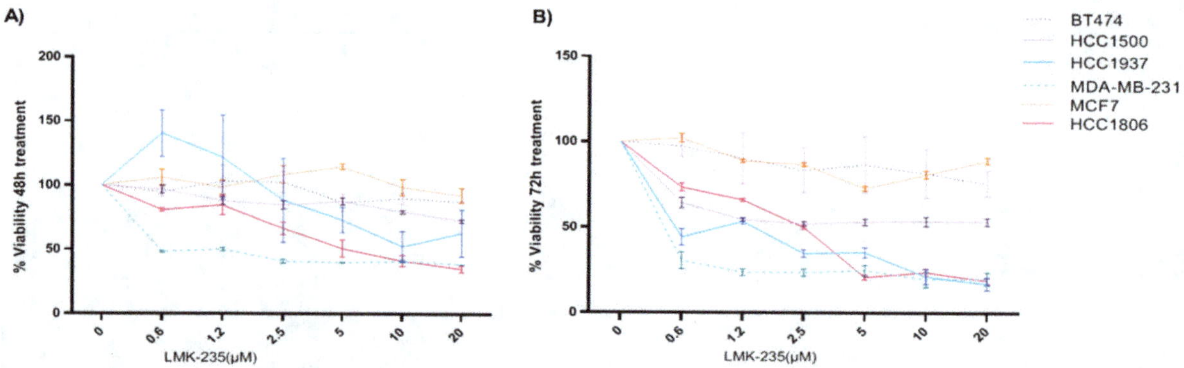

Figure 3. Effects of LMK-235 treatments in BC cell proliferation. Cell proliferation was determined by MTT assay for HCC1500 and HCC1937 (<35 years old) and MDA-MB-231, MCF-7, HCC1806, and BT-474 (>45 years old) cell lines that were treated with LMK-235 (0 to 20 μM) for 48 hours (**A**), 72 h (**B**). Points indicate the mean of at least three independent experiments and the standard deviation.

2.4. *Reduced Migration of Breast Cancer Cell Lines Treated with LMK-235 Measured by Wound-Healing Assay*

Wound-healing assays demonstrated that LMK-235 significantly inhibited migration in HCC1937 (p-value = 0.01), HCC1806 (p-value = 4.9×10^{-7}) and MDA-MB-231 (p-value = 1.2×10^{-3}) breast cancer cell lines after 48 h of treatment. Specifically, we observed ~23% less cell migration in the HCC1937 cell line, ~14.7% for MDA-MB-231, and also HCC1806 cell line showed a substantial reduction. HCC1500 cells treated with LMK-235 presented cell migration reduced by ~5.3%. However, the last cell line exhibited considerable cell death at 48 h of cell treatment making wound-healing analysis difficult. In contrast, breast cancer cell lines MCF-7 and BT474, both from luminal old BC patients, showed insignificant cell migration reduction when cells were treated with LMK-235 (Figure 4).

These results revealed higher cell migration and proliferation reduction in cell lines from triple negative subtypes (MDA-MB-231, HCC1806, and HCC1937), independently of age. However, we observed markedly diminished viability in the young and luminal HCC1500 cell line treated with HDAC5 inhibitor, which could not be detected in the luminal subtypes from older cell lines (MCF7 and BT474).

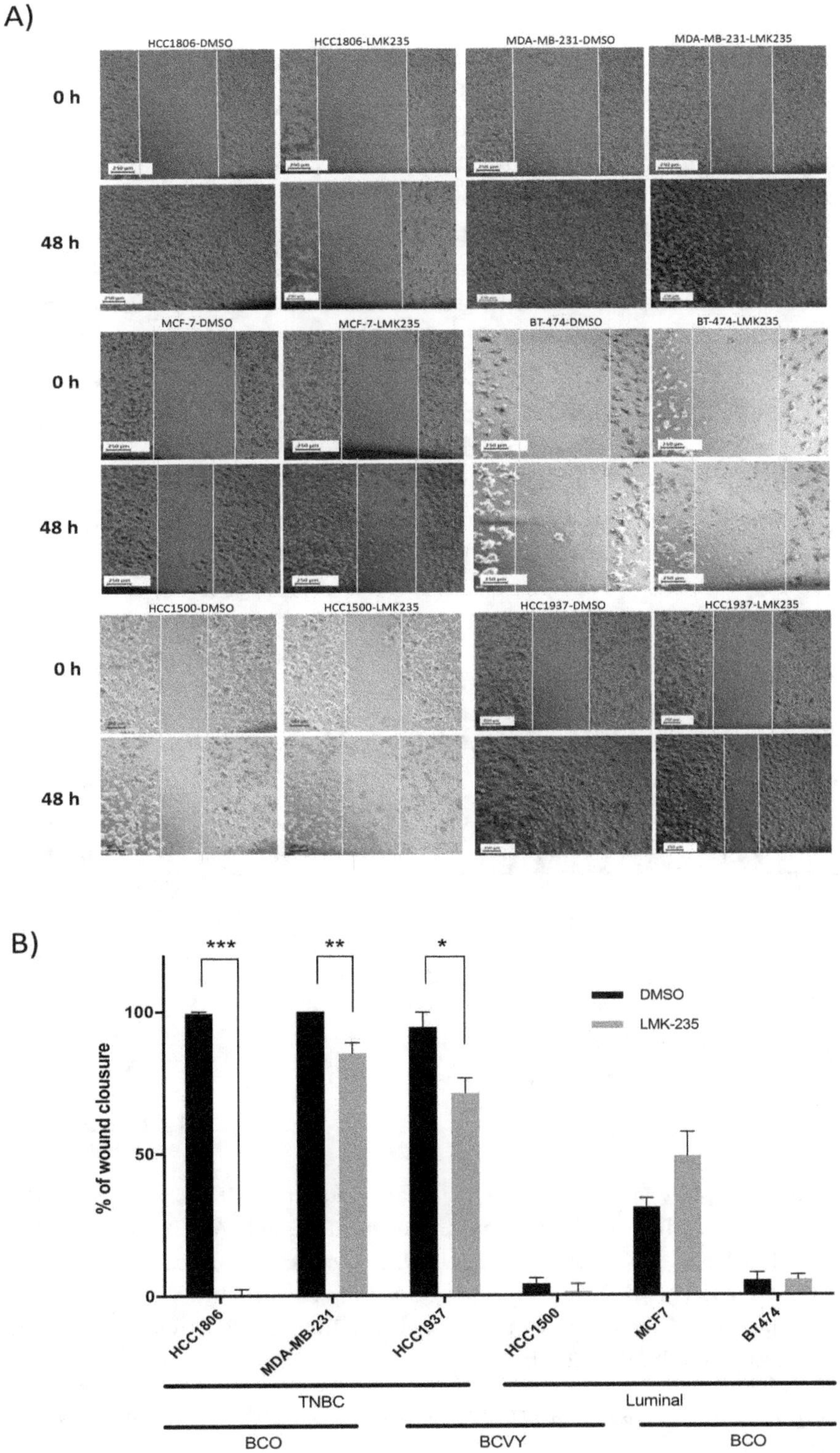

Figure 4. Effects of LMK-235 treatments in BC cell migration. Cell migration was assessed by scratch wound-healing assay after treatment with LMK-235 (20 μM) for 48 h. Images of cell migration at 0 h and 48 h after LMK-235 (20 μM) treatment (**A**); Percentage of wound closure after 48 h of LMK-235 (20 μM) treatment or DMSO/control. Three separate experiments were conducted, and representative results are shown (**B**). Columns mean ± SD of the percentage of wound closure in the three independent experiments. Black bars represent control DMSO cells and grey bars represent cells treated with LMK-235. * $p \leq 0.05$, ** $p \leq 0.01$, *** $p \leq 0.001$ statistically significant. TNBC: Triple negative breast cancer; BCVY: breast cancer in very young women; BCO: Breast cancer in old women.

2.5. Apoptosis AfterLMK-235 Treatment

To confirm the results obtained by MTT, we performed an apoptosis assay by flow cytometry. After 48 h of treatment, similar results to the MTT assay were observed. Results show increasingly early apoptosis in most BC cells lines after 48 h of LMK-235 (10 and/or 20 μM) treatment. Interestingly, and in line with previous proliferation and migration results, the most important increase in apoptosis was observed in triple negative cell lines from both BCVY and BCO. Intriguingly, LMK-235 induced a more profound increase in HCC1500 cell death for higher concentrations than in MTT assay (Figure 5A). These results agree with the wound-healing assay observations, where after 48 h of treatment most of the HCC1500 cells were dead and no wound-healing analysis could be performed.

2.6. Accumulation of Acetyl-H3 After LMK-235 Treatment in Breast Cancer Cell Lines

We observed increased *HDAC5* mRNA expression in all breast cancer cell lines that were treated with LMK-235 (Figure 5B). These results confirm that the HDACi does not act at the mRNA level, but rather at the protein level. LMK-235 induces an increase in mRNA expression as a positive feedback mechanism in order to increase and restore protein expression. Additionally, *HDAC5* expression was higher in control/DMSO conditions for all BC cell lines independently of their response to the HDAC5 inhibitor.

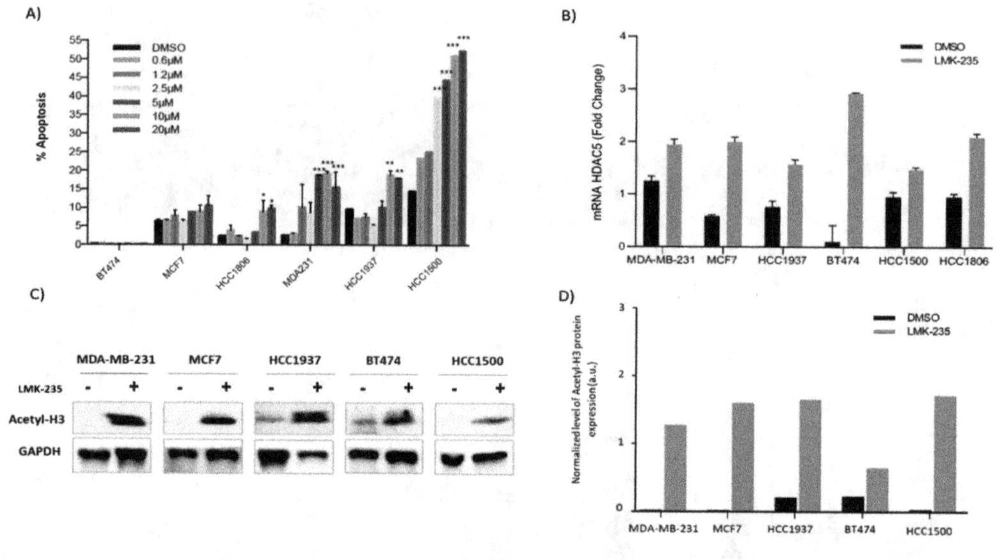

Figure 5. Percentages of apoptosis are shown after treatment with LMK-235 (0.6 to 20 μM) or DMSO for 48 h. Apoptosis was analyzed by triplicated and SD was calculated (**A**); Expression of *HDA5* in breast cancer cell lines treated with LMK-235 (20 μM) and DMSO control (**B**); Accumulation of acetyl-histone H3 after 48 h of LMK-235 (20 μM) treatment in breast cancer cell lines examined by western-blot. The levels of acetyl-histone H3 were determined by western blot. GAPDH was used as a loading control (**C**). Densitometry western bolt analyzed by ImageJ software (**D**). * $p \leq 0.05$, ** $p \leq 0.01$, *** $p \leq 0.001$.

To investigate whether the changes in *HDAC5* mRNA expression are reflected in persistent changes at their protein levels, these were determined in breast cancer cell lines by western-blotting following treatment with LMK-235 (20 μM) for 48 h. The levels of HDAC5 protein were barely detectable for all cell lines, as previously observed in other studies [14,24] that showed the low quantity of HDAC5 protein by western blot (data not shown). Next, we measured HDAC5 activity at the acetylation of lysine residues on histone H3 to determine the inhibitory effect of LMK-235 on HDAC5. Western-blot studies showed accumulation of acetyl-histone H3 in breast cancer cell lines after 48 h of LMK-235 treatment (Figure 5C,D). We observed acetyl-histone H3 accumulation both in luminal breast cancer cell lines (BT474, HCC1500 and MCF7) and in triple negative breast cancer cell lines (HCC1937 and MDA-MB-231). These results demonstrate that LMK-235 specifically inhibits HDACs, which catalyze the removal of acetyl groups from N-acetyl lysine histone residues. Therefore, their inhibition produces an accumulation of acetyl-histones and acetyl-H3 is one of the most extensively modified.

3. Discussion

BCVY can be understood as a unique and different entity from breast cancer in older people, not only because of patients' characteristics (where aspects such as fertility preservation must take into account) but also in its biological and molecular tumor characteristics. Our group has focused for years on the study of these differential molecular characteristics in breast cancer tumors of young and old women. Previous results [23] showed us that *HDAC5* was notably overexpressed in BCVY. We validate this issue analyzing *HDAC5* overexpression in a larger cohort of young patients under 35 years and over 45, as well as studying the correlation of *HDAC5* expression levels with different clinic-pathological features. Additionally, we analyzed the effects of an HDAC5 inhibitor, LMK-235, on apoptosis, proliferation, and migration in breast cancer cell lines.

Histones are acetylated on lysine side chains, which neutralizes lysine's positive charge, leading to open chromatin structure by reducing interaction between histone and negatively charged DNA [25,26]. Thus, histone acetylation increases the accessibility of proteins such as transcription factors to promoters and enhancers, thereby mediating active gene expression. Acetylated histones also function as binding sites for numerous proteins with bromodomains, which often activate gene transcription [25]. In contrast, histone deacetylation is associated with chromatin condensation and transcriptional repression [25]. Analogous to histone methylation, histone acetylation is reversibly controlled by two large enzyme families: histone lysine acetyltransferases (KATs) and HDACs.

Turning to *HDAC5*, high expression has been correlated with poorer prognosis in patients with BC or pancreatic neuroendocrine tumors and has been attributed to oncogenic effects [27,28]. Specifically, *HDAC5* overexpression has been correlated with triple negative BC tumors [14,29]. However, our study showed higher *HDAC5* expression in BCVY than BCO samples. Next, we wonder whether *HDAC5* overexpression was correlated with relapse and survival, and other clinical and pathological data. BCVY patients with *HDAC5* overexpression showed a higher risk of exitus, whereas results were contrary for BCO that showed a significant risk of death when *HDAC5* was repressed. In agreement with these results, higher *HDAC5* expression was observed in BCVY samples that died whereas lower expression was found in BCO patients that die. Our results reinforce the hypothesis that *HDAC5* overexpression in BCVY patients is related with a poor outcome observed in this group of age. BCVY is not a usual diagnosis, so there is a limitation in the number of BCVY samples and the present study is actually the first report that includes one of the highest cohort of BCVY patients in comparison with other larger datasets (ex., TCGA and METABRIC [30,31]).

Next, we evaluated *HDAC5* expression and its correlation with different clinical and pathological features (histologic subtypes, Ki67, tumor size, grade, and axillary affection). We found no correlation between *HDAC*5 expression and clinical features in BCVY. The only meaningful association observed was between *HDAC5* downregulation and higher tumor grades (II and III) in BCO. Higher tumor grades are associated with poorer prognosis and in our study with *HDAC5* repression for BCO, which agrees with survival tendencies observed at this age group where *HDAC5* repression correlates with poorer survival in BCO.

HDAC inhibitors are the most widely investigated epigenetic drugs in clinical studies [32]. In vitro studies suggest that the HDAC5 inhibitor LMK-235 could be a novel therapeutic strategy for BC treatment [14]. We evaluated the inhibitory effect of LMK-235 in breast cancer cell lines from young women and compared it with breast cancer cell lines from older counterparts. Our results demonstrated that LMK-235 induced important reduction in progression, migration, and apoptosis, not only in triple negative young and old but also in luminal young cell lines. Regarding that, we observed important viability reduction under treatment conditions for the cell lines that presented significant differences in the migration assay between control and treatment conditions. These results were observed in triple negative cell lines (from young and old patients). Thus, the reduction in cell viability correlates with a reduction in cell migration under LMK-235 treatment. Interestingly, the luminal cell lines from old patients (BT474 and MCF7) were not affected by LMK-235 inhibitor. However, the luminal young cell line HCC1500 presented intermedium results between triple negative and luminal old cell lines. These results point out a potential breast cancer treatment not only for triple negative breast cancer but also for young patients from different molecular subtypes.

Additionally, LMK-235 response was lower in ER-positive cell lines, except for HCC1500 which presented an intermedium response in comparison with the rest of ER-positive cells, as we previously mentioned. Previous studies found LMK-235 response in triple negative BC cell lines [33–36]. However, our results showed an important response to LMK-235 in the breast cancer cell line from young women that present luminal subtype, as HCC1500. These results suggest an effect of ER in the LMK-235 treatment but must exist other mechanisms in young cell lines that increase the effect of LMK-235, which are not present in older cell lines. There was a pronounced time- and dose-dependent decrease in cell viability and migration and hence an increased apoptosis in all breast cancer cell lines from triple negative subtypes (BCVY and BCO). Furthermore, HCC1500 luminal BCVY cell line presented similar results, showing significant apoptosis rates and reduced cell viability, avoiding the possibility of analyzed migration wound-healing assays. It is worth to mention that LMK-235 treatment induces higher apoptosis in HCC1500 cell line at lower doses in comparison with the rest of cell lines. These results suggest the existence of off-target effects that increase the apoptosis at this cell line, so further studies are required to analyze the underlying mechanisms of LMK-235 inhibitor.

These results reinforce the hypothesis that *HDAC5* is involved in tumorigenesis and cancer progression reducing survival, specifically in BCVY. We propose studying HDAC5 inhibitors like LMK-235 in a larger cohort of breast cancer cell lines from young and old women and from different molecular subtypes in order to evaluate their inhibitory effect. Additionally, cell lines studies show a significant response to HDAC5i of triple negative BCO in addition to all BCVY cell lines independently of their molecular subtype.

4. Materials and Methods

4.1. Patient Selection

All samples included in the study were archived formalin-fixed paraffin-embedded (FFPE) BC tissues stored at the Hospital Clínico Universitario of Valencia, Spain. We selected 60 breast cancer samples from women under 35 years old (BCVY) and 47 samples from women over 45 (BCO). The clinical characteristics of patients are included in Table 1. This study was approved by the Institutional Health INCLIVA-Hospital Clínico Ethics Committee and informed consent was obtained from all subjects. The code of the ethical committee of the Hospital Clínico Universitario of Valencia (Spain) is 2013/128.

All patients' clinical data and tumor pathological characteristics were collected at their first visit and information about relapse and survival on subsequent visits. Tumor size and lymph node involvement were assessed using the eighth edition of the American Joint Committee on Cancer staging manual [37]. Patient clinicopathological data used in this study are shown in Table 1.

4.2. Breast Cancer Cell Lines Culture and Treatment

Breast cancer cell lines were obtained from the American Type Culture Collection (ATCC, Rockville, MD, USA). Cell lines were cultured in RPMI 1640 or DMEM medium supplemented with 1% L-glutamine and 10% fetal bovine serum (GIBCO, New York, NY, USA). The culture conditions were identical in all cell lines: 37 °C and 5% CO_2 (Table 2). Cells were seeded for 24 h before treatment with LMK-235 (Selleck Chemicals, Houston, TX, USA) or DMSO (control) for MTT assay, wound-healing, and apoptosis assay.

Table 2. Cell lines characteristics and culture conditions.

Cell Line	Subtype	Receptor Expression	Tumor Type	Age	Culture Medium	Conditions	Supplements
HCC 1500	Luminal	ER, PR	IDC	32	RPMI	5% CO_2 37 °C	1% L-glu 10% FBS
HCC1937	Basal	EGP2	IDC	24	RPMI	5% CO_2 37 °C	1% L-glu 10% FBS
MDA-MB-231	Basal	EGFR, TGF-β	Carcinoma	51	RPMI	5% CO_2 37 °C	1% L-glu 10% FBS
MCF7	Luminal	ER, IGFBP	IDC	69	RPMI	5% CO_2 37 °C	1% L-glu 10% FBS
BT474	Luminal	ER, PR, HER2	IDC	60	DMEM	5% CO_2 37 °C	1% L-glu 10% FBS
HCC1806	Basal	EGP2	Carcinoma	60	RPMI	5% CO_2 37 °C	1% L-glu 10% FBS 10% FBS

EGP2: Epithelial glycoprotein 2; EGFR: Epidermal growth factor receptor; TGF-β/α: transforming growth factor β/α; ER: Estrogen receptor; PR: Progesterone receptor; HER2: Hormonal estrogen receptor 2; IGFBP: Insulin growth factor binding protein; RPMI: RPMI 1640 medium; FBS: Fetal bovine serum; L-glu: L-glutamine; IDC: Invasive ductal carcinoma.

4.3. Cell Proliferation Assay

The protocol used is based on a colorimetric MTT (3-(4,5-dimethylthiazol-2-yl)-2,5-diphenyltetrazolium bromide) assay. We seeded and cultured 2000 cells in 96-well plates. Next, cells were treated with a specific drug dose, and MTT assay was performed 24, 48, and 72 h after treatment. The absorbance of this colored solution was quantified by measuring at 590 by spectrophotometer. Each experiment was performed in triplicate and repeated at least twice. Average values for triplicates were calculated. Absorbance observed at different drug concentrations was compared with the respective non-treated controls and cell viability was calculated.

4.4. Scratch Wound-Healing Assay

Cells were seeded in six-well plates at a density of 5×10^5 cells/well and incubated overnight until they reached 70% confluence. A pipette tip was used to generate a wound in the cell layer. Cells were then treated with LMK-235 (20 μM). Each experiment was performed in triplicate and repeated at least twice. Images were obtained at 0, 24 and 48 h at the same position and percentage of cell migration was evaluated using ImageJ (LOCI, University of Wisconsin).

4.5. Apoptosis Assay by Flow Cytometry

We plated 100,000 cells in 12-well plates. After 48 h of treatment, trypsinized and floating cells collected from the supernatant were centrifuged and incubated with Annexin V-FITC (BioLegend, San Diego, California, United States) and DAPI for 15 min. Apoptosis was detected using Flow Cytometry BD LSRFortessa™ (BD, Franklin Lake, NJ, USA).

4.6. Western Blot

We then prepared the nuclear protein fraction of breast cancer cell lines using a nuclear extraction kit (Active Motif, Belgium, Germany). A total of 40 μg of protein were resolved by 12% SDS-PAGE and transferred onto nitrocellulose membranes. Membranes were blocked in 5% BSA and hybridized with antibodies against aceyl-H3 (1:1000) and GAPDH (1:1000) as a loading control. Immunoreactive bands were visualized by chemiluminescence (GE Healthcare, Life Science, Oslo, Norway) and captured by Image Quant™ LAS4000 (GE Healthcare, Life Science, Oslo, Norway). The band densities, normalized to the GAPDH, were analyzed with ImageJ software.

4.7. RNA Extraction

Total RNA from BC cell lines was isolated using the High Pure RNA Isolation Kit (Roche, Basel, Switzerland), following the manufacturer's protocol. Total RNA from FFPE samples was isolated using RecoverAll Total Nucleic Acid Isolation Kit (Applied Biosystems™ by Life Technologies™, Carlsbad, CA, USA), following the manufacturer's protocol. RNA concentration was measured using a NanoDrop ND 2000-UV-vis Spectrophotometer (Thermo Fisher Scientific Inc., Wilmington, DE, USA).

4.8. Gene Expression by qRT-PCR

Gene expression of *HDAC5* and *GAPDH* as endogenous control was carried out by quantitative real time-PCR (qRT-PCR) in RNA extracted from FFPE samples. We used the TaqMan®Gene Expression Assays (Applied Biosystems™ by Life Technologies™, Carlsbad, CA, USA). Normalization was done with *GAPDH*. The data were managed using the QuantStudio Desing & Analysis Software v1.4 (Applied Biosystems™ by Life Technologies™, Carlsbad, CA, USA). Relative expression was calculated using the comparative Ct method and obtaining the fold-change value ($\Delta\Delta$Ct).

4.9. Statistical Analysis

All statistical analysis was performed using R Bioconductor (https://www.bioconductor.org/). To determine differences between *HDAC5* expression and breast cancer patients/cells from different ages we performed a Wilcoxon Rank Sum test. Results were considered significant when p-value < 0.05. OS and RFS were performed using follow-up data from BC patients to analyze the prognostic value of *HDAC5* expression in terms of relapse and survival. Patients were divided into three groups according to the distribution of the log10 *HDAC5* Fold change: high expression (> 0.2 log10 Fold change), medium (> -0.2 and <0.2) and low (< -0.2). RFS and OS studies were performed using *survival* R package (https://CRAN.R-project.org/package=survival).

5. Conclusions

Taken together, the results provide insights into the biology of breast cancer in younger women and support our hypothesis that breast tumors of younger women activate molecular pathways related to increased aggressiveness, such as *HDAC5*. Our findings are consistent with those previously published by Li et al. [14], confirming that *HDAC5* promotes proliferation, invasion, and migration in human breast cancer. We also demonstrate that *HDAC5* overexpression in BCVY correlates with lower survival rates.

In our study, we show that targeted treatment with HDAC5 inhibitor LMK-235 reduces migration and proliferation of tumor cells and increases apoptosis in triple negative breast cancer cell lines, as previous results demonstrated, and as a novelty in luminal cell lines from younger BC patients. In summary, our findings show, for the first time, a potential treatment specific for breast cancer affecting very young patients. However, more efforts should be addressed to analyze its therapeutic role.

Author Contributions: G.R., M.T.M. and A.L. conceived the study. G.R., M.T.M., P.E. and M.P.-C. supervised the study. M.T.M. and S.S.O. coordinate and designed all the aspects of the work. S.S.O. and E.T. contributed in experimental and computational analysis. M.A., A.F. and M.N. contributed in the cell lines experiments. E.A. and O.B. contributed in the pathology aspects. A.L., B.B., J.M.C., C.H., I.C. and M.T.M. contributed in clinical patient data selection. S.S.O. and M.T.M. wrote the manuscript. All authors have read and agreed to the published version of the manuscript.

Acknowledgments: We wish to thank all patients and volunteers who gave their consent for inclusion in this study, and the medical staff of the Medical Oncology Unit at the INCLIVA Biomedical Research Institute in Valencia (Spain) for collecting the samples and providing the material for all the analyses. We thank the Cytometry Unit from the Unidad Central de Investigación Médica (UCIM), University of Valencia. The Biomedical Research Centre Network in Cancer (CIBERONC) is a Carlos III Health Institute initiative. We thank INCLIVA Biobank, which is part of the Spanish Hospital Biobanks Network (ReTBioH) for storage and providing samples for the study. Moreover, we thank the private patients' foundation Fundación Le Cadó. We would like also to thank several patients' organizations for their financial support.

References

1. Shapira, N. The potential contribution of dietary factors to breast cancer prevention. *Eur. J. Cancer Prev.* **2017**, *26*, 385–395. [CrossRef] [PubMed]
2. Narod, S.A. Breast cancer in young women. *Nat. Rev. Clin. Oncol.* **2012**, *9*, 460–470. [CrossRef] [PubMed]
3. Anastasiadi, Z.; Lianos, G.D.; Ignatiadou, E.; Harissis, H.V.; Mitsis, M. Breast cancer in young women: An overview. *Updates Surg.* **2017**, *69*, 313–317. [CrossRef] [PubMed]
4. Colleoni, M.; Rotmensz, N.; Robertson, C.; Orlando, L.; Viale, G.; Renne, G.; Luini, A.; Veronesi, P.; Intra, M.; Orecchia, R.; et al. Very young women (<35 years) with operable breast cancer: Features of disease at presentation. *Ann. Oncol.* **2002**, *13*, 273–279. [CrossRef] [PubMed]
5. Parker, J.S.; Mullins, M.; Cheang, M.C.; Leung, S.; Voduc, D.; Vickery, T.; Davies, S.; Fauron, C.; He, X.; Hu, Z.; et al. Supervised risk predictor of breast cancer based on intrinsic subtypes. *J. Clin. Oncol.* **2009**, *27*, 1160–1167. [CrossRef]
6. Han, W.; Kim, S.W.; Park, I.A.; Kang, D.; Kim, S.W.; Youn, Y.K.; Oh, S.K.; Choe, K.J.; Noh, D.Y. Young age: An independent risk factor for disease-free survival in women with operable breast cancer. *BMC Cancer* **2004**, *4*, 82. [CrossRef]
7. Anders, C.K.; Fan, C.; Parker, J.S.; Carey, L.A.; Blackwell, K.L.; Klauber-DeMore, N.; Perou, C.M. Breast carcinomas arising at a young age: Unique biology or a surrogate for aggressive intrinsic subtypes? *J. Clin. Oncol.* **2011**, *29*, e18. [CrossRef]
8. Eckschlager, T.; Plch, J.; Stiborova, M.; Hrabeta, J. Histone Deacetylase Inhibitors as Anticancer Drugs. *Int. J. Mol. Sci.* **2017**, *18*, 1414. [CrossRef]
9. Moser, M.A.; Hagelkruys, A.; Seiser, C. Transcription and beyond: The role of mammalian class I lysine deacetylases. *Chromosoma* **2014**, *123*, 67–78. [CrossRef]
10. Nakagawa, M.; Oda, Y.; Eguchi, T.; Aishima, S.; Yao, T.; Hosoi, F.; Basaki, Y.; Ono, M.; Kuwano, M.; Tanaka, M.; et al. Expression profile of class I histone deacetylases in human cancer tissues. *Oncol. Rep.* **2007**, *18*, 769–774. [CrossRef]
11. Montezuma, D.; Henrique, R.M.; Jeronimo, C. Altered expression of histone deacetylases in cancer. *Crit. Rev. Oncog.* **2015**, *20*, 19–34. [CrossRef]
12. Weichert, W. HDAC expression and clinical prognosis in human malignancies. *Cancer Lett.* **2009**, *280*, 168–176. [CrossRef] [PubMed]
13. Witt, O.; Deubzer, H.E.; Milde, T.; Oehme, I. HDAC family: What are the cancer relevant targets? *Cancer Lett.* **2009**, *277*, 8–21. [CrossRef] [PubMed]
14. Li, A.; Liu, Z.; Li, M.; Zhou, S.; Xu, Y.; Xiao, Y.; Yang, W. HDAC5, a potential therapeutic target and prognostic biomarker, promotes proliferation, invasion and migration in human breast cancer. *Oncotarget* **2016**, *7*, 37966–37978. [CrossRef]
15. Hull, E.E.; Montgomery, M.R.; Leyva, K.J. HDAC Inhibitors as Epigenetic Regulators of the Immune System: Impacts on Cancer Therapy and Inflammatory Diseases. *BioMed Res. Int.* **2016**, *2016*, 8797206. [CrossRef]
16. Thurn, K.T.; Thomas, S.; Moore, A.; Munster, P.N. Rational therapeutic combinations with histone deacetylase inhibitors for the treatment of cancer. *Future Oncol.* **2011**, *7*, 263–283. [CrossRef]
17. Subramanian, S.; Bates, S.E.; Wright, J.J.; Espinoza-Delgado, I.; Piekarz, R.L. Clinical Toxicities of Histone Deacetylase Inhibitors. *Pharmaceuticals* **2010**, *3*, 2751–2767. [CrossRef]
18. Thaler, F.; Minucci, S. Next generation histone deacetylase inhibitors: The answer to the search for optimized epigenetic therapies? *Expert Opin. Drug Discov.* **2011**, *6*, 393–404. [CrossRef]
19. Noureen, N.; Rashid, H.; Kalsoom, S. Identification of type-specific anticancer histone deacetylase inhibitors: Road to success. *Cancer Chemother. Pharmacol.* **2010**, *66*, 625–633. [CrossRef]

20. Marek, L.; Hamacher, A.; Hansen, F.K.; Kuna, K.; Gohlke, H.; Kassack, M.U.; Kurz, T. Histone deacetylase (HDAC) inhibitors with a novel connecting unit linker region reveal a selectivity profile for HDAC4 and HDAC5 with improved activity against chemoresistant cancer cells. *J. Med. Chem.* **2013**, *56*, 427–436. [CrossRef]
21. Pena-Chilet, M.; Martinez, M.T.; Perez-Fidalgo, J.A.; Peiro-Chova, L.; Oltra, S.S.; Tormo, E.; Alonso-Yuste, E.; Martinez-Delgado, B.; Eroles, P.; Climent, J.; et al. MicroRNA profile in very young women with breast cancer. *BMC Cancer* **2014**, *14*, 529. [CrossRef] [PubMed]
22. Oltra, S.S.; Pena-Chilet, M.; Vidal-Tomas, V.; Flower, K.; Martinez, M.T.; Alonso, E.; Burgues, O.; Lluch, A.; Flanagan, J.M.; Ribas, G. Methylation deregulation of miRNA promoters identifies miR124-2 as a survival biomarker in Breast Cancer in very young women. *Sci. Rep.* **2018**, *8*, 14373. [CrossRef] [PubMed]
23. Oltra, S.S.; Peña-Chilet, M.; Flower, K.; Martinez, M.T.; Alonso, E.; Burgues, O.; Lluch, A.; Flanagan, J.M.; Ribas, G. Acceleration in the DNA methylation age in breast cancer tumours from very young women. *Sci. Rep.* **2019**, *9*, 14991. [CrossRef] [PubMed]
24. Kaletsch, A.; Pinkerneil, M.; Hoffmann, M.J.; Jaguva Vasudevan, A.A.; Wang, C.; Hansen, F.K.; Wiek, C.; Hanenberg, H.; Gertzen, C.; Gohlke, H.; et al. Effects of novel HDAC inhibitors on urothelial carcinoma cells. *Clin. Epigenetics* **2018**, *10*, 100. [CrossRef] [PubMed]
25. Haberland, M.; Montgomery, R.L.; Olson, E.N. The many roles of histone deacetylases in development and physiology: Implications for disease and therapy. *Nat. Rev. Genet.* **2009**, *10*, 32–42. [CrossRef]
26. Dawson, M.A.; Kouzarides, T. Cancer epigenetics: From mechanism to therapy. *Cell* **2012**, *150*, 12–27. [CrossRef]
27. Li, A.; Liu, Z.; Li, M.; Zhou, S.; Xu, Y.; Xiao, Y.; Yang, W. Correction: HDAC5, a potential therapeutic target and prognostic biomarker, promotes proliferation, invasion and migration in human breast cancer. *Oncotarget* **2017**, *8*, 30619–30620. [CrossRef]
28. Klieser, E.; Urbas, R.; Stattner, S.; Primavesi, F.; Jager, T.; Dinnewitzer, A.; Mayr, C.; Kiesslich, T.; Holzmann, K.; Di Fazio, P.; et al. Comprehensive immunohistochemical analysis of histone deacetylases in pancreatic neuroendocrine tumors: HDAC5 as a predictor of poor clinical outcome. *Hum. Pathol.* **2017**, *65*, 41–52. [CrossRef]
29. Vasilatos, S.N.; Katz, T.A.; Oesterreich, S.; Wan, Y.; Davidson, N.E.; Huang, Y. Crosstalk between lysine-specific demethylase 1 (LSD1) and histone deacetylases mediates antineoplastic efficacy of HDAC inhibitors in human breast cancer cells. *Carcinogenesis* **2013**, *34*, 1196–1207. [CrossRef]
30. Dawson, S.J.; Rueda, O.M.; Aparicio, S.; Caldas, C. A new genome-driven integrated classification of breast cancer and its implications. *EMBO J.* **2013**, *32*, 617–628. [CrossRef]
31. Curtis, C.; Shah, S.P.; Chin, S.F.; Turashvili, G.; Rueda, O.M.; Dunning, M.J.; Speed, D.; Lynch, A.G.; Samarajiwa, S.; Yuan, Y.; et al. The genomic and transcriptomic architecture of 2,000 breast tumours reveals novel subgroups. *Nature* **2012**, *486*, 346–352. [CrossRef] [PubMed]
32. Ohguchi, H.; Hideshima, T.; Anderson, K.C. The biological significance of histone modifiers in multiple myeloma: Clinical applications. *Blood Cancer J.* **2018**, *8*, 83. [CrossRef] [PubMed]
33. De Cremoux, P.; Dalvai, M.; N'Doye, O.; Moutahir, F.; Rolland, G.; Chouchane-Mlik, O.; Assayag, F.; Lehmann-Che, J.; Kraus-Berthie, L.; Nicolas, A.; et al. HDAC inhibition does not induce estrogen receptor in human triple-negative breast cancer cell lines and patient-derived xenografts. *Breast Cancer Res. Treat.* **2015**, *149*, 81–89. [CrossRef] [PubMed]
34. Jang, E.R.; Lim, S.J.; Lee, E.S.; Jeong, G.; Kim, T.Y.; Bang, Y.J.; Lee, J.S. The histone deacetylase inhibitor trichostatin A sensitizes estrogen receptor alpha-negative breast cancer cells to tamoxifen. *Oncogene* **2004**, *23*, 1724–1736. [CrossRef]
35. Raha, P.; Thomas, S.; Thurn, K.T.; Park, J.; Munster, P.N. Combined histone deacetylase inhibition and tamoxifen induces apoptosis in tamoxifen-resistant breast cancer models, by reversing Bcl-2 overexpression. *Breast Cancer Res.* **2015**, *17*, 26. [CrossRef]
36. Thomas, S.; Thurn, K.T.; Raha, P.; Chen, S.; Munster, P.N. Efficacy of histone deacetylase and estrogen receptor inhibition in breast cancer cells due to concerted down regulation of Akt. *PLoS ONE* **2013**, *8*, e68973. [CrossRef]
37. AJCC. *Cancer Staging Manual Form Supplement*, 8th ed.; American Joint Committee On Cancer (AJCC): Chicago, IL, USA. Available online: https://cancerstaging.org/About/news/Pages/AJCC-8th-Edition-Cancer-Staging-Form-and-Histology-and-Topography-Supplements-Available-Now.aspx (accessed on 5 June 2018).

12

Should all Patients with HR-Positive HER2-Negative Metastatic Breast Cancer Receive CDK 4/6 Inhibitor as First-Line Based Therapy? A Network Meta-Analysis of Data from the PALOMA 2, MONALEESA 2, MONALEESA 7, MONARCH 3, FALCON, SWOG and FACT Trials

Valentina Rossi [1,†], Paola Berchialla [2,†], Diana Giannarelli [3,†], Cecilia Nisticò [4], Gianluigi Ferretti [4], Simona Gasparro [4], Michelangelo Russillo [4], Giovanna Catania [4], Leonardo Vigna [1], Rossella Letizia Mancusi [5], Emilio Bria [6,7], Filippo Montemurro [8], Francesco Cognetti [9] and Alessandra Fabi [4,*]

1 Breast Unit, S. Camillo-Forlanini Hospital of Rome, 00152 Rome, Italy; VRossi@scamilloforlanini.rm.it (V.R.); LVigna@scamilloforlanini.rm.it (L.V.)
2 Department of Clinical and Biological Sciences, University of Turin, 10124 Turin, Italy; paola.berchialla@unito.it
3 Department of Medical Statistics, IRCCS Regina Elena National Cancer Institute, 00128 Rome, Italy; Diana.giannarelli@ifo.gov.it
4 Division of Medical Oncology1, IRCCS Regina Elena National Cancer Institute, 00128 Rome, Italy; cecilia.nistico@ifo.gov.it (C.N.); gianluigi.ferretti@alice.it (G.F.); simona.gasparro@ifo.gov.it (S.G.); michelangelo.russillo@ifo.gov.it (M.R.); giovanna.catania@ifo.gov.it (G.C.)
5 Department of Statistical Sciences, University Tor Vergata of Rome, 00133 Rome, Italy; mncrsl01@uniroma2.it
6 Comprehensive Cancer Center, Fondazione Policlinico Universitario Agostino Gemelli IRCCS, 00168 Rome, Italy; emiliobria@yahoo.it
7 Department of Medical Oncology, Università Cattolica del Sacro Cuore, 00168 Rome, Italy
8 Direzione Day Hospital Oncologico Multidisciplinare, Istituto di Candiolo, FPO-IRCCS, 10060 Candiolo, Italy; Filippo.montemurro@ircc.it
9 Università La Sapienza, 00185 Rome, Italy; francesco.cognetti@ifo.gov.it
* Correspondence: alessandra.fabi@ifo.gov.it
† These authors equally contributed to the statistical analysis.

Abstract: *Background*: We aim to understand whether all patients with hormonal receptor (HR)-positive (+)/human epidermal growth factor receptor-2 (HER2)-negative (−) metastatic breast cancer (MBC) should receive cyclin D-dependent kinase (CDK) 4/6 inhibitor-based therapy as a first-line approach. Methods: A network meta-analysis (NMA) using the Bayesian hierarchical arm-based model, which provides the estimates for various effect sizes, were computed. Results: First-line treatment options in HR+/HER2− MBC, including CDK 4/6 inhibitors combined with aromatase inhibitors (AIs) or fulvestrant (F), showed a significantly longer progression-free survival (PFS) in comparison with AI monotherapy, with a total of 26% progression risk reduction. In the indirect comparison across the three classes of CDK 4/6 inhibitors and F endocrine-based therapies, the first strategy resulted in longer PFS, regardless of specific CDK 4/6 inhibitor (HR: 0.68; 95% CrI: 0.53–0.87 for palbociclib + AI, HR: 0.65; 95% CrI: 0.53–0.79 for ribociclib + AI, HR: 0.63; 95% CrI: 0.47–0.86 for abemaciclib + AI) and patient's characteristics. Longer PFS was also found in patients with bone-only and soft tissues limited disease treated with CDK 4/6 inhibitors. Conclusions: CDK 4/6 inhibitors have similar efficacy when associated with an AI in the first-line treatment of HR+ MBC, and are superior to either F or AI monotherapy, regardless of any other patients or tumor characteristics.

Keywords: palbociclib; ribociclib; abemaciclib; fulvestrant; aromatase inhibitors; metastatic breast cancer

1. Introduction

Hormone receptor (HR)-positive (+) and human epidermal growth factor receptor type (HER2)-negative (−) metastatic breast cancer (MBC) represents the most common invasive cancer subtype in women [1]. Almost two-thirds of women with newly diagnosed MBC have HR+ tumors, and approximately 25% of women with an early HR+ breast cancer diagnosis eventually relapse after adjuvant treatments [2].

As the role of estrogens in etiology and breast cancer progression is well-established, the modification of estrogen activity has represented the treatment of choice in women with HR+ MBC for several years, particularly for those with slowly progressive disease and limited tumor-related symptoms [3]. Selective estrogen receptor modulators (such as tamoxifen) [4], selective estrogen receptor down-regulators (SERDs, like fulvestrant [F]) [5,6] aromatase inhibitors (AIs; such asletrozole [7], anastrazole [8] or exemestane [9]) are the mainstay of anticancer endocrine therapy (ET) [10]. The recent addition of CDK 4/6 inhibitors to standard ET has further improved outcomes in both first- and later-line therapy settings. CDK 4/6 inhibitors act by inactivating the complex CDK-D-type cyclins (CCND), leading to an increase in the retinoblastoma protein (pRb), which negatively regulates E2F transcriptional factors, eventually resulting in the inhibition of cell cycle progression and apoptosis of tumor cells [11].

In the first-line setting, CDK 4/6 inhibitors, which mechanistically work in different ways through estrogen receptor interference, have been studied in combination with AIs in the PALOMA-2 [12], MONALEESA-2 [13], and MONARCH-3 studies in the context of postmenopausal women [14], as well as in premenopausal women, in combination with either tamoxifen or an AI in the MONALEESA-7 study [15]. In particular, palbociclib, ribociclib, and abemaciclib, the three available CDK 4/6 inhibitors, in combination with standard ET, showed progression-free survival (PFS) improvement in phase III trials, and have been approved for use in first and in later lines of therapy in women with HR+HER2− MBC, regardless of menopausal status, age, endocrine sensitivity and type of metastasis [12,16]. Interestingly, although the mechanism of action of these CDK 4/6 inhibitors is similar, they also present some differences. In fact, while palbociclib and ribociclib have a similar chemical structure, abemaciclib is 14-times more potent against CDK 4 compared with CDK 6 and presents a higher selectivity for the complex CDK 4/cyclin D1 [11].

Despite the progress made in efficacy, combination therapy also resulted in increased toxicities, costs, and tighter clinical monitoring for patients [17]. In addition, the improvement in PFS has not yet translated into an increase in overall survival (OS) for all studies focusing on first-line settings [18–20].

Therefore, how and when to incorporate CDK 4/6 inhibitors in the complex management of HR+ HER2− MBC remains one of the main unmet clinical need in this setting [21].

Indeed, single-agent ET yielded a median PFS ranging from 14 to 16 months in the control arms of the first-line trials with CDK 4/6 inhibitors. Thus, the fact that for some patients, the addition of CDK 4/6 inhibitors might be avoided is a debated clinical topic. Moreover, according to the Fulvestrant and Anastrozole Compared in Hormonal Therapy Naive Advanced Breast Cancer (FALCON) trial, comparing F with anastrozole in the same setting, the single-agent F therapy may be a further reasonable option for HR+/HER2− MBC patients who are ET-naïve, especially those with the non-visceral disease. Indeed, the median PFS of 16.6 months reported in the F arm compared with 13.3 months in the anastrozole arm, which was observed in the context of the general population, was even higher in patients without visceral disease (22.3 versus 13.6 months; hazard ratio [HR]: 0.59; 95% CI: 0.42–0.84) [5].

The ongoing studies, which are evaluating predictive markers of endocrine resistance or sensitivity, will probably provide enough evidence for helping in the clinical decision-making and for a better definition of the optimal ET-based strategy for this specific set of luminal breast cancer [22–24].

In the meantime, in our current daily clinical practice, also considering minor or uncertain differences in efficacy between the available CDK 4/6 inhibitors, the choice of first-line ET strategy is essentially based on one of the three CDK 4/6 inhibitors according to their specific toxicity profile and patient comorbidities or preferences.

Considering the lack of formal and reliable comparisons between the three CDK 4/6 inhibitors, in addition to the lower toxicity profile of F, the aim of this systematic review and meta-analysis is the indirect comparison between the combination strategy, including CDK 4/6 inhibitors plus AI [12–15], and F-based therapies for the first-line treatment of HR+/HER2− MBC [5,25–27].

2. Materials and Methods

2.1. Search Strategy and Study Selection

We followed the PRISMA statement for reporting systematic reviews and meta-analysis. Two authors independently examined the abstracts retrieved by a search strategy in electronic databases (MEDLINE, EMBASE, and The Cochrane Central Register of Controlled Trials) from November 2011 to June 2019. We used the following search string ((metastatic breast cancer) AND (CDK 4/6 inhibitor OR endocrine therapy OR aromatase inhibitor OR letrozole OR anastrozole OR exemestane OR tamoxifen OR F OR palbociclib OR everolimus OR ribociclib OR abemaciclib). The research was conducted on 5 June 2019. Proceedings of the American Society of Clinical Oncology (ASCO) Annual Meeting, San Antonio Breast Cancer Annual Symposium, and the European Society of Medical Oncology Annual Meeting were also queried from November 2011 to June 2019 for relevant abstracts. In cases where a report of the same trial was obtained, the most recent results were included (corresponding to longer follow-up). Then, the authors examined full-text articles of potentially eligible studies according to the eligibility criteria. Disagreements on the inclusion of selected trials were resolved in discussions with another author. This article does not contain any studies with human participants or animals performed by any of the authors. It was unnecessary, given the study does not contain any studies with human participants or animals performed by any of the authors.

2.2. Eligibility Criteria

We decided only to include phase III randomized controlled trials (RCTs) that reported the comparison of CDK 4/6 inhibitors plus ET or F plus or less ET versus ET treatment alone as first-line treatment in HR+/HER2− MBC. We also excluded trials with incomplete data or different control arm.

2.3. Outcomes

The primary outcome was PFS, calculated from the date of randomization to the date of progression (defined by the Response Evaluation Criteria in Solid Tumors "RECIST" 1.1 criteria or death). The secondary outcomes were: (1) objective response rate (ORR): defined as the percentage of patients with complete or partial response as per RECIST 1.1 criteria (as assessed in all randomly assigned patients); (2) clinical benefit (CB): defined as a confirmed complete or partial response or stable disease lasting 24 weeks or more; (3) OS: defined as the time from randomization to death from any causes. Subgroup meta-regression analysis was also conducted for PFS indirect comparison according to age, Eastern Cooperative Oncology Group (ECOG) performance status, ethnicity, prior chemotherapy or ET exposure, measurable disease at the time of metastasis occurrence, visceral or bone-only disease, time from the initial diagnosis of breast cancer to metastasis onset.

2.4. Data Collection and Statistical Analysis

A network meta-analysis (NMA) was carried out utilizing the method in the study by Valkenhoef et al. [28], which performed NMA using the Bayesian hierarchical arm-based model and provides estimates for various effect sizes. For PFS, HR and 95% credible interval (CrI) were reported. In addition, ORR and CB rates were reported, and the results were expressed as odds ratios (OR) with their 95% CrI. The NMA plot, in which treatments directly compared were connected with straight line was generated. NMAs on patients' subgroups were also performed. All analyses were performed using R Statistical Software version 3.4.3 along with the gemtc package, which uses Markov chain Monte Carlo (MCMC) techniques through Just Another Gibbs Sampler (JAGS) [29].

3. Results

3.1. Study Selection

Through the search strategy, we identified four phase III trials comparing 1441 patients treated with CDK 4/6 inhibitors (palbociclib, ribociclibor, abemaciclib) in combination with an AI (1106 patients) [12–14], an AI plus ovarian function suppression (OFS; 248 premenopausal patients), or tamoxifen plus OFS (87 premenopausal patients) [15]. Three other phase III randomized controlled trials (RCTs) compared 837 patients treated with F alone (230 patients) or in combination with AI (607 patients) versus a total of 1891 patients treated with AI alone (letrozole 2.5 mg daily or anastrozole 1 mg per day on a continuous schedule), tamoxifen plus OFS (90 premenopausal patients) or AI plus OFS (247 premenopausal) [5,25,27]. The Preferred Reporting Items for Systematic Reviews and Meta-Analyses (PRISMA) flow diagram for study inclusion is shown in Figure 1.

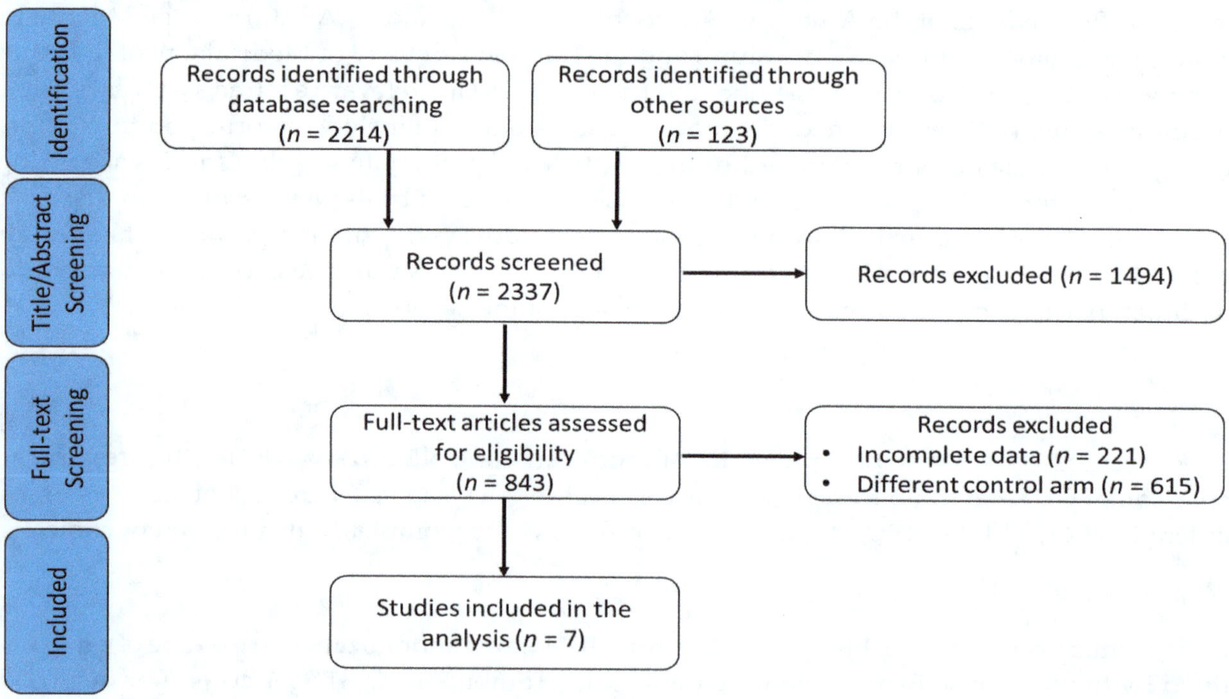

Figure 1. The Preferred Reporting Items for Systematic Reviews and Meta-Analyses (PRISMA) flow chart summarizing the process for the identification of the eligible studies.

3.2. Description of Studies and Patients

Table 1 summarizes the main characteristics and outcomes of each trial. Palbociclib and ribociclib were tested in combination with letrozole 2.5 mg/day in PALOMA-2 and MONALEESA-2, respectively. Abemaciclib was used in combination with anastrozole 1 mg/day (19.9%) or letrozole 2.5 mg/day (79.1%) as per the physician's choice in the MONARCH-3 trial. Furthermore, ribociclib was also studied in premenopausal patients in the context of the MONALEESA-7 trial. Specifically, in this study, ribociclib was combined with tamoxifen plus goserelin (26%) or with letrozole 2.5 mg/day or anastrozole 1 mg/day plus goserelin (74%). Eventually, F alone or in combination with anastrozole 1 mg/day was compared with the AI in the FALCON, Southwest Oncology Group (SWOG), and Fulvestrant and Anastrozole Combination Therapy (FACT) trials. The primary outcome was PFS in all trials (Table 1); secondary outcomes (ORR, CB rate, OS) in all trials were also reported in Table 1, while the NMA core design is shown in Figure 2. The network plot in Figure 2 offers a visual representation of the evidence. Nodes represent treatments, and edges represent the available direct comparisons—that is, they connect treatments that are directly compared in studies.

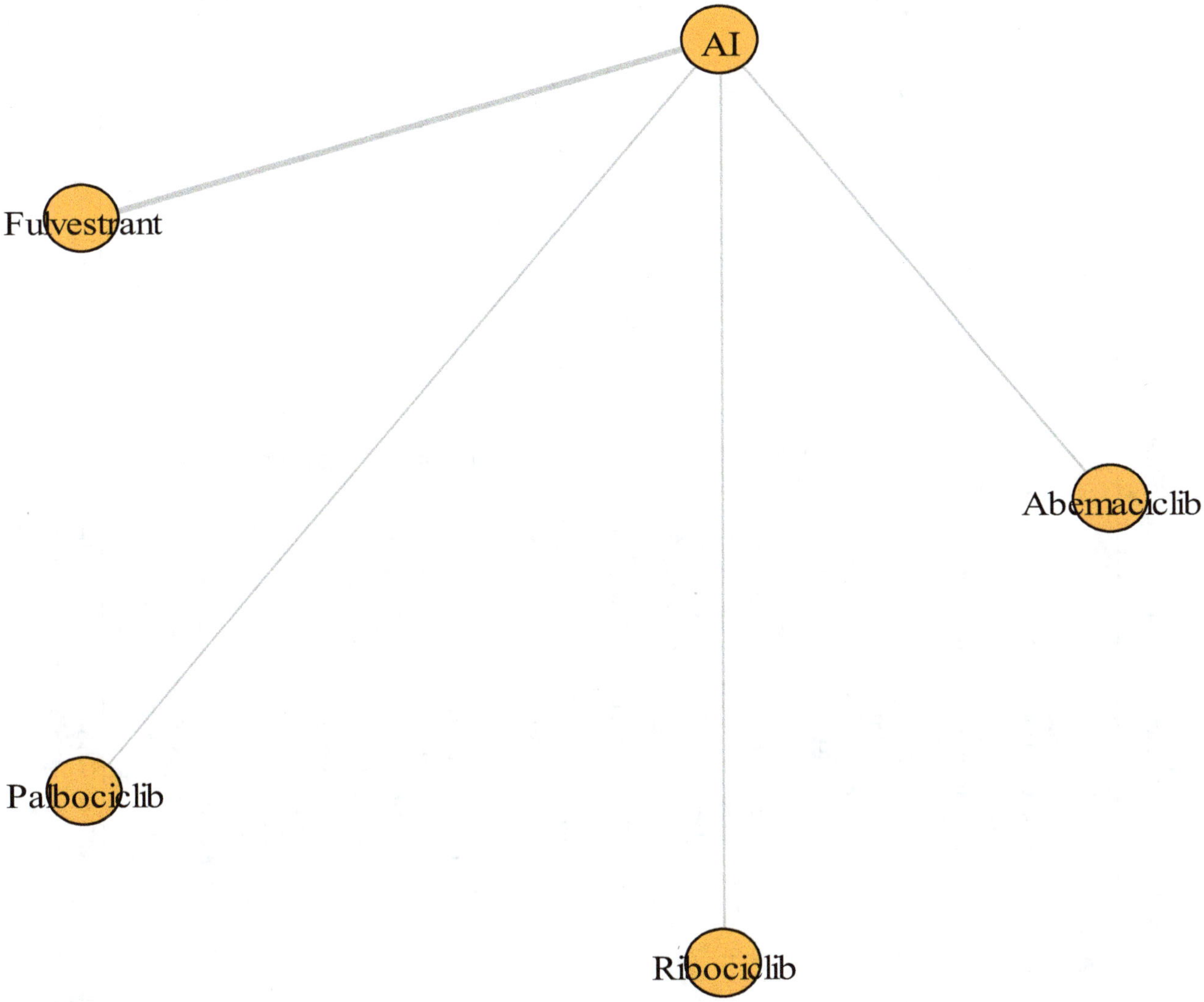

Figure 2. The network meta-analysis design: Network plot of the network meta-analysis. AI: Aromatase inhibitor.

Table 1. Main characteristics and outcomes of the seven eligible trials included for meta-analysis.

Study and First Author	Publication Year	Phase	Setting	Post-Menopausal	RR (%)	CB (%)	Median PFS (months)	Median OS (months)
PALOMA-2 Finn [12]	2016	III	First-line therapy for MBC in patients not treated before for their metastatic disease.	Yes	42.1 vs. 34.7	84.9 vs. 70.3	24.8 vs. 14.5	NR
MONALEESA-2 Hotobagyi [13]	2016 2018	III	First-line therapy for locally advanced and MBC. Patients who had not received previous systemic therapy for advanced disease were eligible. Previous neoadjuvant or adjuvant therapy with a nonsteroidal AI was not allowed unless the disease-free interval was more than 12 months	Yes	40.7 vs. 27.5 42.5 vs. 28.7	79.6 vs. 72.8 79.9 vs. 73.1	NR vs. 14.7 25.3 vs. 16	NR NR vs. 33
MONARCH-3 Goetz [14]	2017	III	First-line therapy for locally advanced and MBC (endocrine therapy in the neoadjuvant or adjuvant setting was permitted if the patient had a disease-free interval 12 months from the completion of endocrine therapy)	Yes	48.2 vs. 34.5	78 vs. 71.5	NR vs. 14.7	NR
MONALEESA-7 Tripathy [15]	2018 2019	III	First-line therapy for locally advanced or MBC (endocrine therapy and chemotherapy in the adjuvant or neoadjuvant setting was permitted, as was up to one line of chemotherapy for advanced disease).	Not (only pre and perimenopausal women were included and treated with goserelin)	41 vs. 30	79 vs. 70	23.8 vs. 13.0	NR NR vs. 40.9
FALCON Robertson [5]	2016	III	First-line therapy for locally advanced or MBC (no previous adjuvant therapy was admitted, only a first-line CHT for metastatic disease was accepted)	Yes	46 vs. 45	78 vs. 74	16.6 vs. 13.8	NR
SWOG Mehta [26]	2012 2019	III	First line for de novo MBC or recurrent MBC after 12 months by the end of adjuvant CHT or HT	Yes	27 vs. 22	73 vs. 70	15 vs. 13.5 15 vs. 13.5	47.7 vs. 41.3 49.8 vs. 42
FACT Bergh [27]	2012	III	First-line therapy in recurrent MBC after or during primary treatment (with or without HT, CHT, RT). Patients treated with an adjuvant AI had to be relapse-free for more than one year after completion of this type of endocrine therapy (30.2% of the patients in the experimental arm were endocrine naive)	Yes (only 3% of patients wer in the premenopausal status and were treated with GnRH agonists)	31.8 vs. 33.6	55 vs. 55.1	10.8 vs. 10.2	37.8 vs. 38.2

AI: aromatase inhibitor; CB: clinical benefit; CHT: chemotherapy; HT: hormonal therapy; MBC: metastatic breast cancer; GnRH, gonadotropin-releasing hormone; NR: not reported; OS: overall survival; PFS: progression-free survival; RR: response rate; RT: radiotherapy.

3.3. Outcomes

3.3.1. Progression-Free Survival

As shown in the indirect comparison between CDK 4/6 inhibitors versus F-based therapies, the first strategy resulted in longer PFS, regardless of the specific CDK 4/6 inhibitor (HR: 0.68; 95% CrI: 0.53–0.87 for palbociclib + AI, HR: 0.65; 95% CrI: 0.53–0.79 for ribociclib + AI, HR: 0.63; 95% CrI: 0.47–0.86 for abemaciclib + AI) (Figure 3; top)

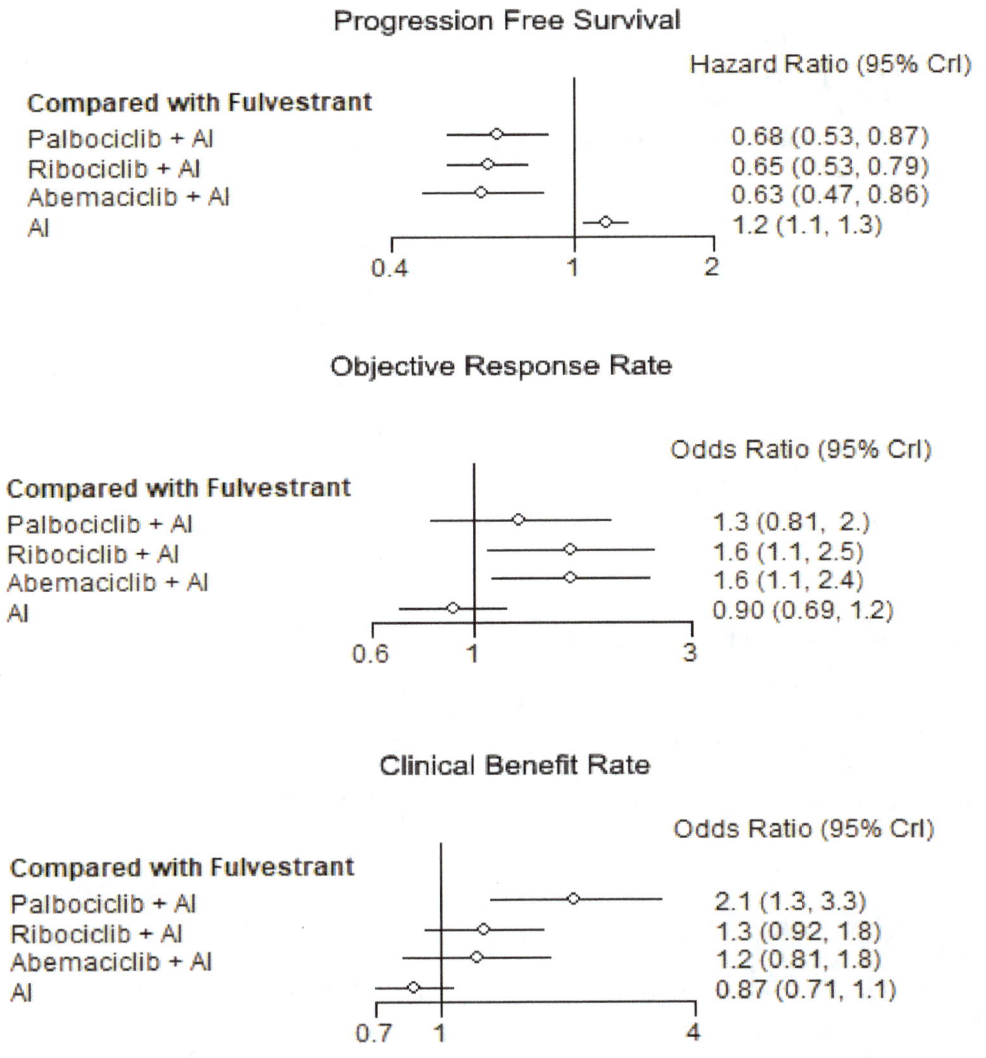

Figure 3. Forest plots with direct comparisons against fulvestrant for progression-free survival, objective response rate, and clinical benefit rate. AI: Aromatase inhibitor.

3.3.2. Objective Response

The CDK 4/6 inhibitors combination strategies resulted in higher RR in indirect comparison with F (OR:1.3; 95% CrI: 0.81–2.0 from palbociclib + AI versus AI: OR:1.6; 95% CrI: 1.1–2.5 from ribociclib + AI versus AI: OR:1.6; 95% CrI: 1.1–2.4 from abemaciclib + AI versus AI). (Figure 3; middle)

3.3.3. Clinical Benefit

The CDK 4/6 inhibitor combination strategies resulted in higher CB in indirect comparison with F (OR: 2.1; 95% CrI: 1.3–3.3 from palbociclib + AI versus AI: OR: 1.3; 95% CrI: 0.92–1.8 from ribociclib + AI versus AI: OR:1.2; 95% CrI: 0.81–1.8 from abemaciclib + AI versus AI). (Figure 3; bottom).

3.3.4. Overall Survival

For overall survival (OS), no indirect comparison by NMA was performed because not all the studies data were completely mature. Indeed, data on OS have been recently reported in the MONALEESE-7 study where the estimated OS at 42 months was 70.2% (95% CI 63.5–76.0) in the CDK 4/6 inhibitor arm versus 46% (95% CI: 32–58.9) in the ET alone arm [18,19] In addition, also the SWOG trial has recently shown the median OS of 49.8 months in 71% of the patients receiving F combination strategy vs. 42 months in 76% of the patients receiving ET monotherapy alone [23].

3.3.5. Safety Profile

The main adverse effects registered in each trial are reported in Table 2.

Table 2. Main adverse effects registered in each trial.

Study	Treatment	AEs	G3 (%)	G4 (%)
PALOMA-2	Palbociclib–letrozole	Any AEs Neutropenia Leukopenia	62.2% 56.1% 24.1%	13.5% 10.4% 0.7%
	Placebo–letrozole	Any AEs Neutropenia	22.1% 0.9%	2.3% 0.5%
MONALEESA-2	Ribociclib–letrozole	Neutropenia Abnormal LFT Leukopenia	52.4% 8.4% 20.1%	9.6% 1.8% 1.2%
	Placebo–letrozole	Abnormal LFT Neutropenia, anemia, arthralgia	2.4% 1.2%	– –
MONARCH-3	Abemaciclib–nonsteroidal AI	Any AEs Neutropenia Leukopenia ALT increase	51.7% 22.0% 8.3% 6.1%	6.7% 1.8% 0.3% 0.3%
	Placebo–nonsteroidal AI	Any AEs Neutropenia	22.4% 0.6%	2.5% 0.6%
MONALEESA-7	Ribociclib group	Any AEs Neutropenia Leukopenia	63% 51% 13%	14% 10% 1%
	Placebo group	Any AEs Neutropenia	26% 3%	4% 1%
FALCON Robertson	Fulvestrant	Arthralgia (17%) Hot flush, fatigue, nausea (11%) Back pain (9%)		
	Anastrozole	Arthralgia, hot flush, nausea (10%)		
SWOG Mehta	Anastrozole	Musculoskeletal pain, fatigue, hot flashes, mood alterations, GI symptoms	15% (each 1–4%)	
	Anastrozole–fulvestrant	Musculoskeletal pain, fatigue, hot flashes, mood alterations, GI symptoms	13% (each 1–4%)	
FACT Bergh	Anastrozole	GI symptoms (25.2%) Joint disorders (27.6%) Hot flashes (13.8%)		
	Anastrozole–fulvestrant	GI symptoms (28.9%) Joint disorders (26.6%) Hot flashes (24.6%)		

ALT: alanine aminotransferase; AE: adverse event; AI: aromatase inhibitor; GI: gastrointestinal; G3: grade 3; G4: grade 4; LFT: liver function test.

3.4. Subgroup Analyses

Table 3 summarizes the main patient's characteristic according to subgroups analysis in each trial. Subgroup NMA among the three classes of CDK 4/6 inhibitors and F is reported in Figure 4.

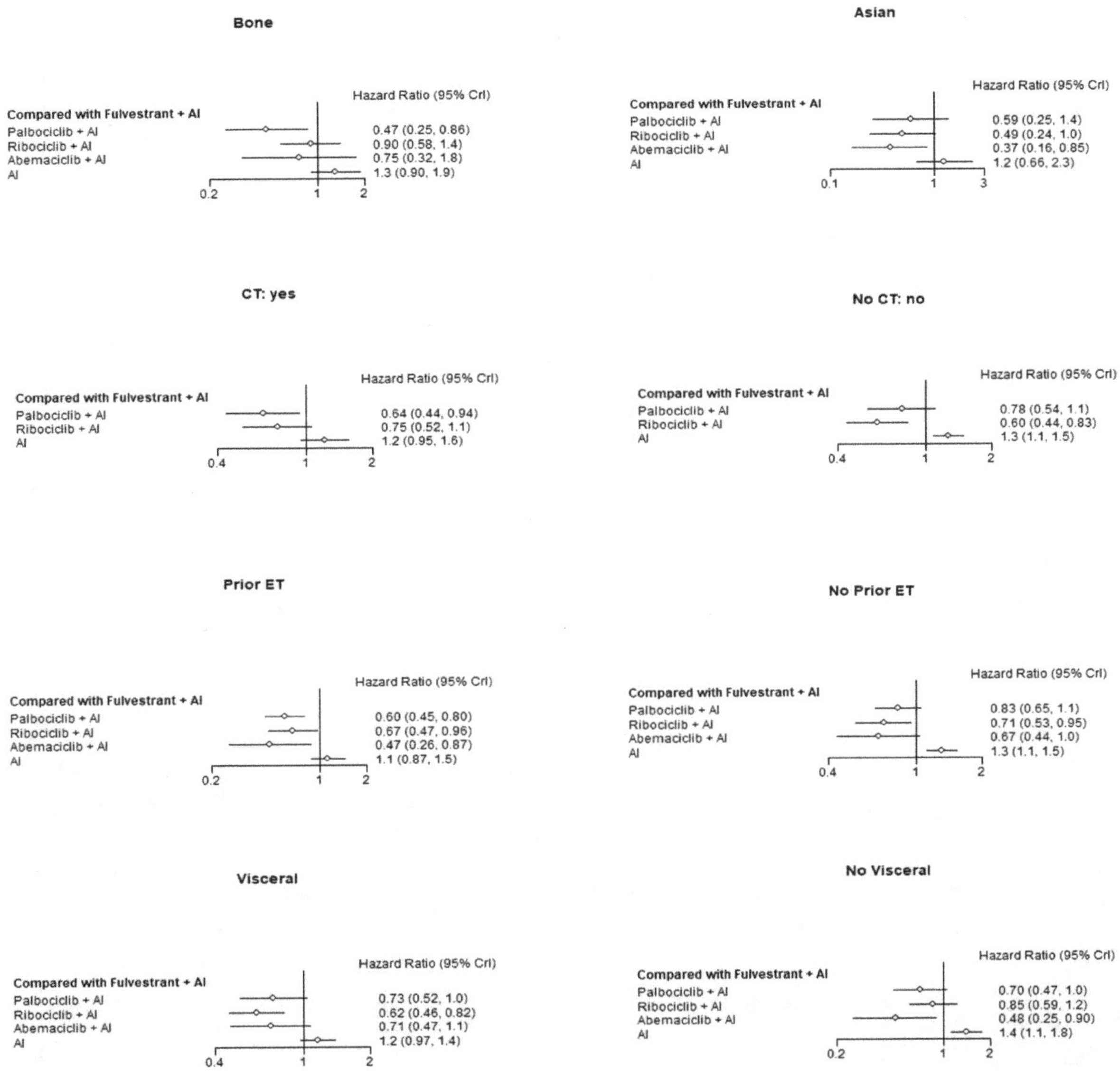

Figure 4. Forest plot on treatment effect for progression-free survival by subgroups in the indirect comparison between CDK 4/6 inhibitors, aromatase inhibitors, and fulvestrant. AI: Aromatase inhibitor; CT: Chemotherapy; ET: Endocrine therapy.

For PFS analysis of the seven selected phase III RCTs [5,12–15,25,27] according to prespecified subgroups, a total of 2278 patients were in the CDK 4/6 inhibitors or fulvestrant arm and a total of 1891 patients were in ET arm alone. Among them, 335 patients in the CDK 4/6 inhibitors and 337 patients in ET arms alone were premenopausal. The indirect comparison between CDK 4/6 inhibitors combination strategies and F-based therapies showed quite consistent PFS improvements in favor of CDK 4/6 inhibitors in all subgroups. With reference to the most important NMA aim, compared with F-based therapy, the CDK 4/6 inhibitor combination strategy was associated with PFS improvement also in patients with disease limited to the bone or in non-visceral sites. Although no statistically significant difference emerged among the three classes of inhibitors in indirect comparison, NMA results also suggested a different potential tropism among them, which should be further investigated in prospective clinical trials.

Table 3. Main characteristics of the patients included in the randomized trials evaluated for the present network meta-analysis.

Characteristics	PALOMA-2, n (%)		MONALEESA-2, n (%)		MONARCH-3, n (%)		MONALEESA-7, n (%)		FALCON [a], n (%)		SWOG [b], n (%)		FACT4, n (%)	
	L. + Palb.	L.	L. + Rib.	L.	L or A. + Abem.	L. or A.	Rib. + T or nAIs	T or nAIs	F.	A.	F.+ A.	A.	F. + A.	A.
No. of patients	444	222	334	334	328	165	335	337	230	232	345	349	258	256
Age:														
• Median (range), years	62(3089)	61 (28–88)	62 (23–91)	63 (29–88)	63 (38–87)	63 (32–88)	43 (25–58)	45 (29–58)	64 (38–87)	62 (36–90)	65 (36–91)	65 (27–92)	65 (33–86)	63 (36–90)
• <65 years	263 (59.2)	141 (63.5)	NR	NR	NR	NR	NR	NR	NR	NR	NR	NR	124 (48.1)	145 (56.6)
• ≥65 years	181 (40.8)	81 (36.5)	NR	NR	NR	NR	NR	NR	108 (47)	91 (39)	NR	NR	134 (51.9)	111 (43.3)
Ethnicity:														
• White	344 (77.5)	172 (77.5)	269 (80.5)	280 (83.8)	186 (56.7)	102 (61.8)	187 (56)	201 (60)	175 (76)	174 (75)	NR	NR	242 (93.8)	237 (92.6)
• Asian	65 (14.6)	30 (13.5)	28 (8.4)	23 (6.9)	103 (31.4)	45 (27.3)	99 (30)	99 (29)	36 (16)	34 (15)	NR	NR	4 (1.6)	2 (0.8)
• Black	8 (1.8)	3 (1.4)	10 (3.0)	7 (2.1)	NR	NR	10 (3)	9 (3)	NR	NR	NR	NR	1 (0.4)	2 (0.8)
• Other	27 (6.1)	17 (7.7)	27 (8.1)	24 (7.2)	11 (3.4)	7 (4.2)	39 (12)	28 (8)	19 (8)	24 (10)	NR	NR	11 (4.3)	15 (5.9)
Hormone receptor status:														
• ER+, PgR+	NR	NR	NR	NR	255 (77.7)	127 (77.0)	290 (87)	288 (85)	175 (76)	179 (77)	NR	NR	193 (74.8)	195 (76.2)
• ER+, PgR−	NR	NR	NR	NR	70 (21.3)	36 (21.8)	NR	NR	44 (19)	43 (19)	NR	NR	60 (23.3)	51 (19.9)
• Unknown	NR	NR	NR	NR	NR	NR	NR	NR	10(4)	7 (3)	NR	NR	4 (1.6)	6 (2.3)
• ER−PgR+	NR	NR	NR	NR	NR	NR	NR	NR	1 (<1)	3 (1)	NR	NR	1 (0.4)	4 (1.6)
Performance status:														
• ECOG 0	257 (57.9)	102 (45.9)	205 (61.4)	202 (60.5)	192 (58.5)	104 (63.0)	245 (73)	255 (76)	117 (51)	115 (50)	NR	NR	NR	NR
• ECOG 1	178 (40.1)	117 (52.7)	129 (38.6)	132 (39.5)	136 (41.5)	61 (37.0)	87 (26)	78 (23)	106 (46)	105 (45)	NR	NR	NR	NR
• ECOG 2	9 (2.0)	3 (1.4)	NR	NR	NR	NR	0	1 (<1)	7 (3)	12 (5)	NR	NR	NR	NR
• ECOG > 2	NR	NR	NR	NR	NR	NR	NR	NR	NR	NR	NR	NR	NR	NR
• Unavailable	NR	NR	NR	NR	NR	NR	3 (1)	3 (1)	NR	NR	NR	NR	NR	NR

Table 3. *Cont.*

Characteristics	PALOMA-2, n (%)		MONALEESA-2, n (%)		MONARCH-3, n (%)		MONALEESA-7, n (%)		FALCON [a], n (%)		SWOG [b], n (%)		FACT4, n (%)	
	L. + Palb.	L.	L. + Rib.	L.	L or A. + Abem.	L. or A.	Rib. + T or nAIs	T or nAIs	F.	A.	F.+ A.	A.	F. + A.	A.
Disease stage:														
• I	51 (11.5)	30 (13.5)	NR	NR	NR	NR	NR	NR	NR	NR	NR	NR	NR	NR
• II	137 (30.9)	68 (30.6)	NR	NR	NR	NR	NR	NR	NR	NR	NR	NR	NR	NR
• III	72 (16.2)	39 (17.6)	1 (0.3)	3 (0.9)	NR	NR	NR	NR	NR	NR	NR	NR	NR	NR
• IV	138 (31.1)	72 (32.4)	333 (99.7)	331 (99.1)	NR	NR	NR	NR	202 (88)	200 (86)	NR	NR	245 (95)	242 (94.5)
• Unknown	36 (8.1)	1 (0.5)	NR	NR	NR	NR	NR	NR	NR	NR	NR	NR	NR	NR
Site of metastasis:														
• Bone only	103 (23.2)	48 (21.6)	69 (20.1)	78 (23.4)	70 (21.3)	39 (23.6)	81 (24)	78 (23)	24 (10)	24 (10)	76 (22.0)	75 (21.5)	63 (24.4)	71 (27.7)
• Visceral	214 (48.2)	110 (49.5)	197 (59.0)	196 (58.7)	172 (52.4)	89 (53.9)	193 (58)	188 (56)	135 (59)	119 (51)	167 (48.4)	181 (51.9)	134 (51.9)	124 (48.4)
• Non- visceral	230 (51.8)	112 (50.5)	NR	NR	NR	NR	NR	NR	60 (26)	81 (35)	102 (29.6)	93 (26.6)	195 (28.1)	NR
• Lymph nodes	NR	NR	133 (39.8)	123 (36.8)	NR	NR	142 (42)	158 (47)	NR	NR	NR	NR	NR	NR
• Other	NR	NR	45 (12.9)	33 (9.9)	86 (26.2)	37 (22.4)	8 (2)	8(2)	11 (4)	8 (4)	NR	NR	1 (0.4)	1 (0.4)
Measurable disease:														
• Yes	NR	NR	NR	NR	267 (81.4)	130 (78.8)	NR	NR	193 (84)	196 (84)	188 (54.5)	188 (53.9)	129 (50.0)	113 (44.1)
• No	NR	NR	NR	NR	61 (18.6)	35 (21.2)	NR	NR	NR	NR	157 (45.5)	161 (46.1)	129 (50.0)	143 (55.9)
Disease-free interval:														
• *De novo*	167 (37.6)	81 (36.5)	114 (34.1)	113 (33.8)	NR	NR	136 (41)	134 (40)	NR	NR	NR	NR	NR	NR
• ≤12 months	99 (22.3)	48 (21.6)	4 (1.2)	10 (3.0)	NR	NR	23 (7)	13 (4)	NR	NR	NR	NR	14 (5.4)	18 (7.0)
• >12 months	178 (40.1)	93 (41.9)	216 (64.7)	210 (62.9)	NR	NR	176 (53)	190 (56)	NR	NR	NR	NR	85 (32.9)	78 (30.5)
• Unknown	NR	NR	NR	1 (0.3)	NR	NR	NR	NR	NR	NR	NR	NR	NR	NR

Table 3. *Cont.*

Characteristics	PALOMA-2, n (%)		MONALEESA-2, n (%)		MONARCH-3, n (%)		MONALEESA-7, n (%)		FALCON [a], n (%)		SWOG [b], n (%)		FACT4, n (%)	
	L. + Palb.	L.	L. + Rib.	L.	L or A. + Abem.	L. or A.	Rib. + T or nAIs	T or nAIs	F.	A.	F.+ A.	A.	F. + A.	A.
No. of disease sites														
• 0	NR	NR	2 (0.6)	1 (0.3)	NR	NR	1 (<1)	NR	NR	NR	NR	NR	NR	NR
• 1	138 (31.1)	66 (29.7)	100 (29.9)	117 (35.0)	96 (29.3)	47 (28.5)	112 (33)	117 (35)	NR	NR	NR	NR	NR	NR
• 2	117 (26.4)	52 (23.4)	118 (35.3)	103 (30.8)	76 (23.2)	42 (25.5)	106 (32)	99 (29)	NR	NR	NR	NR	NR	NR
• 3	112 (25.2)	61 (27.5)	114 (34.1)	113 (33.8)	154 (47)[2]	75 (45.5)[2]	116 (35)	121 (36)	NR	NR	NR	NR	NR	NR
• ≥4	77 (17.3)	43 (19.4)	NR	NR	NR	NR	NR	NR	NR	NR	NR	NR	NR	NR
Prior chemotherapy:														
• Adjuvant	180 (40.5)	89 (40.1)	146 (43.7)	145 (43.4)	125 (38.1)	66 (40.0)	138 (41)	138 (41)	35 (15)	27 (12)	103 (29.9)	129 (37.0)	108 (41.9)	127 (49.6)
• Neoadjuvant	54 (12.2)	32 (14.4)	*	*	*	*	*	*	11 (5)	16 (7)	NR	NR	NR	NR
• Palliative	NR	NR	NR	NR	NR	NR	47 (14)	47 (14)	36 (16)	43 (19)	NR	NR	NR	NR
• None	NR	NR	NR	NR	203 (61.9)	99 (60.0)	150 (45)	152 (45)	NR	NR	242 (70.1)	220 (63.0)	NR	NR
Prior hormonal therapy:														
• Adjuvant	249 (56.1)	126 (56.8)	175 (52.4)	171 (51.2)	150 (45.7)	80 (48.5)	127 (38)	141 (42)	2 (1)	1 (<1)	139 (40.3)	141 (40.4)	180 (69.8)	168 (65.6)
• Neoadjuvant	NR		*	*										
• None	NR	NR	NR	NR	178 (54.3)	85 (51.5)	208 (62)	196 (58)	NR	NR	206 (59.7)	208 (59.6)	NR	NR
Type of adjuvant ET:														
• Tamoxifen	209 (47.1)	98 (44.1)	140 (41.9)	145 (43.4)	NR	NR	NR	NR	NR	NR	NR	NR	NR	NR
• Anastrozole	56 (12.6)	29 (13.1)	47 (14.1)	42 (12.6)	NR	NR	NR	NR	NR	NR	NR	NR	NR	NR
• Letrozole	36 (8.1)	16 (7.2)	34 (10.2)	25 (7.5)	NR	NR	NR	NR	NR	NR	NR	NR	NR	NR
• Exemestane	30 (6.8)	13 (5.9)	19 (5.7)	25 (7.5)	NR	NR	NR	NR	NR	NR	NR	NR	NR	NR
• Other	NR	NR	8 (2.4)	7 (2.1)	NR	NR	NR	NR	NR	NR	NR	NR	NR	NR

[a] The experimental arm consisted of F 500 mg intramuscular injection; on days 0, 14, 28, then every 28 days thereafter. [b] The experimental arm consisted of F 500 mg on day 1 and 250 mg on days 14 and 28 and monthly thereafter. * Patients included among those of the adjuvant setting. L: letrozole; Palb.: palbociclib; Rib: Ribociclib; A: anastrozole; Abe: abemaciclib; T: tamoxifen; nAIs: non-steroidal aromatase inhibitors; F: fulvestrant; NR: not reported; ECOG: Eastern Cooperative Oncology Group; ER: estrogen receptor; PgR: progesteron receptor; +: positive.

4. Discussion

HR+/HER2− BC is the most common subtype of this disease, representing approximately 60–70% of all breast tumors [1]. For many years, the sequential use of ET was the preferred approach in HR+ MBC patients due to its effectiveness and favorable toxicity profile [3,30,31]. The recent introduction of new combinations of ET plus CDK 4/6 or phosphatidylinositol 3-kinases (PI3K) inhibitors led to further clinical improvement in HR+ MBC patients [30,31]. Regarding the first-line setting, several randomized phase III clinical trials clearly demonstrated that the three highly selective CDK 4/6 inhibitors (palbociclib, ribociclib, abemaciclib) significantly improve ORR and CB and prolong PFS when combined with an AI or tamoxifen, both in pre- and post-menopausal women [12–15].

Although clinical outcomes are very similar for the three CDK 4/6 inhibitors and are not influenced by classic clinical and pathological factors, several differences were recognized concerning their toxicity profile and mechanism of action. In the patients who received the combination CDK 4/6 inhibitor plus ET, a higher incidence of hematologic adverse events occurred compared to control groups. The most common hematologic adverse events with grade 3 or 4 were neutropenia (43% vs. 1%), leucopenia (20% vs. 0.4%), anemia (5% vs. 1%), and thrombocytopenia (2% vs. 0.1%) [32]. Despite the high incidence of neutropenia reported in the RCTs, a higher incidence of febrile neutropenia was not recorded, which is evident just in 1.3% of patients. Unlike palbociclib and ribociclib, abemaciclib caused low-grade diarrhea and transaminase elevation, readily managed with conventional medications or dose reduction [17]. On the other hand, data suggest that abemaciclib has distinct single-agent activity at the molecular level, which could reflect its unique effects and toxicity profile [33]. For example, abemaciclib, but not ribociclib or pabociclib, is a potent inhibitor of kinases other than CDK 4/6, including CDK1/cyclin B, which appears to cause arrest in the G2 phase of the cell cycle, and CDK2/cyclin E/A, which is implicated in resistance to palbociclib. Whereas ribociclib and palbociclib induce cytostasis, and cells adapt to these drugs within 2–3 days of exposure, abemaciclib induces cell death and durably blocks cell proliferation. Abemaciclib is active even in pRB-deficient cells in which CDK 4/6 inhibition by palbociclib or ribociclib is completely ineffective [34]. In luminal tumors, some useful biomarkers are being studied to identify the best target treatment combined with anti-hormonal therapy and which can then determine the ideal choice for activity rather than toxicity. Recently, the *PI3K* mutation presented in progressive luminal tumors from the first-line treatment with AI showed a significant benefit in PFS when associated with F [35].

Against this background, knowing whether these three agents can be interchangeable remains an urgent unmet clinical need [21,32,36,37]. Thus, a better understanding of molecular differences is a relevant challenge since it could be informative for their right use in the clinical setting. Additionally, since there are no comparative data between CDK 4/6 inhibitors and F, the hormonal agent approved in endocrine-naïve patients with MBC for first-line setting, the identification of the most suitable HR+ MBC patients who can benefit most from the less toxic F-based-therapy is still a significant challenge [5,21]. Herein, we performed a meta-analysis, including only data from phase III RCTs available concerning the same clinical scenario. This approach allows the synthesis of a large body of evidence while retaining the benefits of randomization within each trial. Hence, we use this indirect comparison method to investigate whether F-based ET could still play a role in some specific subgroup of patients with HR+ MBC in the first-line setting

In this meta-analysis, we found that CDK 4/6 inhibitors produced significant improvement in ORR, CB, and PFS in all patients with HR+ MBC in comparison with F-based therapies. Furthermore, these results were independent of age, race, performance status, disease site, prior chemotherapy, prior ET, disease-free interval after adjuvant treatment, menopausal status, type of CDK 4/6 inhibitor or expression of the progesterone receptor. Interestingly, significant PFS improvement in favor of CDK 4/6 inhibitors was observed even in patients with bone-only disease and in non-visceral disease. Due to the lack of convincing efficacy criteria to prefer one or the other CDK 4/6 inhibitor, the choice should rely on the toxicity profile. It must be remembered, however, that no direct comparison has ever been performed between the three CDK 4/6 inhibitors to allow an appropriate selection in the clinic.

Our meta-analysis has several limitations suggesting caution in interpreting the results. First, it is not based on individual patient data but was conducted considering the HR and 95% CIs of each study extracted. Moreover, for some subgroups, the HRs were not reported in all studies, particularly in F-based trials. In addition, the number of trials was relatively limited, preventing formal comparisons among all treatment strategies for each group. Second, and this is a well-known caveat of studies with F, not all the included studies with this compound used the now considered standard dose (500 mg monthly plus an additional dose of 500 mg for 15 days during the first month) [25,27]. The CONFIRM trial has revealed a superior activity of 500 mg when compared with 250 mg of F in terms of PFS and OS [6]. Therefore, the non-standard F dose used in some trials may partially bias our findings. Third, while the four RCTs [12–15] including CDK 4/6 inhibitors are rather homogenous in terms of inclusions criteria and patient characteristics, the greater heterogeneity observed in F-based studies [5,25,27] inevitably affected the pooled meta-analyses results. For instance, the line of therapy, metastatic sites, tumor burden, prior anti-estrogen drugs, and anti-estrogen treatment sequence, previous endocrine therapies sensitivity were also heterogeneous. Notably, F was more effective in endocrine-naïve patients without the visceral disease [5]. As demonstrated in Table 1, the FALCON trial exclusively included those patients who had never been exposed to ET, both in the metastatic and early settings. By contrast, a percentage ranging from 40 to 65% of patients included in the remaining trials were previously exposed to ET in the adjuvant or neoadjuvant settings. In addition, F efficacy in "bone-only" limited disease was not established in all studies [27]. Finally, for peri and premenopausal patients, we cannot rule out the possibility that the administered luteinizing hormone-releasing hormone analog (LHRHa) may affect the final estimation, as LHRHa itself was reported as an effective endocrine approach in breast cancer. Moreover, the limited number of peri or premenopausal patients in F-based studies makes a comparison between F and CDK 4/6 inhibitor ET strategies unreliable in this setting of patients. Specifically, while the FALCON and SWOG trials were enrolled merely post-menopausal patients, in the FACT trial, premenopausal patients were also included and were treated with GnRHa. Unfortunately, they only represented 3.1% of the experimental arm. Although previous reviews and meta-analyses of treatments in MBC patients have been conducted, many of these studies focus on population different from the current study. For example, Ayyagari et al. explored the safety and efficacy of only two CDK 4/6 inhibitors (palbociclib and ribociclib) in postmenopausal women after progression on a non-steroidal AI [35]. Ding et al. also conducted a similar NMA, focusing on the results of all three CDK4/6 inhibitors in phase II and III trials both in the first and second lines; however, the analysis did not include a direct comparison with F in first-line treatment [32]. Finally, El Rassy et al. investigated which CDK4/6 inhibitor was more effective in patients with luminal breast cancer, but their study was limited by the small sample size and lack of studies on F (1 included) [36]. Therefore, our study specifically focused on the results of phase III studies in the first-line setting and comprised an indirect comparison with first-line F. In addition, the present meta-analysis includes recently published data that were not included in previous reviews, in particular, the results of MONALEESA-7 on premenopausal women [32,36,37]. Despite the differences in study design and specific limitations, the results of our and previous NMAs are consistent in reporting the improved clinical outcomes obtained with CDK4/6 inhibitors compared with monotherapy [32,36,37].

5. Conclusions

In conclusion, the results of this meta-analysis confirm that CDK 4/6 inhibitors have similar efficacy when associated with an AI in the first-line treatment of HR+ MBC, and are superior to either F or AI monotherapy, regardless of any other patients or tumor characteristics. Though all CDK 4/6 inhibitors resulted associated with similar outcomes, the differences in toxicity profile, drug interactions, and patient preferences seem to be the main factors to be considered in the clinical decision-making process. Interestingly, CDK 4/6 inhibitors with AI resulted in more effective than F-based therapies even in patients with the bone-limited disease and, what is more, in patients without visceral disease involvement. Hence, the use of F in the first-line setting is destined to be abandoned as a single agent, and its right place in HR+ MBC patients management needs to be urgently refined. Based on preclinical and early clinical trial results, its mechanism of action and pharmacokinetic properties make it an ideal backbone for combination therapies contributing to overcome or delaying endocrine resistance. Rational combinations with other therapies, such as *PI3K* inhibitors, HER2-directed therapies, and immunotherapy, are being explored. The emerging data also suggest a potential use of CDK4/6-targeted approaches in neoadjuvant settings (Supplementary Table S1). Different clinical trials are also ongoing to assess the safety and efficacy of CDK4/6 inhibitors alone or in combination with chemotherapy in different groups of patients. These trials, together with future comparative studies and biomarker analyses, are indispensable to better select patients who derive the greatest benefit from a specific class of CDK 4/6 inhibitors.

Author Contributions: Conceptualization—V.R. and A.F. Methodology—P.B., D.G., V.R. and A.F. Software—P.B. and D.G. Formal Analysis—P.B. and D.G. Resources—V.R., A.F., P.B. and D.G. Data Curation—P.B. and D.G. Writing—Original Draft Preparation—V.R. and A.F. Writing—Review & Editing—V.R., P.B., D.G., C.N., G.F., S.G., M.R., G.C., L.V., R.L.M., E.B., F.M., F.C. and A.F.

Acknowledgments: Editorial assistance was provided by Luca Giacomelli, Ambra Corti and Aashni Shah (Polistudium SRL). This assistance was supported by internal funds.

References

1. Sorlie, T.; Perou, C.M.; Tibshirani, R.; Aas, T.; Geisler, S.; Johnsen, H.; Hastie, T.; Eisen, M.B.; van de Rijn, M.; Jeffrey, S.S.; et al. Gene expression patterns of breast carcinomas distinguish tumor subclasses with clinical implications. *Proc. Natl. Acad. Sci. USA* **2001**, *98*, 10869–10874. [CrossRef] [PubMed]
2. Gonzalez-Angulo, A.M.; Morales-Vasquez, F.; Hortobagyi, G.N. Overview of resistance to systemic therapy in patients with breast cancer. *Adv. Exp. Med. Biol.* **2007**, *608*, 1–22. [CrossRef] [PubMed]
3. Rugo, H.S.; Rumble, R.B.; Macrae, E.; Barton, D.L.; Connolly, H.K.; Dickler, M.N.; Fallowfield, L.; Fowble, B.; Ingle, J.N.; Jahanzeb, M.; et al. Endocrine therapy for hormone receptor-positive metastatic breast cancer: American Society of Clinical Oncology Guideline. *J. Clin. Oncol.* **2016**, *34*, 3069–3103. [CrossRef] [PubMed]
4. Kiang, D.T.; Kennedy, B.J. Tamoxifen (antiestrogen) therapy in advanced breast cancer. *Ann. Intern. Med.* **1977**, *87*, 687–690. [CrossRef]
5. Robertson, J.F.R.; Bondarenko, I.M.; Trishkina, E.; Dvorkin, M.; Panasci, L.; Manikhas, A.; Shparyk, Y.; Cardona-Huerta, S.; Cheung, K.L.; Philco-Salas, M.J.; et al. Fulvestrant 500 mg versus anastrozole 1 mg for hormone receptor-positive advanced breast cancer (FALCON): An international, randomised, double-blind, phase 3 trial. *Lancet* **2016**, *388*, 2997–3005. [CrossRef]
6. Di, L.A.; Jerusalem, G.; Petruzelka, L.; Torres, R.; Bondarenko, I.N.; Khasanov, R.; Verhoeven, D.; Pedrini, J.L.; Smirnova, I.; Lichinitser, M.R.; et al. Results of the CONFIRM phase III trial comparing fulvestrant 250 mg with fulvestrant 500 mg in postmenopausal women with estrogen receptor-positive advanced breast cancer. *J. Clin. Oncol.* **2010**, *28*, 4594–4600. [CrossRef]
7. Mouridsen, H.; Gershanovich, M.; Sun, Y.; Perez-Carrion, R.; Boni, C.; Monnier, A.; Apffelstaedt, J.; Smith, R.; Sleeboom, H.P.; Jaenicke, F.; et al. Phase III study of letrozole versus tamoxifen as first-line therapy of advanced breast cancer in postmenopausal women: Analysis of survival and update of efficacy from the International Letrozole Breast Cancer Group. *J. Clin. Oncol.* **2003**, *21*, 2101–2109. [CrossRef]
8. Nabholtz, J.M. Advanced breast cancer updates on anastrozole versus tamoxifen. *J. Steroid Biochem. Mol. Biol.* **2003**, *86*, 321–325. [CrossRef]
9. Paridaens, R.J.; Dirix, L.Y.; Beex, L.V.; Nooij, M.; Cameron, D.A.; Cufer, T.; Piccart, M.J.; Bogaerts, J.; Therasse, P. Phase III study comparing exemestane with tamoxifen as first-line hormonal treatment of metastatic breast cancer in postmenopausal women: The European Organisation for Research and Treatment of Cancer Breast Cancer Cooperative Group. *J. Clin. Oncol.* **2008**, *26*, 4883–4890. [CrossRef]
10. Mauri, D.; Pavlidis, N.; Polyzos, N.P.; Ioannidis, J.P. Survival with aromatase inhibitors and inactivators versus standard hormonal therapy in advanced breast cancer: Meta-analysis. *J. Natl. Cancer Inst.* **2006**, *98*, 1285–1291. [CrossRef]

11. Schettini, F.; De Santo, I.; Rea, C.G.; De Placido, P.; Formisano, L.; Giuliano, M.; Arpino, G.; De Laurentiis, M.; Puglisi, F.; De Placido, S.; et al. CDK 4/6 inhibitors as single agent in advanced solid tumors. *Front. Oncol.* **2018**, *8*, 608. [CrossRef] [PubMed]
12. Finn, R.S.; Martin, M.; Rugo, H.S.; Jones, S.; Im, S.A.; Gelmon, K.; Harbeck, N.; Lipatov, O.N.; Walshe, J.M.; Moulder, S.; et al. Palbociclib and letrozole in advanced breast cancer. *N. Engl. J. Med.* **2016**, *375*, 1925–1936. [CrossRef]
13. Hortobagyi, G.N.; Stemmer, S.M.; Burris, H.A.; Yap, Y.S.; Sonke, G.S.; Paluch-Shimon, S.; Campone, M.; Petrakova, K.; Blackwell, K.L.; Winer, E.P.; et al. Updated results from MONALEESA-2, a phase III trial of first-line ribociclib plus letrozole versus placebo plus letrozole in hormone receptor-positive, HER2-negative advanced breast cancer. *Ann. Oncol.* **2018**, *29*, 1541–1547. [CrossRef] [PubMed]
14. Goetz, M.P.; Toi, M.; Campone, M.; Sohn, J.; Paluch-Shimon, S.; Huober, J.; Park, I.H.; Trédan, O.; Chen, S.C.; Manso, L.; et al. MONARCH 3: Abemaciclibas initial therapy for advanced breast cancer. *J. Clin. Oncol.* **2017**, *35*, 3638–3646. [CrossRef] [PubMed]
15. Tripathy, D.; Im, S.A.; Colleoni, M.; Franke, F.; Bardia, A.; Harbeck, N.; Hurvitz, S.A.; Chow, L.; Sohn, J.; Lee, K.S.; et al. Ribociclib plus endocrine therapy for premenopausal women with hormone-receptor-positive, advanced breast cancer (MONALEESA-7): A randomised phase 3 trial. *Lancet Oncol.* **2018**, *19*, 904–915. [CrossRef]
16. Cristofanilli, M.; Turner, N.C.; Bondarenko, I.; Ro, J.; Im, S.A.; Masuda, N.; Colleoni, M.; DeMichele, A.; Loi, S.; Verma, S.; et al. Fulvestrant plus palbociclib versus fulvestrant plus placebo for treatment of hormone-receptor-positive, HER2-negative metastatic breast cancer that progressed on previous endocrine therapy (PALOMA-3): Final analysis of the multicentre, double-blind, phase 3 randomised controlled trial. *Lancet Oncol.* **2016**, *17*, 425–439. [CrossRef]
17. Spring, L.M.; Zangardi, M.L.; Moy, B.; Bardia, A. Clinical management of potential toxicities and drug interactions related to cyclin-dependent kinase 4/6 inhibitors in breast cancer: Practical considerations and recommendations. *Oncologist* **2017**, *22*, 1039–1048. [CrossRef]
18. Turner, N.C.; Slamon, D.J.; Ro, J.; Bondarenko, I.; Im, S.A.; Masuda, N.; Colleoni, M.; DeMichele, A.; Loi, S.; Verma, S.; et al. Overall survival with palbociclib and fulvestrant in advanced breast cancer. *N. Engl. J. Med.* **2018**, *379*, 1926–1936. [CrossRef]
19. Hurvitz, S.A.; Im, S.A.; Lu, Y.S.; Colleoni, M.; Franke, F.A.; Bardia, A.; Harbeck, N.; Chow, L.W.C.; Sohn, J. Phase III MONALEESA-7 trial of premenopausal patients with HR+/HER2− advanced breast cancer (ABC) treated with endocrine therapy ± ribociclib: Overall survival (OS) results. *J. Clin. Oncol.* 2019. [CrossRef]
20. Im, S.A.; Lu, Y.S.; Bardia, A.; Harbeck, N.; Colleoni, M.; Franke, F.; Chow, L.; Sohn, J.; Lee, K.S.; Campos-Gomez, S.; et al. Overall survival with ribociclib plus endocrine therapy in breast cancer. *N. Engl. J. Med.* **2019**, *381*, 307–316. [CrossRef]
21. van Ommen-Nijhof, A.; Konings, I.R.; van Zeijl, C.J.J.; Uyl-de Groot, C.A.; van der Noort, V.; Jager, A.; Sonke, G.S.; SONIA Study Steering Committee. Selecting the optimal position of CDK 4/6 inhibitors in hormone receptor-positive advanced breast cancer – the SONIA study: Study protocol for a randomized controlled trial. *BMC Cancer* **2018**, *18*, 1146. [CrossRef] [PubMed]
22. Cristofanilli, M.; DeMichele, A.; Giorgetti, C.; Turner, N.C.; Slamon, D.J.; Im, S.A.; Masuda, N.; Verma, S.; Loi, S.; Colleoni, M.; et al. Predictors of prolonged benefit from palbociclib plus fulvestrant in women with endocrine-resistant hormone receptor-positive/human epidermal growth factor receptor 2-negative metastatic breast cancer in PALOMA-3. *Eur. J. Cancer* **2018**, *104*, 21–31. [CrossRef] [PubMed]
23. O'Leary, B.; Cutts, R.J.; Liu, Y.; Hrebien, S.; Huang, X.; Fenwick, K.; André, F.; Loibl, S.; Loi, S.; Garcia-Murillas, I.; et al. The genetic landscape and clonal evolution of breast cancer resistance to palbociclib plus fulvestrant in the PALOMA-3 trial. *Cancer Discov.* **2018**, *8*, 1390–1403. [CrossRef] [PubMed]
24. O'Leary, B.; Hrebien, S.; Morden, J.P.; Beaney, M.; Fribbens, C.; Huang, X.; Liu, Y.; Bartlett, C.H.; Koehler, M.; Cristofanilli, M.; et al. Early circulating tumor DNA dynamics and clonal selection with palbociclib and fulvestrant for breast cancer. *Nat. Commun.* **2018**, *9*, 896. [CrossRef] [PubMed]
25. Mehta, R.S.; Barlow, W.E.; Albain, K.S.; Vandenberg, T.A.; Dakhil, S.R.; Tirumali, N.R.; Lew, D.L.; Hayes, D.F.; Gralow, J.R.; Livingston, R.B.; et al. Combination anastrozole and fulvestrant in metastatic breast cancer. *N. Engl. J. Med.* **2012**, *367*, 435–444. [CrossRef]

26. Mehta, R.S.; Barlow, W.E.; Albain, K.S.; Vandenberg, T.A.; Dakhil, S.R.; Tirumali, N.R.; Lew, D.L.; Hayes, D.F.; Gralow, J.R.; Linden, H.H.; et al. Overall survival with fulvestrant plus anastrozole in metastatic breast cancer. *N. Engl. J. Med.* **2019**, *380*, 1226–1234. [CrossRef]
27. Bergh, J.; Jonsson, P.E.; Lidbrink, E.K.; Trudeau, M.; Eiermann, W.; Brattström, D.; Lindemann, J.P.; Wiklund, F.; Henriksson, R. FACT: An open-label randomized phase III study of fulvestrant and anastrozole in combination compared with anastrozole alone as first-line therapy for patients with receptor-positive postmenopausal breast cancer. *J. Clin. Oncol.* **2012**, *30*, 1919–1925. [CrossRef]
28. Van Valkenhoef, G.; Lu, G.; de Brock, B.; Hillege, H.; Ades, A.E.; Welton, N.J. Automating network meta-analysis. *Res. Synth. Methods* **2012**, *3*, 285–299. [CrossRef]
29. Van Valkenhoef, G. GEMTC: Network Meta-Analysis Using Bayesian Methods. R package version 0.8-2. Available online: https://rdrr.io/cran/gemtc/ (accessed on 25 October 2019).
30. Vidula, N.; Rugo, H.S. Emerging data on improving response to hormone therapy: The role of novel targeted agents. *Expert Rev. Anticancer Ther.* **2018**, *18*, 3–18. [CrossRef]
31. Başaran, G.A.; Twelves, C.; Dieras, V.; Cortés, J.; Awada, A. Ongoing unmet needs in treating estrogen receptor-positive/HER2-negative metastatic breast cancer. *Cancer Treat. Rev.* **2018**, *63*, 144–155. [CrossRef]
32. Ding, W.; Li, Z.; Wang, C.; Ruan, G.; Chen, L.; Tu, C. The CDK 4/6 inhibitor in HR-positive advanced breast cancer: A systematic review and meta-analysis. *Medicine (Baltimore)* **2018**, *97*, e10746. [CrossRef] [PubMed]
33. Corona, S.P.; Generali, D. Abemaciclib: A CDK 4/6 inhibitor for the treatment of HR+/. *Drug Des. Devel. Ther.* **2018**, *12*, 321–330. [CrossRef] [PubMed]
34. Mills, C.E. Omics profiling of CDK 4/6 inhibitors reveals functionally important secondary targets of abemaciclib. In Proceedings of the Visualizing and Quantifying Drug Distribution in Tissue II, San Francisco, CA, USA, 14 March 2018; SPIE: Bellingham, WA, USA, 2018.
35. André, F.; Ciruelos, E.; Rubovszky, G.; Campone, M.; Loibl, S.; Rugo, H.S.; Iwata, H.; Conte, P.; Mayer, I.A.; Kaufman, B.; et al. Alpelisib for *PIK3CA*-mutated, hormone receptor–positive advanced breast cancer. *N. Engl. J. Med.* **2019**, *380*, 1929–1940. [CrossRef] [PubMed]
36. Ayyagari, R.; Tang, D.; Patterson-Lomba, O.; Zhou, Z.; Xie, J.; Chandiwana, D.; Dalal, A.A.; Niravath, P.A. Progression-free survival with endocrine-based therapies following progression on non-steroidal aromatase inhibitor among postmenopausal women with hormone receptor positive, human epidermal growth factor receptor-2 negative metastatic breast cancer: A network meta-analysis. *Curr. Med. Res. Opin.* **2018**, *34*, 1645–1652. [CrossRef] [PubMed]
37. El, R.E.; Bakouny, Z.; Assi, T.; Kattan, J. Different inhibitors for the same target in metastatic luminal breast cancer: Is there any difference? *Future Oncol.* **2018**, *14*, 891–895. [CrossRef]

13

Clinical Significance of Lymph-Node Ratio in Determining Supraclavicular Lymph-Node Radiation Therapy in pN1 Breast Cancer Patients Who Received Breast-Conserving Treatment (KROG 14-18)

Jaeho Kim [1,†], Won Park [2,†], Jin Hee Kim [1,*], Doo Ho Choi [2], Yeon-Joo Kim [3], Eun Sook Lee [3], Kyung Hwan Shin [4], Jin Ho Kim [4], Kyubo Kim [5], Yong Bae Kim [6], Sung-Ja Ahn [7], Jong Hoon Lee [8], Mison Chun [9], Hyung-Sik Lee [10], Jung Soo Kim [11] and Jihye Cha [12]

1 Department of Radiation Oncology, Dongsan Medical Center, Keimyung University School of Medicine, Daegu 42601, Korea; rainfield@naver.com

2 Department of Radiation Oncology, Samsung Medical Center, Sungkyunkwan University School of Medicine, Seoul 06351, Korea; wonro.park@samsung.com (W.P.); dohochoi@hanmail.net (D.H.C.)

3 Center for Breast Cancer, Research Institute and Hospital, National Cancer Center, Goyang 10408, Korea; jane2000md@gmail.com (Y.-J.K.); eslee@ncc.re.kr (E.S.L.)

4 Department of Radiation Oncology, Seoul National University College of Medicine, Seoul 03080, Korea; radiat@snu.ac.kr (K.H.S.); jinho.kim.md@gmail.com (J.H.K.)

5 Department of Radiation Oncology, Ewha Womans University Mokdong Hospital, Ewha Womans University School of Medicine, Seoul 07804, Korea; kyubokim.ro@gmail.com

6 Department of Radiation Oncology, Yonsei Cancer Center, Yonsei University College of Medicine, Seoul 03722, Korea; ybkim3@yuhs.ac

7 Department of Radiation Oncology, Chonnam National University Medical School, Gwangju 61469, Korea; ahnsja@chonnam.ac.kr

8 Department of Radiation Oncology, St. Vincent's Hospital, The Catholic University of Korea College of Medicine, Seoul 06591, Korea; koppul@catholic.ac.kr

9 Department of Radiation Oncology, Ajou University School of Medicine, Suwon 16499, Korea; chunm@ajou.ac.kr

10 Department of Radiation Oncology, Dong-A University Hospital, Dong-A University School of Medicine, Busan 49201, Korea; hyslee@dau.ac.kr

11 Department of Radiation Oncology, Chonbuk National University Medical School, Jeonju 54907, Korea; jskim@chonbuk.ac.kr

12 Department of Radiation Oncology, Wonju Severance Christian Hospital, Wonju 26426, Korea; lukanus@yonsei.ac.kr

* Correspondence: jhkim@dsmc.or.kr

† These two authors contributed equally to this work.

Abstract: This study evaluated the clinical significance of the lymph-node ratio (LNR) and its usefulness as an indicator of supraclavicular lymph-node radiation therapy (SCNRT) in pN1 breast cancer patients with disease-free survival (DFS) outcomes. We retrospectively analyzed the clinical data of patients with pN1 breast cancer who underwent partial mastectomy and taxane-based sequential adjuvant chemotherapy with postoperative radiation therapy in 12 hospitals (n = 1121). We compared their DFS according to LNR, with a cut-off value of 0.10. The median follow-up period was 66 months (range, 3–112). Treatment failed in 73 patients (6.5%) and there was no significant difference in DFS between the SCNRT group and non-SCNRT group. High LNR (>0.10) showed significantly worse DFS in both univariate and multivariate analyses (0.010 and 0.033, respectively). In a subgroup analysis, the effect of SCNRT on DFS differed significantly among patients with LNR > 0.10 (p = 0.013). High LNR can be used as an independent prognostic factor for pN1 breast cancer patients treated with partial mastectomy and postoperative radiotherapy. It may also be useful in deciding whether to perform SCNRT to improve DFS.

Keywords: breast cancer; radiotherapy; lymph-node ratio; disease-free survival

---

1. Introduction

In addition to surgery, chemotherapy and radiotherapy are both important in curative breast cancer treatment. Radiotherapy has a significant role in the removal of microscopic tumor cells from remnant breast tissue after breast-conserving surgery [1]. Radiotherapy is used to treat not only the remaining breast tissue, but also the tumor cells in the regional lymphatic system, including the axillar and internal mammary lymph nodes. This prevents locoregional failure in patients with breast-conserving surgery and lymph-node metastasis after axillary-lymph-node dissection. It can also reduce distant metastasis [2]. The Danish Breast Cancer Cooperative Group reported the benefits of radiation therapy targeting the supraclavicular area in high-risk breast cancer patients [3,4]. The current guidelines generally recommend that elective nodal irradiation (ENI) be applied to the regional lymphatics as well as the whole breast in locally advanced breast cancer [5–7].

The use of ENI in pathological N1 breast cancer patients is still controversial. Taxane-based chemotherapy has been used as an effective adjuvant therapy for breast cancer for decades, reducing the importance of elective nodal irradiation in low-risk breast cancer [8–10]. There is no consensus on whether ENI should be administered to patients with a low risk of regional lymphatic metastasis, such as those with N1 breast cancer [6,11–13]. The current National Comprehensive Cancer Network (NCCN) guidelines also recommend that ENI be strongly considered in N1 breast cancer [14].

In a study based on existing Korean Radiation Oncology Group (KROG) 14-18 data, supraclavicular lymph-node radiation therapy (SCNRT) was ineffective in N1 breast cancer patients undergoing taxane-based chemotherapy [15]. However, several studies have reported that various risk factors affect the outcomes of patients with N1 breast cancer, and claimed that ENI can be beneficial in patients with N1 breast cancer, depending on the risk factors present [16–18]. The lymph-node ratio (LNR), defined as the proportion of positive axillary lymph nodes among the total number of axillary lymph nodes removed, is recognized as one of these risk factors. Although the absolute number of axillary lymph nodes affected by metastasis is associated with a poor prognosis in the American Joint Committee on Cancer (AJCC) guidelines, axillary-lymph-node dissection techniques may differ across different institutions [19]. Therefore, the number of lymph nodes removed may differ, even when patients have the same numbers of metastatic lymph nodes [20]. Several studies have investigated whether LNR can be used to ensure more accurate nodal staging [19–21]. In a previous single-center retrospective study that examined the relationship between LNR and SCNRT, LNR was found to have utility as an indicator of the suitability of SCNRT [22]. Against this background, it was investigated whether LNR can be used as an index of the suitability of SCNRT in multicenter studies.

2. Materials and Methods

2.1. *Study Design and Patients*

In this study, the records of patients diagnosed with N1 breast cancer who underwent breast-conserving surgery between January 2006 and December 2010 at one of 12 hospitals that are members of KROG were examined. Patients who underwent Adriamycin/Taxol (AT) chemotherapy and post-lumpectomy radiotherapy for N1 breast cancer within this period were included in this study. The eligibility criteria were patients with N1 breast cancer who underwent breast-conserving surgery and axillary-lymph-node dissection, who completed postoperative AT chemotherapy and radiotherapy as planned, and for whom information regarding the pathological features of the tumor was available.

The exclusion criteria were patients who received neoadjuvant chemotherapy or chemotherapy other than AT, had a previous history of malignancy, or were male. Patients with fewer than 10 dissected lymph nodes in total were also excluded from the study to ensure accurate lymph node evaluation. The Institutional Review Board of each participating hospital approved the current study.

The patient data collected were age; the pathological features of each tumor, such as the tumor size, number of tumors, and resection margin; number of positive lymph nodes; histological grade; presence of lymphovascular invasion; and expression status of the estrogen receptor (ER), progesterone receptor (PR), and human epidermal growth factor receptor 2 (HER2). Positivity for ER or PR was defined as an Allred score of 3–8 on immunohistochemistry (IHC). HER2 positivity was defined as either 3+ on IHC staining or 2+ on IHC with a positive fluorescence in situ hybridization or chromogenic in situ hybridization signal. The molecular subtype of each breast cancer was categorized as follows: ER+ or PR+, and HER2− (luminal A); ER+ or PR+, and HER2+ (luminal B); ER−, PR−, and HER2+ (HER2 enriched); or ER−, PR−, and HER2− (triple negative). The optimal cut-off value for LNR was determined with an analysis of the area under the curve (AUC) of a receiver-operating characteristic (ROC) curve. A value of 0.10, for which the sensitivity and specificity were highest, was chosen as the optimal cut-off point for LNR.

2.2. Treatments

In this study, patients who had undergone more than 10 lymph-node dissections after axillary-lymph-node dissection were evaluated. The patients were treated with adjuvant chemotherapy consisting of doxorubicin and cyclophosphamide, followed by paclitaxel or docetaxel, and then by the appropriate adjuvant hormone therapy based on the presence of hormone receptors and the HER2 receptor. All patients underwent whole-breast irradiation (WBI) and tumor-bed boost, and SCNRT was selected according to each institution's policy or physician's preference.

The dose of irradiation for the whole breast was 45.0–60.4 Gy at 1.8–3.0 Gy per fraction and the dose for the tumor bed was 4.0–19.8 Gy at 1.8–4.0 Gy per fraction. The radiation dose to the supraclavicular lymph nodes (SCN) was 45.0–50.4 Gy at 1.8–2.0 Gy per fraction. The borders of each field of WBI or WBI+SCNRT were defined differently in the 12 hospitals according to each institutional policy. The axillary lymph nodes were not intentionally irradiated, but level I and a proportion of level II axillary lymph nodes were covered during WBI while a proportion of the level II and level III axillary lymph nodes and the SCN were irradiated during SCNRT. The inclusion of the internal mammary lymph node in the radiation field was determined according to each hospital's policy, considering the location of the primary tumor, pathologic findings, and status of the metastatic lymph nodes.

2.3. Follow-Up and Endpoints

Disease-free survival (DFS) was defined as the time from the date of diagnosis to any recurrence. The patients were followed up on every 3–6 months after surgery with history and physical examinations in each hospital. Mammography was performed every 12 months. Additional imaging studies were performed in patients with suspicious clinical signs or symptoms.

2.4. Statistical Analysis

Data were analyzed with SPSS ver. 20.0 for Windows (SPSS Inc., Chicago, IL, USA). The Kaplan–Meier method was used to analyze disease-free survival (DFS) and statistical significance was determined with a log-rank test. Cox's stepwise regression analysis was used for the multivariable analysis. Statistically significant variables in the univariate analysis ($p < 0.05$) were included in the Cox's regression model. Statistical significance was set at $p < 0.05$.

3. Results

The characteristics of the patients with pN1 breast cancer are summarized in Table 1. In total, 1121 patients satisfied the inclusion criteria for this study and were enrolled. Among them, 745 patients did not undergo SCNRT and 376 patients did undergo SCNRT. The presence of an extensive intraductal component (EIC), lymphovascular invasion (LVI), number of positive lymph nodes, LNR, and the presence of an extracapsular extension (ECE) occurred significantly more frequently in the SCNRT group than in the non-SCNRT group. LNR was statistically independent of other prognostic factors, such as age, type of surgery, T stage, resection margin, LVI, molecular subtype, and histological grade.

Table 1. Patient characteristics.

Characteristics		**Number of Patients (%)**		***p* Value**
		Non-SCNRT (*n* = 745)	**SCNRT (*n* = 376)**	
Age (years)	≤45	442 (59.3)	221 (58.8)	0.859
	>45	303 (40.7)	155 (41.2)	
OP site	Left	343 (46.0)	193 (51.3)	0.094
	Right	402 (54.0)	183 (48.7)	
Pathology	IDC	702 (94.2)	346 (92.0)	0.157
	Others	43 (5.8)	30 (8.0)	
T stage	T1	388 (52.1)	181 (48.1)	0.282
	T2	351 (47.1)	192 (51.1)	
	T3	6 (0.8)	2 (0.5)	
	T4	0 (0.0)	1 (0.3)	
Number of tumors	Single	615 (82.6)	318 (84.6)	0.392
	Multiple	130 (17.4)	58 (15.4)	
Resection margin	Clear	682 (92.2)	351 (93.9)	0.588
	Less than 1 mm	51 (6.9)	20 (5.3)	
	Positive	7 (0.9)	3 (0.8)	
	Unknown	5	2	
EIC	(−)	344 (71.2)	225 (63.9)	0.025
	(+)	139 (28.8)	127 (36.1)	
	Unknown	262	24	
LVI	(−)	360 (49.0)	81 (24.0)	<0.001
	(+)	375 (51.0)	256 (76.0)	
	Unknown	10	39	
HG	I or II	452 (61.9)	235 (63.0)	0.725
	III	278 (38.1)	138 (37.0)	
	Unknown	15	3	
Anti-HER2 therapy	(−)	678 (91.0)	339 (90.2)	0.644
	(+)	67 (9.0)	37 (9.8)	
Dissected LNs	<20	456 (61.2)	245 (65.2)	0.197
	≥20	289 (38.8)	131 (34.8)	
Number of positive LNs	1	509 (68.5)	121 (32.2)	<0.001
	2	161 (21.7)	145 (38.6)	
	3	73 (9.8)	110 (29.3)	
	Unknown	2	0	
LNR	≤0.10	599 (80.6)	189 (50.3)	<0.001
	>0.10	144 (19.4)	187 (49.7)	
	Unknown	2	0	
ECE	(−)	369 (52.4)	92 (31.8)	<0.001
	(+)	335 (47.6)	197 (68.2)	
	Unknown	41	87	
Hormone therapy	(−)	172 (23.1)	86 (22.9)	0.917
	(+)	571 (76.9)	290 (77.1)	
	Unknown	2	0	
Molecular subtype	Luminal A	498 (67.0)	247 (65.7)	0.19
	Luminal B	71 (9.5)	49 (13.0)	
	HER2-enriched	53 (7.1)	17 (4.5)	
	Triple negative	122 (16.4)	63 (16.8)	
	Unknown	1	0	

Abbreviations: SCNRT, supraclavicular lymph node radiation therapy; OP, operation; IDC, invasive ductal carcinoma; EIC, extensive intraductal component; LVI, lymphovascular invasion; HG, histologic grade; HER2, human epidermal growth factor receptor 2; LNR, lymph-node ratio; ECE, extracapsular extension.

The median follow-up time was 66 months (range, 3–112). The overall 5-year DFS was 93.7%. The 5-year DFS in the subgroup was 92.8% in the SCNRT group and 94.1% in the non-SCNRT group. The patterns of failure are shown in Table 2. Distant metastasis was the major pattern of failure, and regional recurrence limited to the SCN occurred in less than 1% of the total patients.

Table 2. Patterns of failure.

Outcome	No. Patients (%)
Follow-up (months)	
Median (range)	66 (3–112)
Patterns of failure	
NED	1048 (93.5)
LR only	8 (0.7)
RR only	5 (0.4)
DM only	45 (4.0)
LR + DM	1 (0.1)
RR + DM	11 (1.0)
LR + RR + DM	3 (0.3)

Abbreviations: NED, no evidence of disease; LR, local recurrence; RR, regional recurrence; DM, distant metastasis.

A univariate analysis of DFS showed that T stage, LVI, histological grade, luminal type, and LNR were significant factors affecting DFS. In a multivariate analysis of these factors, T stage, LVI, histological grade, and LNR significantly affected DFS (Tables 3 and 4).

A subgroup analysis according to SCNRT was performed to analyze the risk of recurrence according to differences in LNR. In this analysis, the risk of recurrence differed significantly according to LNR in the non-SCNRT group, but there was no such difference in the SCNRT group (Figure 1). The use of SCNRT reduced the difference in the incidence of recurrence according to LNR.

Table 3. Univariate analysis of disease-free survival.

Characteristics		No. (%)	5-Year DFS	*p* Value
T stage	T1	569 (50.7)	97.1	<0.001
	T2–4	552 (49.2)	90.2	
Number of tumors	Single	933 (83.2)	93.9	0.953
	Multiple	188 (16.8)	93.1	
Resection margin	≥1 mm	1033 (92.1)	93.8	0.634
	<1 mm	81 (7.2)	92.5	
EIC	(−)	569 (50.8)	94.8	0.213
	(+)	266 (23.7)	91.8	
LVI	(−)	441 (39.3)	97.0	0.001
	(+)	631 (56.3)	91.4	
HG	I or II	687 (61.3)	96.1	<0.001
	III	416 (37.1)	89.9	
LNR	≤0.10	788 (70.3)	94.9	0.010
	>0.10	331 (29.5)	90.8	
ECE	(−)	461 (41.1)	92.7	0.110
	(+)	532 (47.5)	94.9	
Molecular Subtype	Lumimal A	463 (41.3)	96.0	0.008
	Non-luminal A	657 (58.6)	82.1	

Abbreviations: EIC, extensive intraductal component; LVI, lymphovascular invasion; HG, histologic grade; LNR, lymph-node ratio; ECE, extracapsular extension.

Table 4. Multivariate analysis of disease-free survival.

Characteristics		Cox Regression Model		*p* Value
		Hazard Ratio	95% CI	
T stage	T1 vs. T2–4	2.628	1.489–4.638	0.001
LVI	(−) vs. (+)	1.92	1.071–3.441	0.028
HG	I or II vs. III	2.288	1.349–3.880	0.002
LNR	≤0.10 vs. >0.10	1.689	1.043–2.737	0.033
Molecular subtype	Luminal A vs. non-luminal A	1.029	0.695–2.121	0.496

Abbreviations: LVI, lymphovascular invasion; HG, histologic grade; LNR, lymph-node ratio.

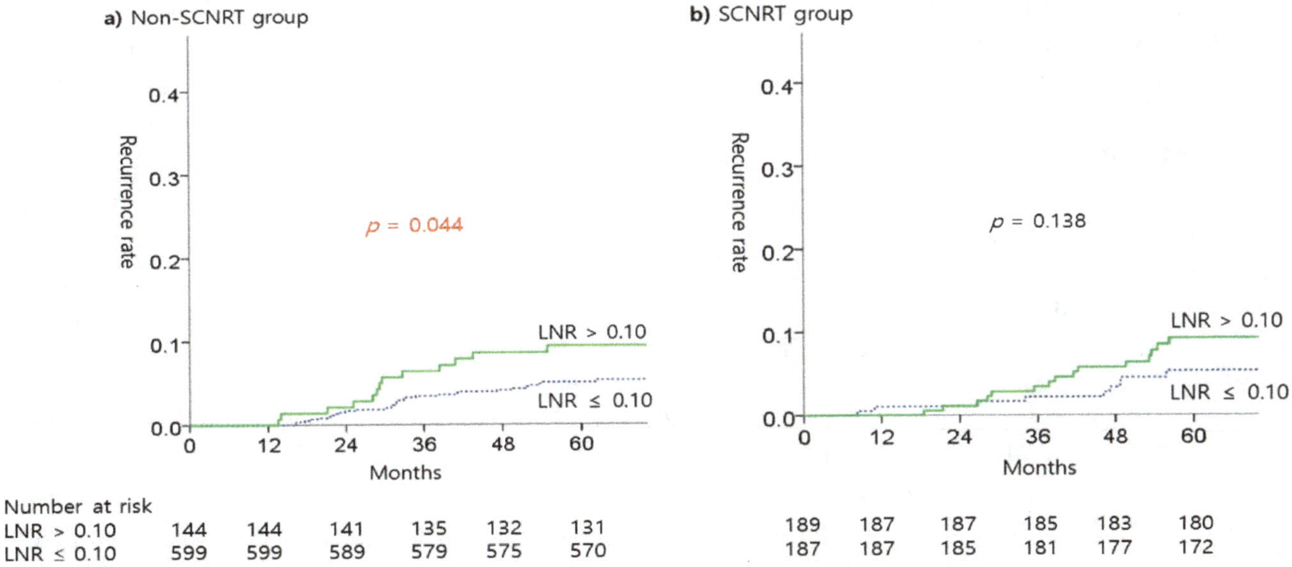

Figure 1. Kaplan-Meier estimates of recurrent rate according to LNR in SCNRT treatment subgroups.

4. Discussion

Although many studies have reported that ENI is not required by patients with pN0 breast cancer, it is widely accepted that postoperative locoregional radiation therapy reduces locoregional recurrence and mortality in patients with lymph-node-positive breast cancer [23]. However, its effectiveness in N1 breast cancer patients treated with systemic chemotherapy is still unclear [24,25]. In this context, the NCCN guidelines recommend the use of SCNRT in patients with N1 breast cancer as for level of evidence IIB [14].

Appropriate chemotherapy for breast cancer patients not only prevents systemic metastasis of the cancer, but also reduces the risk of locoregional recurrence [26]. The recurrence rate after treatment has been steadily declining with the development of surgical and adjunct therapies, and questions about the utility of SCNRT for early breast cancer patients have begun to emerge [27]. The frequency of adverse effects, such as lymphedema, increases when SCNRT is used with systemic chemotherapy. A previous study based on the KROG 14–18 patient data used in the present study showed that SCNRT was unnecessary in the N1 patient group and increased adverse effects [15,28]. In the case of another side effect, brachial plexopathy, the risk showed 1.3% in the conventional 50 Gy SCNRT group, but the risk was increased with adjuvant chemotherapy or total dose over 50 Gy to the brachial plexus [29].

Although the risk is low, treatment failure in N1 breast cancer occurs in regional and distant areas, and may be related to microscopic tumor cells in the regional lymphatic system, which can be removed with SCNRT. SCNRT still plays an important role in breast cancer treatment within this context. This may justify the use of SCNRT in selected patients with high-risk N1 breast cancer, rather than in all patient groups. Using SCNRT for N1 breast cancer is an interesting issue in the field of radiation oncology, and several studies have recommended that SCNRT be performed after various risk factors are considered, but not in all patient groups [17,18]. SCNRT can entail radiation side effects, such as lymphedema, brachial plexopathy, and radiation pneumonitis, so it should not be performed for small potential benefits alone. The benefits of SCNRT and its adverse effects in N1 breast cancer patients are highly controversial, and are affected by other modalities, such as the chemotherapy regimen and tumor characteristics. Therefore, its benefits should be clarified in a prospective study.

In this study, the utility of LNR was investigated as a factor to be considered in selecting SCNRT as a treatment for N1 breast cancer patients. Several studies have reported that nodal staging using LNR can predict the prognosis more effectively than conventional AJCC nodal staging [19,20,30]. In patients with N1 breast cancer with a relatively small number of metastatic lymph nodes, the prognosis can vary according to the total number of dissected lymph nodes, even in patients with the same number of metastatic lymph nodes. Therefore, this study investigated whether the utility of SCNRT can be estimated from LNR. This study was conducted with KROG 14–18 patients, and previous studies using the same patient group showed that SCNRT was ineffective in N1 breast cancer patients [15]. In the present study, it was demonstrated that SCNRT may be beneficial in patients with high LNRs, despite the use of taxane-based chemotherapy.

This study had several limitations. In addition to the limitations of all retrospective studies, there was no definitive standard according to which all institutions decided whether or not to administer SCNRT. Similarly, internal mammary node irradiation was also applied without clear criteria, which blurred the conclusions of this study. The difficulty in evaluating adverse effects was another limitation of this study. It is well known that SCNRT induces lymphedema. According to preliminary findings reported by Coen et al., the addition of regional lymph-node radiotherapy significantly increased the risk of lymphedema from 1.8% to 8.9% ($p = 0.0001$) [28]. When considering the use of SCNRT, clinicians should weigh the potential benefits of SCNRT in disease control against the increased risk of lymphedema. A previous study based on existing KROG 14–18 data showed that lymphedema occurred in 16.6% of patients after WBI+ and SCNRT, but in only 10.7% of patients after WBI alone ($p = 0.04$) [15]. To compare the benefits of SCNRT, a prospective study is required to establish more precise criteria. In this study, regional recurrence in the SCN, which is the main target of SCNRT, occurred in only 1% of patients. This is a very low recurrence rate upon which to base the claim that SCNRT should be performed in all patients. It is difficult to accept that SCNRT should be used to control recurrence, which occurs in only 1% of patients, given its adverse effects mentioned above. This study has shown that SCNRT also significantly reduced the risk of distant metastasis, as well as regional lymph-node recurrence. This may be because SCNRT controls the tumor burden in the SCN region, which may be the seed bed of distant metastases. Distant metastasis is the main failure pattern in N1 breast cancer patients, so this study has demonstrated that SCNRT has some therapeutic benefits over and above the control of regional recurrence. Lastly, the fact that there are characteristic differences between SCNRT group and non-SCNRT group is a weakness of the study. These characteristics are significantly higher in the SCNRT group and are generally known as poor prognosis factors, such as LVI, LNR, and ECE [13]. Despite these poor prognosis factors in the SCNRT group, there was no difference in recurrence rate between the two groups and it can be interpreted as indicating the effect of SCNRT.

Despite the several limitations described above, this multicenter study suggests that the use of SCNRT in patients receiving taxane-based chemotherapy may be beneficial if SCNRT is performed selectively. The study is important because it offers another direction of selective SCNRT for N1 breast cancer. Selective SCNRT can reduce unnecessary radiation exposure in N1 breast cancer patients and reduce the recurrence rate in appropriate patients, with a more patient-specific treatment.

5. Conclusions

In this DFS analysis, the patients with high LNR (>0.10) showed benefit with DFS outcomes by SCNRT. This study has shown that LNR can be used as an independent prognostic factor in patients with N1 breast cancer and as a useful index when determining whether to perform SCNRT. However, we did not establish whether the benefits of this treatment are sufficient to risk the associated adverse effects. Prospective studies are required to examine these issues.

Author Contributions: Conceptualization, J.H.K. (Jin Hee Kim); data curation, W.P., J.H.K. (Jin Hee Kim), D.H.C., Y.-J.K., E.S.L., K.H.S., J.H.K. (Jin Ho Kim), K.K., Y.B.K., S.-J.A., J.H.L., M.C., H.-S.L., J.S.K., J.C.; writing—original draft preparation, J.K.; writing—review and editing, W.P.; supervision, J.H.K. (Jin Hee Kim).

References

1. Early Breast Cancer Trialists' Collaborative Group. Effect of radiotherapy after breast-conserving surgery on 10-year recurrence and 15-year breast cancer death: Meta-analysis of individual patient data for 10,801 women in 17 randomised trials. *Lancet* **2011**, *378*, 1707–1716. [CrossRef]
2. Arriagada, R.; Rutqvist, L.E.; Mattsson, A.; Kramar, A.; Rotstein, S. Adequate locoregional treatment for early breast cancer may prevent secondary dissemination. *J. Clin. Oncol.* **1995**, *13*, 2869–2878. [CrossRef] [PubMed]
3. Overgaard, M.; Hansen, P.S.; Overgaard, J.; Rose, C.; Andersson, M.; Bach, F.; Kjaer, M.; Gadeberg, C.C.; Mouridsen, H.T.; Jensen, M.B.; et al. Postoperative radiotherapy in high-risk premenopausal women with breast cancer who receive adjuvant chemotherapy. Danish Breast Cancer Cooperative Group 82b Trial. *N. Engl. J. Med.* **1997**, *337*, 949–955. [CrossRef]
4. Overgaard, M.; Jensen, M.B.; Overgaard, J.; Hansen, P.S.; Rose, C.; Andersson, M.; Kamby, C.; Kjaer, M.; Gadeberg, C.C.; Rasmussen, B.B.; et al. Postoperative radiotherapy in high-risk postmenopausal breast-cancer patients given adjuvant tamoxifen: Danish Breast Cancer Cooperative Group DBCG 82c randomised trial. *Lancet* **1999**, *353*, 1641–1648. [CrossRef]
5. Budach, W.; Matuschek, C.; Bolke, E.; Dunst, J.; Feyer, P.; Fietkau, R.; Krug, D.; Piroth, M.D.; Sautter-Bihl, M.L.; Sedlmayer, F.; et al. DEGRO practical guidelines for radiotherapy of breast cancer V: Therapy for locally advanced and inflammatory breast cancer, as well as local therapy in cases with synchronous distant metastases. *Strahlenther. Onkol.* **2015**, *191*, 623–633. [CrossRef]
6. Whelan, T.J.; Olivotto, I.A.; Levine, M.N. Regional Nodal Irradiation in Early-Stage Breast Cancer. *N. Engl. J. Med.* **2015**, *373*, 1878–1879. [CrossRef]
7. Brackstone, M.; Fletcher, G.G.; Dayes, I.S.; Madarnas, Y.; SenGupta, S.K.; Verma, S. Locoregional therapy of locally advanced breast cancer: A clinical practice guideline. *Curr. Oncol.* **2015**, *22* (Suppl. 1), S54–S66. [CrossRef]
8. Henderson, I.C.; Berry, D.A.; Demetri, G.D.; Cirrincione, C.T.; Goldstein, L.J.; Martino, S.; Ingle, J.N.; Cooper, M.R.; Hayes, D.F.; Tkaczuk, K.H.; et al. Improved outcomes from adding sequential Paclitaxel but not from escalating Doxorubicin dose in an adjuvant chemotherapy regimen for patients with node-positive primary breast cancer. *J. Clin. Oncol.* **2003**, *21*, 976–983. [CrossRef]
9. Mamounas, E.P.; Bryant, J.; Lembersky, B.; Fehrenbacher, L.; Sedlacek, S.M.; Fisher, B.; Wickerham, D.L.; Yothers, G.; Soran, A.; Wolmark, N. Paclitaxel after doxorubicin plus cyclophosphamide as adjuvant chemotherapy for node-positive breast cancer: Results from NSABP B-28. *J. Clin. Oncol.* **2005**, *23*, 3686–3696. [CrossRef] [PubMed]
10. Early Breast Cancer Trialists' Collaborative Group. Comparisons between different polychemotherapy regimens for early breast cancer: Meta-analyses of long-term outcome among 100,000 women in 123 randomised trials. *Lancet* **2012**, *379*, 432–444. [CrossRef]
11. Recht, A.; Bartelink, H.; Fourquet, A.; Fowble, B.; Haffty, B.G.; Harris, J.R.; Kurtz, J.; McCormick, B.; Olivotto, I.A.; Rutqvist, L.; et al. Postmastectomy radiotherapy: Questions for the twenty-first century. *J. Clin. Oncol.* **1998**, *16*, 2886–2889. [CrossRef]
12. Recht, A.; Edge, S.B.; Solin, L.J.; Robinson, D.S.; Estabrook, A.; Fine, R.E.; Fleming, G.F.; Formenti, S.; Hudis, C.; Kirshner, J.J.; et al. Postmastectomy radiotherapy: Clinical practice guidelines of the American Society of Clinical Oncology. *J. Clin. Oncol.* **2001**, *19*, 1539–1569. [CrossRef]
13. Lee, S.; Park, I.H.; Park, S.; Sohn, J.; Jeong, J.; Ahn, S.G.; Lee, I.J.; Lee, H.K.; Lee, S.A.; Park, W.; et al. Meeting Highlights: The Second Consensus Conference for Breast Cancer Treatment in Korea. *J. Breast Cancer* **2017**, *20*, 228–233. [CrossRef] [PubMed]

14. National Comprehensive Cancer Network. NCCN Clinical Practice Guidelines in Oncology: Breast cancer (version 1.2019). Fort Washington, PA: National Comprehensive Cancer Network; c2017. Available online: https://www.nccn.org/professionals/physician_gls/pdf/breast.pdf (accessed on 16 May 2019).
15. Kim, H.; Park, W.; Yu, J.I.; Choi, D.H.; Huh, S.J.; Kim, Y.-J.; Lee, E.S.; Lee, K.S.; Kang, H.S.; Park, I.H.; et al. Prognostic Impact of Elective Supraclavicular Nodal Irradiation for Patients with N1 Breast Cancer after Lumpectomy and Anthracycline Plus Taxane-Based Chemotherapy (KROG 1418): A Multicenter Case-Controlled Study. *Cancer Res. Treat.* **2017**, *49*, 970–980. [CrossRef] [PubMed]
16. Yu, J.I.; Park, W.; Huh, S.J.; Choi, D.H.; Lim, Y.H.; Ahn, J.S.; Yang, J.H.; Nam, S.J. Determining which patients require irradiation of the supraclavicular nodal area after surgery for N1 breast cancer. *Int. J. Radiat. Oncol. Biol. Phys.* **2010**, *78*, 1135–1141. [CrossRef] [PubMed]
17. Yu, J.I.; Park, W.; Choi, D.H.; Huh, S.J.; Nam, S.J.; Kim, S.W.; Lee, J.E.; Kil, W.H.; Im, Y.H.; Ahn, J.S.; et al. Prognostic Modeling in Pathologic N1 Breast Cancer Without Elective Nodal Irradiation After Current Standard Systemic Management. *Clin. Breast Cancer* **2015**, *15*, e197–e204. [CrossRef]
18. Kong, M.; Hong, S.E. Predictive factors for supraclavicular lymph node recurrence in N1 breast cancer patients. *Asian Pac. J. Cancer Prev.* **2013**, *14*, 2509–2514. [CrossRef] [PubMed]
19. Vinh-Hung, V.; Nguyen, N.P.; Cserni, G.; Truong, P.; Woodward, W.; Verkooijen, H.M.; Promish, D.; Ueno, N.T.; Tai, P.; Nieto, Y.; et al. Prognostic value of nodal ratios in node-positive breast cancer: A compiled update. *Future Oncol.* **2009**, *5*, 1585–1603. [CrossRef] [PubMed]
20. Ahn, S.H.; Kim, H.J.; Lee, J.W.; Gong, G.Y.; Noh, D.Y.; Yang, J.H.; Jung, S.S.; Park, H.Y. Lymph node ratio and pN staging in patients with node-positive breast cancer: A report from the Korean breast cancer society. *Breast Cancer Res. Treat.* **2011**, *130*, 507–515. [CrossRef]
21. Megale Costa, L.J.; Soares, H.P.; Gaspar, H.A.; Trujillo, L.G.; Santi, P.X.; Pereira, R.S.; de Santana, T.L.; Pinto, F.N.; del Giglio, A. Ratio between positive lymph nodes and total dissected axillaries lymph nodes as an independent prognostic factor for disease-free survival in patients with breast cancer. *Am. J. Clin. Oncol.* **2004**, *27*, 304–306. [CrossRef]
22. Kim, J.; Kim, J.H.; Kim, O.B.; Oh, Y.K.; Park, S.G. Clinical significance of the lymph node ratio in N1 breast cancer. *Radiat. Oncol. J.* **2017**, *35*, 227–232. [CrossRef]
23. Early Breast Cancer Trialists' Collaborative Group. Effects of radiotherapy and of differences in the extent of surgery for early breast cancer on local recurrence and 15-year survival: An overview of the randomised trials. *Lancet* **2005**, *366*, 2087–2106. [CrossRef]
24. Reddy, S.G.; Kiel, K.D. Supraclavicular nodal failure in patients with one to three positive axillary lymph nodes treated with breast conserving surgery and breast irradiation, without supraclavicular node radiation. *Breast J.* **2007**, *13*, 12–18. [CrossRef]
25. Strom, E.A.; Woodward, W.A.; Katz, A.; Buchholz, T.A.; Perkins, G.H.; Jhingran, A.; Theriault, R.; Singletary, E.; Sahin, A.; McNeese, M.D. Clinical investigation: Regional nodal failure patterns in breast cancer patients treated with mastectomy without radiotherapy. *Int. J. Radiat. Oncol. Biol. Phys.* **2005**, *63*, 1508–1513. [CrossRef]
26. Early Breast Cancer Trialists' Collaborative Group. Effects of chemotherapy and hormonal therapy for early breast cancer on recurrence and 15-year survival: An overview of the randomised trials. *Lancet* **2005**, *365*, 1687–1717. [CrossRef]
27. Lai, S.F.; Chen, Y.H.; Kuo, W.H.; Lien, H.C.; Wang, M.Y.; Lu, Y.S.; Lo, C.; Kuo, S.H.; Cheng, A.L.; Huang, C.S. Locoregional recurrence risk for postmastectomy breast cancer patients with T1-2 and one to three positive lymph nodes receiving modern systemic treatment without radiotherapy. *Ann. Surg. Oncol.* **2016**, *23*, 3860–3869. [CrossRef]
28. Coen, J.J.; Taghian, A.G.; Kachnic, L.A.; Assaad, S.I.; Powell, S.N. Risk of lymphedema after regional nodal irradiation with breast conservation therapy. *Int. J. Radiat. Oncol. Biol. Phys.* **2003**, *55*, 1209–1215. [PubMed]
29. Galecki, J.; Hicer-Grzenkowicz, J.; Grudzień-Kowalska, M.; Michalska, T.; Załucki, W. Radiation-induced brachial plexopathy and hypofractionated regimens in adjuvant irradiation of patients with breast cancer—A review. *Acta Oncol.* **2006**, *45*, 280–284. [CrossRef] [PubMed]

Impact of Overdiagnosis on Long-Term Breast Cancer Survival

Jean Ching-Yuan Fann [1], King-Jen Chang [2], Chen-Yang Hsu [3], Amy Ming-Fang Yen [4], Cheng-Ping Yu [5,6], Sam Li-Sheng Chen [4], Wen-Hung Kuo [2], László Tabár [7] and Hsiu-Hsi Chen [3,8,*]

1 Department of Health Industry Management, College of Healthcare Management, Kainan University, Taoyuan 338, Taiwan; jeanfann@ntu.edu.tw
2 Department of Surgery, National Taiwan University Hospital, Taipei 100, Taiwan; kingjen@ntu.edu.tw (K.-J.C.); brcancer@gmail.com (W.-H.K.)
3 Graduate Institute of Epidemiology and Preventive Medicine, College of Public Health, National Taiwan University, Taipei 100, Taiwan; bacilli65@gmail.com
4 School of Oral Hygiene, College of Oral Medicine, Taipei Medical University, Taipei 110, Taiwan; amyyen@tmu.edu.tw (A.M.-F.Y.); samchen@tmu.edu.tw (S.L.-S.C.)
5 Department of Pathology and Graduate Institute of Pathology and Parasitology, Tri-Service General Hospital, National Defense Medical Center, Taipei 114, Taiwan; cpyupath@yahoo.com.tw
6 Graduate Institute of Life Sciences, National Defense Medical Center, Taipei 114, Taiwan
7 Department of Mammography, Falun Central Hospital, 791823 Falun, Sweden; laszlo@mammographyed.com
8 Innovation and Policy Center for Population Health and Sustainable Environment, College of Public Health, National Taiwan University, Taipei 100, Taiwan
* Correspondence: chenlin@ntu.edu.tw

Abstract: Elucidating whether and how long-term survival of breast cancer is mainly due to cure after early detection and effective treatment and therapy or overdiagnosis resulting from the widespread use of mammography provides a new insight into the role mammography plays in screening, surveillance, and treatment of breast cancer. Given information on detection modes, the impact of overdiagnosis due to mammography screening on long-term breast cancer survival was quantitatively assessed by applying a zero (cured or overdiagnosis)-inflated model design and analysis to a 15-year follow-up breast cancer cohort in Dalarna, Sweden. The probability for non-progressive breast cancer (the zero part) was 56.14% including the 44.34% complete cure after early detection and initial treatment and a small 11.80% overdiagnosis resulting from mammography screening program (8.94%) and high awareness (2.86%). The 15-year adjusted cumulative survival of breast cancer was dropped from 88.25% to 74.80% after correcting for the zero-inflated part of overdiagnosis. The present findings reveal that the majority of survivors among women diagnosed with breast cancer could be attributed to the cure resulting from mammography screening and accompanying effective treatment and therapy and only a small fraction of those were due to overdiagnosis.

Keywords: overdiagnosis; mammography screening; invasive breast cancer; zero-inflated Poisson regression model

---

1. Introduction

While the prognosis of breast cancer (BC) has been substantially improved due to early detection of breast cancer attributed to the widespread use of mammography, the issue of overdiagnosis resulting from mammography screening has been debated over the past decade [1–5]. As these overdiagnosed cases are biologically indolent and non-progressive they would have never progressed to clinical phase and caused death due to breast cancer during the patients' lifetime, implying that any treatment was unnecessary and would not have been administered had screening not been applied to these women [6–10].

The previous studies on the extent of overdiagnosis were estimated by excess incidence due to screening compared with background incidence derived from randomized control trials or predicted incidence extrapolated from previous unexposed epochs, making allowance for lead-time [2,9,11,12]. Note that these previous methods, while estimating the proportion of overdiagnosis, require individual normal and incident breast cancer data and also a strong assumption of lead-time distribution. These traditional approaches cannot be used for assessing the impact of overdiagnosis on long-term survival when only information on breast cancer cases and deaths from breast cancer is available.

Here, we propose a new approach to estimating overdiagnosis using information on the survival of breast cancer detected by different modalities (detection modes) together with prognostic factors with the premise that overdiagnosis of BC would not result in deaths from breast cancer. However, the survivors of these overdiagnosed BCs are often indistinguishable from those with of non-overdiagnosed BC cases but without potential of dying from breast cancer due to effective initial treatment and therapy, namely the completely cured. Both types are regarded as non-progressive BC with zero-probability of dying from BC but have manifestly different causes. To distinguish the completely cured patients from overdiagnosed ones requires information on detection mode such as screen-detected cases, interval cancers, and cancers in non-participants. The overestimation of cumulative survival due to the zero-probability of dying from breast cancer resulting from overdiagnosis would be expected if these overdiagnosed cases cannot not be separated from the completely cured.

Moreover, the non-progressive BCs indicated above would also be mixed up with progressive BC patients still alive at each specific follow-up timepoint. Whether and when these progressive cases would die from BC is highly dependent on subsequent treatments and therapies and prognostic factors [13–18]. However, only relying on these prognostics may not be sufficient to distinguish between progressive and non-progressive BC because excellent survival tumors with good prognostic factors may also be a consequence of overdiagnosis due to mammography [19].

The aim of this study is therefore to apply the zero-inflated regression model to estimate the proportion of overdiagnosis resulting from mammography screening separated from the proportion of the completely cured due to effective treatment and therapy. We also assess the cumulative survival after correction for the zero-inflated part of overdiagnosis.

2. Materials and Methods

2.1. Study Subjects and Design

We quantified the respective contributions of overdiagnosis attributable to mammography and cures due to early detection and effective treatment by using a cohort composed of 1346 patients diagnosed with invasive BC at Falun Central Hospital of Dalarna County in Sweden in two periods with available information on prognostic factors, from 1996 to 1998 and from 2006 to 2010, in combination with a zero-inflated model design and analysis. The main reason of selecting two periods is mainly due to available information on immunohistochemical (IHC) markers, particularly HER2, which had not been widely tested before 2005. The period of 1996–1998 was a pilot phase for collecting such information. The two cohorts were followed over time until the end of 2010. Note that breast cancer service screening program with mammography has been offered since 1985 at the close of the Swedish Two-county randomized controlled trial [20].

In addition to longitudinal follow-up data, the current study design illustrated in Figure 1 is based on the concept of the zero-inflated model for solving the problem of being unable to distinguish between overdiagnosed cases from cured cases due to effective treatment and therapies as mentioned in the introduction. All diagnosed breast cancers are classified into three types according to the potential for progression and the cure after initial treatment. The top left circle represents overdiagnosed cases (blue) with zero probability of dying from breast cancer mainly resulting from mammography screening. The dotted box is composed of those breast cancers with potential of progression, which are further divided into two types, the cured after initial treatment (green) and the cured after subsequent therapies during 15-year follow-up (red). The final column is the estimated attributable proportions among three types of survivors of breast cancer. If there is a lack of information on detection mode it is very difficult to distinguish the cured from the overdiagnosed. The screened cohort together with the collection of these prognostic factors provide an opportunity to distinguish overdiagnosis from the cured. The derivation of percentages among breast cancer cases delineated in Figure 1 is elaborated in the Statistical Analysis section and Appendix

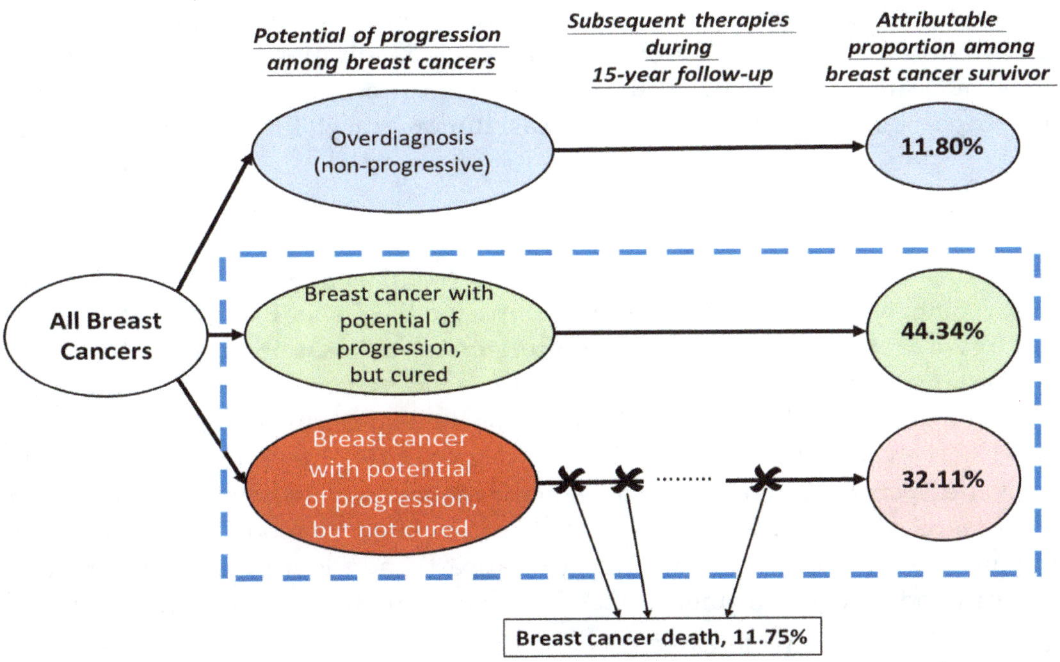

Figure 1. Study design for estimating the proportion of breast cancer survivors attributed to overdiagnosis, the completely cured after initial treatment, and the curation after subsequent therapies during 15-year follow-up.

2.2. *Detection Mode Related to Curation and Overdiagnosis*

There are three detection modes, screen-detected cases, interval cancers, and cancers from non-participants or outside the age ranges of screening. Here we assume overdiagnosis of BC due to mammography screening can only result from screen-detected cases as they were detected though mammography. Interval cancers after the exposure to a previous screen with negative findings were detected either through possible self-referral of patients or due to the presence of symptoms and signs. Cancers from non-participants or outside screening were diagnosed due to the presence of symptom and signs. In this sense, interval cancers would enhance awareness of being diagnosed as BC compared to cancers from non-participants. This can be supported by the fact that interval cancers have higher survival than cancers from non-participants [21]. Suppose treatment and therapies were administered to three groups according to the indication for the choice of treatment modality based on significant prognostic factors. The difference of zero probability on death from BC between screen-detected cancers and interval cancers would provide information on excess zeros due to overdiagnosis resulting from mammography. The difference of zero probability between interval cancers and cancers from non-participant offers information on overdiagnosis due to increased awareness. Details of the calculation are given in the statistical section.

2.3. Prognostic Factors

We collected factors responsible for progressive BCs including conventional tumor attributes (size, lymph node involvement, and histological grade), three immunohistochemical markers (ER, PR, HER2), triple negative (defined by these three IHC markers), surgical treatment and adjuvant therapy. Conventional tumor attributes have been collected since the dawn of the service screening. Surgical treatment (breast-conserving surgery, mastectomy, or others), and adjuvant therapy (radiotherapy, chemotherapy, or hormone therapy) had been collected since 1996.

Data on tumor phenotypes related to IHC markers including ER, PR and HER2 status were collected retrospectively for the period of 1996 to 1998 by standard antibody staining in the largest invasive tumor component for each patient and was described in full in previous studies [22]. The antibodies (supplier, type, dilution) used for staining are delineated as follows: ER (clone SP1; Ventana Medical Systems, Tucson, AZ, USA; 1:200 dilution), PR (clone PgR 636; Dako, Glostrup, Denmark; 1:50 dilution), and HER2 (code A 0485; Dako; 1:250 dilution). The cut-off point for ER and PR positivity is nuclear staining >10% of tumor cells. The criteria of HER2 positivity was offered by manufacturer. Triple negative BC is defined as a breast tumor with all ER, PR, and HER2 being negative.

2.4. Statistical Analysis

Descriptive data are presented with frequency and percentage. For categorical data, the chi-square test was used to compare the difference between groups and the Fisher Exact test was used if any count was less than 5. We first applied the Poisson regression model assuming the number of BC deaths follows a Poisson distribution. We estimated follow-up women years from the date of diagnosis as BC to the date of death from BC, loss of follow-up, or the end of this study as the offset in Poisson regression model. The value of deviance divided by degree of freedom provides an indicator to assess the extent of over-dispersion and under-dispersion for the specified Poisson regression model. For the elucidation of overdiagnosis in BC, we applied the zero-inflated Poisson (ZIP) regression model [23], which is a mixture of a Poisson regression model (count part) and a logistic regression model (zero part) as derived in Appendix A. The former model (Poisson regression model, count part) was used to evaluate the prognostic factors for progressive BCs. The prognostic factors included three conventional tumor attributes and treatment and therapies (surgery, chemotherapy, radiotherapy, hormone therapy). The latter model (logistic regression model, zero part) was used to estimate the probability of zero part (including overdiagnosis cases or cure after initial treatment and therapies) for non-progressive BCs. We used the detection mode of cancers as covariates to distinguish two types in the zero part (Appendix A). We then used the regression coefficients of logistic regression part in the ZIP model to calculate the probability of zero among all BCs and respective probabilities of zero by detection mode as detailed in Appendix A. The probability of overdiagnosis due to mammography screening and enhanced awareness is calculated as follows:

$$\begin{gathered}\text{The probability of overdiagnosis due to mammography screening} = \\ ((\text{The probability of zero for screen-detected - the probability of zero for interval cancer}) \\ \times \text{The probability of zero among all BCs})\end{gathered} \tag{1}$$

$$\begin{gathered}\text{The probability of overdiagnosis due to awareness} \\ = ((\text{the probability of zero for interval cancers - the probability of zero for cancers from non-participants}) \\ \times \text{the probability of zero among all BCs})\end{gathered} \tag{2}$$

$$\text{The probability of cure due to treatment} = \text{The probability of zero among all BCs - }((1) + (2)) \tag{3}$$

We further derive 15-year cumulative survival curves with and without correcting for overdiagnosis by using the hazard rate derived from the ZIP model and the corresponding figure from the conventional Poisson regression model without considering overdiagnosis as described in

Appendix A). Two-sided p-value less than 0.05 was treated as statistical significance. All analyses were conducted with SAS version 9.4 (SAS Institute, Cary, NC, USA).

2.5. Ethics Approval

This study was approved by the Joint Institutional Review Board of Taipei Medical University (TMU-JIRB, approval numbers N201607008).

3. Results

Table 1 shows the frequencies of age at diagnosis, first generation prognostic factors (tumor size, node status, histologic malignancy grade), IHC markers (ER, PR, HER2, triple negative), and treatment and therapies by BC death. The distribution of age at diagnosis was similar between women who died from BC and those who did not. The distributions of tumor size, status of node involvement, histological grade, ER, PR, triple negative, surgery, and hormonal therapy were significantly different (p-value < 0.05) according to BC death. Women who had tumor size larger than 20 mm, positive nodes, grade 3, ER(−), PR(−), and triple negative were more likely to die from BC.

Table 1. The distribution of age at diagnosis, conventional tumor attributes, IHC markers (ER, PR, HER2, Triple negative), mammographic appearance, and treatment by status of breast cancer death.

Variable/Level	Breast Cancer Death				p-Value
	No (n = 1228)	%	Yes (n = 118)	%	
Age at diagnosis					0.345
<50	202	92.7	16	7.3	
50–69	596	91.8	53	8.2	
70+	430	89.8	49	10.2	
Size *, mm					<0.001
1–9	233	98.3	4	1.7	
10–14	273	96.1	11	3.9	
15–19	260	95.2	13	4.8	
20–29	263	87.4	38	12.6	
≥30	155	83.8	30	16.2	
Nodes *					<0.001
Negative	805	95.4	39	4.6	
Positive	390	87.2	57	12.8	
Grade *					<0.001
1	284	97.3	8	2.7	
2	633	93.6	43	6.4	
3	263	85.4	45	14.6	
ER *					<0.001
Negative	174	84.1	33	15.9	
Positive	990	94.6	57	5.4	
PR *					<0.001
Negative	448	87.3	65	12.7	
Positive	714	96.6	25	3.4	
HER2 *					0.8771
Negative	1018	92.9	78	7.1	
Positive	149	92.5	12	7.5	
Triple negative *					<0.0001
Yes	115	81.6	26	18.4	
No	1046	94.2	64	5.8	

Table 1. *Cont.*

Variable/Level	Breast Cancer Death				*p*-Value
	No (*n* = 1228)	%	Yes (*n* = 118)	%	
Surgery *					<0.0001
MA	452	87.8	63	12.2	
BCS	538	95.9	23	4.1	
Others	238	88.1	32	11.9	
Chemotherapy					0.2018
Yes	270	89.4	32	10.6	
No	958	91.8	86	8.2	
Radiotherapy					0.8979
Yes	632	91.3	60	8.7	
No	596	91.1	58	8.9	
Tamoxifen					0.0061
Yes	480	93.9	31	6.1	
No	748	89.6	87	10.4	

Abbreviations: ER: estrogen receptor; HER2: human epidermal growth factor receptor 2; IHC markers: immunohistochemical markers; PR: progesterone receptor; BCS: breast conserving surgery; MA: mastectomy. * 66 subjects had no information on tumor size (44 survivors, 22 deaths), 55 subjects had no information on nodal involvement (33 survivors, 22 deaths), 70 subjects had no information on histological grade (48 survivors, 22 deaths), 92 subjects had no information on ER status (64 survivors, 28 deaths), 94 subjects had no information on PR status (66 survivors, 28 deaths), 89 subjects had no information on HER2 status (61 survivors, 28 deaths), 95 subjects had no information on triple negative status (67 survivors, 28 deaths).

Table 2 shows that conventional tumor attributes were significant predictors in both univariate and multivariable models. The crude RR was significantly higher for tumor with size 20–29 mm (9.32; 95% CI, 3.33–26.13) and 30 mm+ (13.65; 95% CI, 4.81–38.74) compared with size 1–9 mm, tumor with node positive (3.70; 95% CI, 2.46–5.57) compared with node negative, tumor with grade 3 (2.97; 95% CI, 1.99–4.43) compared with grade 1/2, and triple negative (3.32; 95% CI, 2.11–5.24) compared with non-triple negative cancers. In the multivariable analysis, tumor with size 20–29 mm (aRR = 2.63; 95% CI, 1.38–5.02) and 30+ mm (aRR = 2.39; 95% CI, 1.19–4.80) were at greater risk than those with size 1–9 mm. Positive node led to an elevated risk (aRR = 1.86; 95% CI, 1.18–2.94) as opposed to negative node after adjusting for variables related to treatment such as surgery, chemotherapy, radiotherapy, and hormonal therapy. Interpretation of effect size on treatment and therapies should be taken with great caution as they are not a reflection of efficacy of treatment and therapies but an indication for treatment and therapies according to tumor attributes. These accounted for the findings that those with mastectomy and radiotherapy had higher hazard of dying from breast cancer and insignificant effective chemotherapies and tamoxifen therapy even after adjustment for other significant prognostic factors.

The value of deviance divided by the degree of freedom, an indicator for assessing the level of over-dispersion, was about 0.46–0.59 in the univariate model and 0.49 in the multivariable model. As this value was less than 1, it strongly suggests the problem of under-dispersion (excess zeros).

We used data with complete information (n = 1233) on conventional tumor attributes, variables related to surgery and adjuvant therapy, and detection mode of BCs for the ZIP model analysis. The larger the value of odds ratio (OR), the higher probability to be cured after initial treatment or overdiagnosis. The larger the value of relative risk (RR), the higher the risk of dying from BC. Table 3 shows the estimated parameters, ORs, and RRs for the ZIP model.

Tumor size, node status, grade were significant factors related to risk of dying from BC after considering treatment. Compared with non-participants and outside screening of BCs, screen detected cancers and interval cancers were with higher odds (OR = 2.38, 95% CI: 0.97–5.85 and OR = 1.23, 95% CI: 0.48–3.17, respectively) of being zero.

Table 2. The univariate and multivariable analysis of Poisson regression model for predicting breast cancer death by conventional tumor attributes and other predictors.

Variable/Level	Univariate			Multivariable		
	cRR (95% CI)	p-Value	Deviance/df.	aRR (95% CI)	p-Value	Deviance/df.
Tumor size, mm		<0.001	0.46		<0.001	
10–14 vs. 1–9	2.53 (0.80–7.93)			1.01 (0.45–2.24)		
15–19 vs. 1–9	3.12 (1.02–9.56)			1.12 (0.52–2.43)		
20–29 vs. 1–9	9.32 (3.33–26.13)			2.63 (1.38–5.02)		
30+ vs. 1–9	13.65 (4.81–38.74)			2.39 (1.19–4.80)		
Node (+) vs. (−)	3.70 (2.46–5.57)	<0.001	0.46	1.86 (1.18–2.94)	0.007	
Grade 3 vs. 1/2	2.97 (1.99–4.43)	<0.001	0.48	1.32 (0.84–2.07)	0.228	0.49
Triple negative Yes vs. No	3.32 (2.11–5.24)	<0.001	0.47	1.53 (0.89–2.63)	0.132	
Surgery MA vs. BCS	4.02 (2.49–6.48)	<0.001	0.55	2.79 (1.56–4.98)	<0.001	
Chemotherapy Yes vs. no	1.58 (1.05–2.37)	0.027	0.59	0.83 (0.51–1.38)	0.474	
Radiotherapy Yes vs. no	0.71 (0.50–1.02)	0.063	0.59	1.39 (0.82–2.37)	0.215	
Tamoxifen Yes vs. no	0.96 (0.64–1.45)	0.849	0.59	0.89 (0.56–1.42)	0.633	

Abbreviations: aRR: adjusted relative risk; cRR: crude relative risk; df.: degree of freedom; MA: Mastectomy; BCS: Breast-conserving surgery.

The probability of zero part among all non-progressive BC was 56.14%. The corresponding probabilities for screen detected cancer, interval cancer, and refuser/outside screening cancers were 66.42%, 50.50%, and 45.40% respectively, which gave 8.94% overdiagnosis due to mammography screening and 2.86% due to high awareness for those interval cancers but exposed to mammography screening based on the equation (1) and (2). The probability of zero due to the curation resulting from early detection and effective treatment was 44.34% (Figure 1, green).

The 15-year prognosis-adjusted cumulative survival of BC after correcting for overdiagnosis fell from 88.25% (Figure 2, cross mark) to 74.80% (Figure 2, hollow circle) after further adjustment for prognostic factors in the count part of progressive BC (Figure 1, red). The 15-year survival rate among 43.86% progressive BC after subsequent treatments and adjuvant therapies was 32.11% after adjustment for significant prognostic factors (Figure 1, pink).

Table 3. The regression coefficient of Zero-inflated Poisson regression model and overdiagnosis rate.

Variable	Regression Coefficient	S.E.	RR/OR (95% CI)	p-Value
Count Part			**RR**	
Intercept	−6.216	0.830		
Size, mm				0.015
10–14 vs. 1–9	1.307	0.808	3.69 (0.76–18.01)	
15–19 vs. 1–9	1.348	0.802	3.85 (0.80–18.53)	
20–29 vs. 1–9	2.329	0.769	10.26 (2.27–46.33)	
30+ vs. 1–9	2.246	0.791	9.45 (2.01–44.49)	
Node (+) vs. (−)	0.877	0.315	2.40 (1.30–4.45)	0.005
Grade 3 vs. 1/2	0.484	0.276	1.62 (0.94–2.79)	0.080
Surgery MA vs. BCS	0.651	0.360	1.92 (0.95–3.88)	0.071
Triple Negative Yes vs. No	0.914	0.311	2.49 (1.36–4.59)	0.003
Chemotherapy Yes vs. No	−0.238	0.319	0.79 (0.42–1.47)	0.456
Radiotherapy Yes vs. No	0.210	0.367	1.23 (0.60–2.53)	0.568
Tamoxifen Yes vs. No	−0.054	0.281	0.95 (0.94–1.64)	0.847
Zero Part			**OR**	
Intercept	−0.185	0.381		
Detection mode				0.041
SD vs. RF	0.867	0.459	2.38(0.97–5.85)	
IC vs. RF	0.205	0.484	1.23(0.48–3.17)	

Abbreviations: S.E.: Standard error; MA: Mastectomy; BCS: Breast-conserving surgery; SD: screen detected cancer; IC: interval cancer; RF: refuser & outside screening cancers.

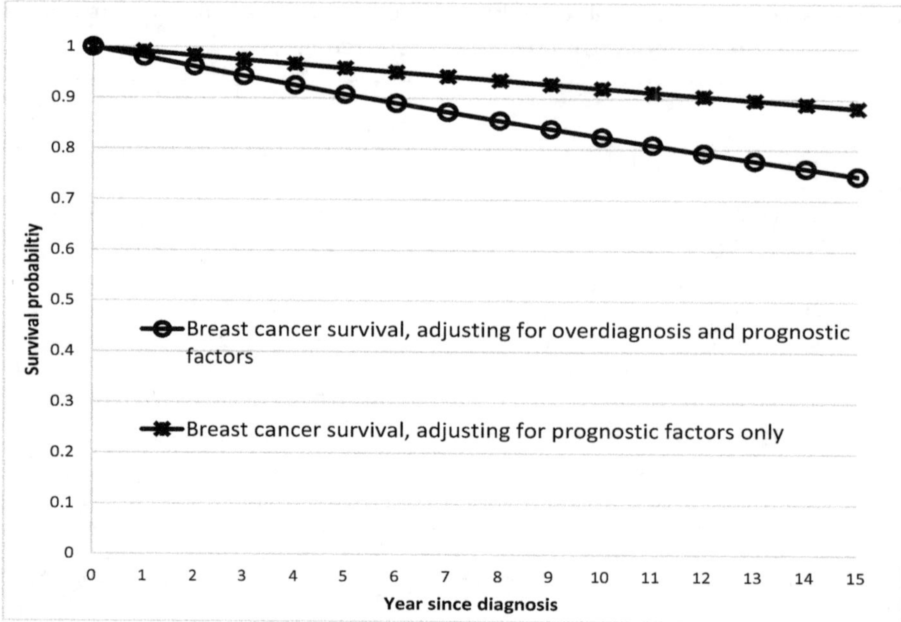

Figure 2. Cumulative survival of breast cancer-based models with and without considering overdiagnosis.

4. Discussion

The long-term prognosis of BC has been substantially improved over the past three decades due to early detection, mainly through mammographic screening. However, the harm of overdiagnosis is a concomitant risk of the benefit of mammography screening and it has now become a debatable issue and concern for population-based mammography screening over the past decade [1–5]. For breast cancer cases with overdiagnosis, there is 0% probability of dying from BC and treatment is unnecessary for them. It may also result in the overestimation of cumulative survival attributed to effective treatment and therapies in accompany with early detection of mammography screening. The survival of BC would thus be artificially inflated if such zero-inflated overdiagnosis is included. Estimating the quantity of overdiagnosis separated from the cured due to treatment is intractable but indispensable and can be truly a reflection of early detection and effective treatment and therapy. Our novel approach with the zero-inflated design and model for separating the cured from the overdiagnosed provides a solution but the conventional statistical model could not distinguish the completed cured after initial treatment (green, Figure 1) and the curation after subsequent therapies during 15-year follow-up (red, Figure 1). From the viewpoint of methodology, the use of the zero-inflated model enables us to separate the zero part with potential of progression but completely cured after initial treatment from the non-zero part with potential of progression but cured after subsequent therapies during 15-year follow-up particularly when tumor attributes related to breast cancer progression were considered in the non-zero (progressive) part.

In addition to the assessment of the impact of overdiagnosis on long-term survival, our proposed zero-inflated model also provides an insight into the proportion of overdiagnosis resulting from mammography screening that has been well studied in previous studies using excess incidence approach with lead-time adjustment [2,9,11,12]. After reviewing the primary articles that estimated the overdiagnosis level in European population-based mammography screening programs, Puliti et al. found that the rates of overdiagnosis of invasive BCs due to mammography screening varied from 0 to 54% [11]. Morrel et al. reported lower estimated baseline incidence resulted in higher level of overdiagnosis (42% vs. 30%) [24]. They also reported that longer lead-time (5 years vs. 2.5 years) contributed to lower extent of overdiagnosis (42% vs. 51%) [24]. Different background incidence rates and the assumption of lead-time distribution may account for such a wide range of estimates on overdiagnosis reported before. Several studies reported that the overdiagnosis rate was different by age [25,26]. In addition to the disparity in the methodology of lead-time adjustment and the extent of mammography screening, variation of overdiagnosis across age may also be explained by the fact that background incidence rate and the distribution of lead-time also vary with age [2,9,11,12].

Our proposed alternative approach to evaluating the extent of overdiagnosis dispenses with background incidence of BC and the assumption of lead-time distribution. We only used empirical data on BCs with available information on detection mode, treatment and therapies, and prognostic factors collected from an organized service screening program after population-based randomized controlled trial on mammography screening since 1977 in Falun (also known as Dalarna now, and Kopparberg in the 1990s), Sweden [27]. This empirical data is well suited to estimate the overdiagnosis from mammography screening and enhanced awareness as the attendance rate of mammography screening was over 80% and women in this county were also with high awareness of being diagnosed as BC through interval cancers [4,6]. Information on BCs with various detection modes is therefore useful for separating the completed cured from overdiagnosis.

It is very interesting to note that the probability of being zero part among interval cancers was higher than refuser/outside screening BCs. The difference might result from high awareness of detecting BCs through interval cancers because they had been exposed to mammography screening. Our result showed about 3% overdiagnosis due to enhanced awareness of detecting BC through interval cancers.

There are two limitations of the current study. Although the application of ZIP enables us to estimate the attributable proportions of three types of breast cancer survivors, personalized prediction for three types cannot be achieved without more updated information on molecular and imaging biomarkers can be included in the zero part and non-zero part, respectively. The second is related to the validation of this zero-inflated model by the application of the proposed model together with the estimated parameters to independent prospective follow-up data of this cohort in the future and also to data outside this country. We therefore strongly suggest here that our proposed zero-inflated model had better be applied to other countries in Europe where mammography screening programs have been widely served since the 1990s and the screening rate was also high in order to see whether and how the cure, overdiagnosis, and the survival of progressive BCs vary with different service screening programs. We also suggest that our model can be applied to regions with lower mammography screening rates and lower awareness of detecting BC in contrast to the current data with high careening rate and enhanced awareness in order to test the generalizability of our proposed zero-inflated regression.

5. Conclusions

In conclusion, the zero-inflated model design is a novel approach to correcting cumulative survival of early-detected BC inflated due to the zero part of overdiagnosis. Application of this model to the Dalarna breast cancer service screening program revealed that, among all breast cancers detected from this program, there were 76% survivors (44% completely cured and 32% still alive) due to early detection of mammography and effective treatment after 15 years of follow-up and overdiagnosis accounted for 12% of survivors.

Author Contributions: Study concept and design: H.-H.C.; Acquisition and interpretation of data: W.-H.K., C.-P.Y., K.-J.C., L.T.; Literature search: K.-J.C., W.-H.K., C.-P.Y., J.C.-Y.F.; Drafting of the manuscript: J.C.-Y.F., C.-Y.H., K.-J.C., H.-H.C.; Critical revision of the manuscript for important intellectual content: L.T., K.-J.C., H.-H.C.; Statistical analysis: C.-Y.H., J.C.-Y.F., S.L.-S.C., A.M.-F.Y.; Obtained funding: S.L.-S.C., A.M.-F.Y., H.-H.C.; Administrative, technical, or material support: A.M.-F.Y., S.L.-S.C.

Acknowledgments: This work was financially supported by the "Innovation and Policy Center for Population Health and Sustainable Environment (Population Health Research Center, PHRC), College of Public Health, National Taiwan University" from The Featured Areas Research Center Program within the framework of the Higher Education Sprout Project by the Ministry of Education (MOE) in Taiwan.

Appendix A Zero-Inflated Poisson Regression Model

Let Y denote the random variable representing the observed counts of breast cancer death. The effect of demographic factors, tumor attributes, IHC (immunohistochemical markers), type of treatments and therapies for progressive BCs can be evaluated by using Poisson regression model specified as follows. The number of breast cancer death (Y) following Poisson distribution, the probability of having observation on $Y = y$ (say 118 death cases in Table 1) is written as follows:

$$\Pr(Y = y; \mu) = \frac{e^{-\mu}\mu^{y}}{y!},\ y = 0, 1, 2, \ldots, \mu > 0. \tag{A-1}$$

The Poisson model can be extended to the zero-inflated Poisson (ZIP) model to account for the zero part (non-progressive BC), including the completely cured and over-diagnosis as diagrammed in Figure 1. By in introducing the mixture probability, say π, of being non-progressive (zero-part) extended from (1), the ZIP is specified by:

$$Pr(Y = y; \mu,\ \pi) = \begin{cases} \pi + (1-\pi)e^{-\mu} \text{ when } y = 0 \\ (1-\pi)\frac{e^{-\mu}\mu^{y}}{y!} \text{ when } y = 1, 2, 3\ldots \end{cases} \tag{A-2}$$

$$\mu > 0,\ 0 \leq \pi \leq 1$$

The probability of having the observation on breast cancer death (y = 1,2, ...) for progressive BCs is thus $(1-\pi)\frac{e^{-\mu}\mu^{y}}{y!}$, subject to the premise that the women must belong to the progressive breast cancer type with the probability specified by $(1-\pi)$. For women who would not die from breast cancer (y = 0), there are two possibilities, the zero part (complete cure and over-diagnosis) and progressive ones but who haven't died at the specified follow-up time. The former is specified by the probability π and the latter is thus the product of the complement scenario and survival probability written as $(1-\pi)\ e^{-\mu}$. Based on such a specification of the ZIP model, the effect of detection mode denoted by two dummy variables, SD and IC as follows:

$$\text{logit}(\pi) = \log\left(\frac{\pi}{1-\pi}\right) = \gamma_0 + \gamma_1 SD + \gamma_2 IC \tag{A-3}$$

For a screen-detected subject, the vector of covariate is specified as (SD = 1, IC = 0) and the vector of (SD = 0, IC = 1) is thus for an interval cancer case. Due to our use of refuser as the reference group, the covariate vector of (SD = 0, IC = 0) is specified for such type of case. The probability for being zero (non-progressive BC) is thus:

$$\pi_i = \frac{\exp(\gamma_0 + \gamma_1 SD_i + \gamma_2 IC_i)}{1 + \exp(\gamma_0 + \gamma_1 SD_i + \gamma_2 IC_i)} \tag{A-4}$$

The probability of being zero among all BCs without considering the covariate of detection mode was estimated as 56.14% using only the intercept term. Following the same rationale, the probability of being zero (non-progressive breast cancer) with the incorporation of detection mode was estimated as 66.42% for screen-detected, 50.50% for interval cancer, and 45.40% for cancers form non-participants or outside screening. According to the Equation (1) and (2) in the text of statistical section, 8.94% and 2.86% were estimated for over-diagnosis resulting from mammography and enhanced awareness, respectively.

In order to compare two cumulative survival curves as shown in Figure 2, we need to derive two annual death rates by using the ZIP model (λ) and the conventional Poisson model (λ′). For the ZIP model, number of breast cancer death is originated from the non-zero part with the following regression form:

$$\log(\mu) = \log(PY) + \beta_0 + \beta_1 x_1 + \beta_2 x_2 \ldots + \beta_p x_p \tag{A-5}$$

The average counts of breast cancer death, say μ, which can be further decomposed into the product of death rate (λ) and the person-year of the breast cancer cases under follow up (*PY*), is written as $\mu = \lambda \times PY$. By using log link, the association between average number of breast cancer death and breast cancer death rates and observed person-years is decomposed into log(μ) = log(λ) + log(*PY*). Breast cancer cases with certain characteristics such as large tumor size, higher grade of malignancy, positive lymph node involvement, triple negative cancer, etc., may have unfavorable prognosis and a higher rate of progression to breast cancer death. We denote these characteristics including demographic factors, tumor attributes, IHC markers, type of treatments and detection modes of a breast cancer case by vector $\boldsymbol{X}$ ($\boldsymbol{X} = (X_1, X_2, X_3, \ldots, X_p)$). The effect of these P characteristics on breast cancer case fatality rate can be incorporated by using log function written as follows:

$$\log(\lambda) = \beta_0 + \beta_1 x_1 + \beta_2 x_2 \ldots + \beta_p x_p, \tag{A-6}$$

Based on the adjusted death rate derived from equation (A-6), the prognosis-adjusted survival with the ZIP model is derived by using $S(t) = \exp\{-\lambda \times t\}$ where t is the follow-up time (in years) and $S(t)$ is the survival function for cumulative survival making allowance for overdiagnosis.

A similar logic can be applied to deriving prognosis-adjusted annual death rates (λ′) using the conventional Poisson regression model without considering the zero-inflated part in the light of $S'(t) = \exp\{-\lambda' \times t\}$ where t is the follow-up time (in years) and $S'(t)$ is the survival function. The comparison of prognosis-adjusted 15-year cumulative survival between the model with and without adjusting for over-diagnosis was made and plotted in the Figure 2 of the main text.

References

1. Nelson, H.D.; Tyne, K.; Naik, A.; Bougatsos, C.; Chan, B.K.; Humphrey, L. Screening for breast cancer: An update for the US Preventive Services Task Force. *Ann. Intern. Med.* **2009**, *151*, 727–737. [CrossRef] [PubMed]
2. Independent UK Panel on Breast Cancer Screening. The benefits and harms of breast cancer screening: An independent review. *Lancet* **2012**, *380*, 1778–1786. [CrossRef]
3. Myers, E.R.; Moorman, P.; Gierisch, J.M.; Havrilesky, L.J.; Grimm, L.J.; Ghate, S.; Davidson, B.; Mongtomery, C.R.; Crowley, M.J.; McCrory, D.; et al. Benefits and Harms of Breast Cancer Screening: A Systematic Review. *JAMA* **2015**, *314*, 1615–1634. [CrossRef] [PubMed]
4. Chen, H.H.; Yen, A.M.F.; Fann, J.C.Y.; Gordon, P.; Chen, S.L.S.; Chiu, S.Y.H.; Hsu, C.Y.; Chang, K.J.; Lee, W.C.; Yeoh, K.G.; et al. Clarifying the debate on population-based screening for breast cancer with mammography: A systematic review of randomized controlled trials on mammography with Bayesian meta-analysis and causal model. *Medicine* **2017**, *96*, e5684. [CrossRef] [PubMed]
5. Brawley, O.W. Accepting the existence of breast cancer Overdiagnosis. *Ann. Intern. Med.* **2017**, *166*, 364–365. [CrossRef] [PubMed]
6. Duffy, S.W.; Agbaje, O.; Tabár, L.; Vitak, B.; Bjurstam, N.; Björneld, L.; Myles, J.P.; Warwick, J. Estimates of overdiagnosis from two trials of mammographic screening for breast cancer. *Breast Cancer Res.* **2005**, *7*, 258–265. [CrossRef] [PubMed]
7. Moss, S. Overdiagnosis in randomized controlled trials of breast cancer screening. *Breast Cancer Res.* **2005**, *7*, 230–234. [CrossRef] [PubMed]
8. Zackrisson, S.; Ancersson, I.; Janzon, L.; Manjer, J.; Garne, J.P. Rate of over-diagnosis of breast cancer 15 years after end of Malmo mammographic screening trial: Follow-up study. *BMJ* **2006**, *332*, 689–692. [CrossRef] [PubMed]

9. Biesheuvel, C.; Barratt, A.; Howard, K.; Houssami, N.; Irwig, L. Effects of study methods and biases on estimates of invasive breast cancer overdetection with mammography screening: A systematic review. *Lancet Oncol.* **2007**, *8*, 1129–1138. [CrossRef]
10. EUROSCREEN Working Group. Summary of the evidence of breast cancer service screening outcomes in Europe and first estimate of the benefit and harm balance sheet. *J. Med. Screen* **2012**, *19* (suppl. 1), 5–13. [CrossRef] [PubMed]
11. Puliti, D.; Duffy, S.W.; Miccinesi, G.; De Koning, H.; Lynge, E.; Zappa, M.; Paci, E. Overdiagnosis in mammographic screening for breast cancer in Europe: A literature review. *J. Med. Screen* **2012**, *19* (suppl. 1), 42–56. [CrossRef] [PubMed]
12. Coldman, A.; Phillips, N. Incidence of breast cancer and estimates of overdiagnosis after the initiation of a population-based mammography screening program. *CMAJ* **2013**, *185*, E498. [CrossRef] [PubMed]
13. Tabár, L.; Fagerberg, G.; Chen, H.H.; Duffy, S.W.; Gad, A. Tumour development, histology and grade of breast cancers: Prognosis and progression. *Int. J. Cancer* **1996**, *66*, 413–419. [CrossRef]
14. Chen, H.H.; Duffy, S.W.; Tabár, L. A mover-stayer mixture of Markov chain models for the assessment of dedifferentiation and tumour progression in breast cancer. *J. Appl. Stat.* **1997**, *24*, 265–278. [CrossRef]
15. Tabár, L.; Chen, H.H.; Duffy, S.W.; Krusemo, U.B. Primary and adjuvant therapy, prognostic factors and survival in 1053 breast cancers diagnosed in a trial of mammography screening. *Jpn. J. Clin. Oncol.* **1999**, *29*, 608–616. [CrossRef] [PubMed]
16. Fitzgibbons, P.L.; Page, D.L.; Weaver, D.; Thor, A.D.; Allred, D.C.; Clark, G.M.; Ruby, S.G.; O'Malley, F.; Simpson, J.F.; Connolly, J.L.; et al. Prognostic factors in breast cancer. College of American Pathologists Consensus Satement 1999. *Arch. Pathol. Lab. Med.* **2000**, *24*, 966–978.
17. Parise, C.A.; Caggiano, V. Breast cancer survival defined by ER/PR/HER2 subtypes and a surrogate classification according to tumor grade and immunohistochemical biomarkers. *J. Cancer Epidemiol.* **2014**, *2014*, 469251. [CrossRef] [PubMed]
18. Dent, R.; Trudeau, M.; Pritchard, K.I.; Hanna, W.M.; Kahn, H.K.; Sawka, C.A.; Lickley, L.A.; Rawlinson, E.; Sun, P.; Narod, S.A. Triple-negative breast cancer: Clinical features and patterns of recurrence. *Clin. Cancer Res.* **2007**, *13*, 4429–4434. [CrossRef] [PubMed]
19. Norad, S.A.; Valentini, A.; Nofech-Mozed, S.; Sun, P.; Hanna, W. Tumour characterisitcs among women with very low-risk breast cancer. *Breast Cancer Res. Treat.* **2012**, *134*, 1241–1246.
20. Swedish Organised Service Screening Evaluation Group. Effect of mammographic service screening on stage at presentation of breast cancer in Sweden. *Cancer* **2007**, *109*, 2205–2212. [CrossRef] [PubMed]
21. Biesheuvel, C.; Czene, K.; Orgeás, C.C.; Hall, P. The role of mammography screening attendance and detection mode in predicting breast cancer survival-is there added prognostic value? *Cancer Epidemiol.* **2011**, *35*, 545–550. [CrossRef] [PubMed]
22. Tot, T. Auxillary lymph node status in unifocal, multifocal, and diffuse breast carcinomas: Differences are related to macrometastatic disease. *Ann. Surg. Oncol.* **2012**, *19*, 3395–3401. [CrossRef] [PubMed]
23. Bohning, D. Zero-inflated Poisson models and C. A. MAN.: A tutorial collection of evidence. *Biom. J.* **1988**, *40*, 833–843. [CrossRef]
24. Morrel, S.; Barratt, A.; Irwig, L.; Howard, K.; Biesheuvel, C.; Armstrong, B. Estimates of overdiagnosis of invasive breast cancer associated with screening mammography. *Cancer Causes Control.* **2012**, *21*, 275–282. [CrossRef] [PubMed]
25. Zahl, P.H.; Strand, B.H.; Maehlen, J. Incidence of breast cancer in Norway and Sweden during introduction of nationwide screening: Prospective cohort study. *BMJ* **2004**, *328*, 921–924. [CrossRef] [PubMed]
26. Jonsson, H.; Johansson, R.; Lenner, P. Increased incidence of invasive breast cancer after the introduction of service screening with mammography in Sweden. *Int. J. Cancer* **2005**, *117*, 842–847. [CrossRef] [PubMed]
27. Tabár, L.; Gad, A.; Ljungquist, U.; Holmberg, L.H.; Kopparberg County Project Group; Fagerberg, C.J.G.; Baldetorp, L.; Gröntoft, O.; Lundström, B.; Månson, J.C.; et al. Reduction in mortality from breast cancer after mass screening with mammography. Randomised trial from the Breast Cancer Screening Working Group of the Swedish National Board of Health and Welfare. *Lancet* **1985**, *1*, 829–832.

15

Cytoplasmic Cyclin E is an Independent Marker of Aggressive Tumor Biology and Breast Cancer-Specific Mortality in Women over 70 Years of Age

Simon J. Johnston [1,2], Binafsha M. Syed [1,3], Ruth M. Parks [1], Cíntia J. Monteiro [1,2], Joseph A. Caruso [4], Andrew R. Green [1], Ian O. Ellis [1], Kelly K. Hunt [5], Cansu Karakas [6], Khandan Keyomarsi [6] and Kwok-Leung Cheung [1,*]

1 Nottingham Breast Cancer Research Centre, School of Medicine, The University of Nottingham, Nottingham NG7 2RD, UK; simon.johnston@cantab.net (S.J.J.); binafsha.syed@lumhs.edu.pk (B.M.S.); ruth.parks@nottingham.ac.uk (R.M.P.); cintiamonteiro@yahoo.com.br (C.J.M.); andrew.green@nottingham.ac.uk (A.R.G.); ian.ellis@nottingham.ac.uk (I.O.E.)

2 Gene Regulation Laboratory, School of Pharmacy, The University of Nottingham, Nottingham NG7 2RD, UK

3 Medical Research Centre, Liaquat University of Medical and Health Sciences, Jamshoro 76080, Pakistan

4 Department of Pathology, University of California, San Francisco, CA 94143, USA; joseph.caruso2@ucsf.edu

5 Department of Breast Surgical Oncology, The University of Texas MD Anderson Cancer Center, Houston, TX 77030, USA; khunt@mdanderson.org

6 Department of Experimental Radiation Oncology, The University of Texas MD Anderson Cancer Center, Houston, TX 77030, USA; cansu_karakas@yahoo.com (C.K.); kkeyomar@mdanderson.org (K.K.)

* Correspondence: kl.cheung@nottingham.ac.uk

Abstract: Multi-cohort analysis demonstrated that cytoplasmic cyclin E expression in primary breast tumors predicts aggressive disease. However, compared to their younger counterparts, older patients have favorable tumor biology and are less likely to die of breast cancer. Biomarkers therefore require interpretation in this specific context. Here, we assess data on cytoplasmic cyclin E from a UK cohort of older women alongside a panel of >20 biomarkers. Between 1973 and 2010, 813 women ≥70 years of age underwent initial surgery for early breast cancer, from which a tissue microarray was constructed ($n = 517$). Biomarker expression was assessed by immunohistochemistry. Multivariate analysis of breast cancer-specific survival was performed using Cox's proportional hazards. We found that cytoplasmic cyclin E was the only biological factor independently predictive of breast cancer-specific survival in this cohort of older women (hazard ratio (HR) = 6.23, 95% confidence interval (CI) = 1.93–20.14; $p = 0.002$). At ten years, 42% of older patients with cytoplasmic cyclin E-positive tumors had died of breast cancer versus 8% of negative cases ($p < 0.0005$). We conclude that cytoplasmic cyclin E is an exquisite marker of aggressive tumor biology in older women. Patients with cytoplasmic cyclin E-negative tumors are unlikely to die of breast cancer. These data have the potential to influence treatment strategy in older patients.

Keywords: breast cancer; cyclin E; older patients; biomarker; tumor biology; prognosis; survival

1. Introduction

The prognosis for patients with primary breast cancer is a function of disease extent at presentation and tumor biology. Time-dependent factors, including metastatic involvement of draining axillary lymph nodes (stage) and the size of the primary tumor, indicate disease extent, while the degree of differentiation (grade) is used as a surrogate for biological aggressiveness. These histopathology-assessed features are classically combined into the Nottingham Prognostic Index (NPI) [1].

Due to comorbidities, older patients with primary breast cancer are more likely to die of non-breast cancer-related causes when compared to their younger counterparts [2,3]. Furthermore, tumors in older patients have distinct biological characteristics that are linked to favorable outcome, such as a higher proportion and degree of hormone receptor (estrogen receptor (ER) and/or progesterone receptor (PR)) positivity, and low histological grade and Ki67 proliferative index [4,5]. Biomarkers that may influence treatment strategy therefore require interpretation in the specific clinical and biological context of older women.

Recent developments in risk stratification, such as tumor gene expression profiling (e.g., Oncotype Dx and MammaPrint), have focused on the biology of the primary tumor, based on the premise that this reflects the biology of presumed micrometastatic deposits [6,7]. Adjuvant therapy is then selected according to risk category with the aim of preventing these deposits from developing into clinically detectable metastases, thus avoiding disease relapse.

We have previously shown that tumor biology in older (>70 years) versus younger primary breast cancer cohorts can be distinguished by immunohistochemistry (IHC) using a panel of biomarkers, including ER, PR, HER2, Ki67, Bcl2, BRCA1, BRCA2, E-Cadherin, EGFR, LKB1, MDM2, MDM4, MUC1, p53, VEGF and cytokeratin markers of luminal and basal disease [4]. Differential expression of age-associated biomarkers clustered tumors from older patients into six groups with distinct clinical outcomes.

The current study focuses on the role of G1/S-specific cyclin-E1 (cyclin E) as a biological marker of aggressive disease, and on its prognostic significance in the context of older women with primary breast cancer.

In normal dividing cells, cyclin E promotes the transition from G1 to S phase by activating cyclin-dependent kinase 2 (CDK2) [8]. In breast cancer cells, tumor-specific proteolytic processing of cyclin E generates hyperactive low molecular weight (LMW) isoforms [9]. In contrast to full length cyclin E, for which prognostic data have been equivocal, LMW isoforms are highly prognostic in primary breast cancer patients [10–12]. As they lack a portion of the amino-terminus containing a nuclear localization sequence, LMW isoforms of cyclin E preferentially accumulate in the cytoplasm where they evade nuclear FBW-7 ubiquitin ligase that would otherwise increase their turnover [13].

In previous work using an antibody named C-19 that interacts with the carboxyl-terminus of cyclin E (present in both full length and LMW isoforms of cyclin E), we showed that transgenic mouse models with mammary gland expression of LMW cyclin E developed mammary tumors positive only for cytoplasmic cyclin E [14]. Furthermore, cytoplasmic cyclin E bound to its catalytic subunit, CDK2, in the cytoplasm of tumor cells [14]. The biological functions of cytoplasmic, LMW cyclin E are summarized in Figure 1.

These critical findings on the biological functions of LMW cyclin E paved the way for a pivotal study on the use of cytoplasmic expression of cyclin E (c-cyclin E) by IHC to predict recurrence in patients with primary breast cancer [15]. Combined analysis of 2494 tumors from four cohorts of patients (from the UK and the USA, covering all age groups) presenting with primary breast cancer demonstrated that c-cyclin E staining is highly prognostic. These data included the current UK cohort of older women (median age 76, versus 53–62 years in all cohorts, $p < 0.0001$).

We now present data on c-cyclin E exclusively from the Nottingham cohort. This paper is distinct from the multi-cohort study as it focuses only on the older population and assesses the role of c-cyclin E against a large panel of more than 20 disease markers. Findings are interpreted in the specific biological and clinical context of primary breast cancer in older women, and the implications for risk stratification and treatment decision-making in older patients are discussed.

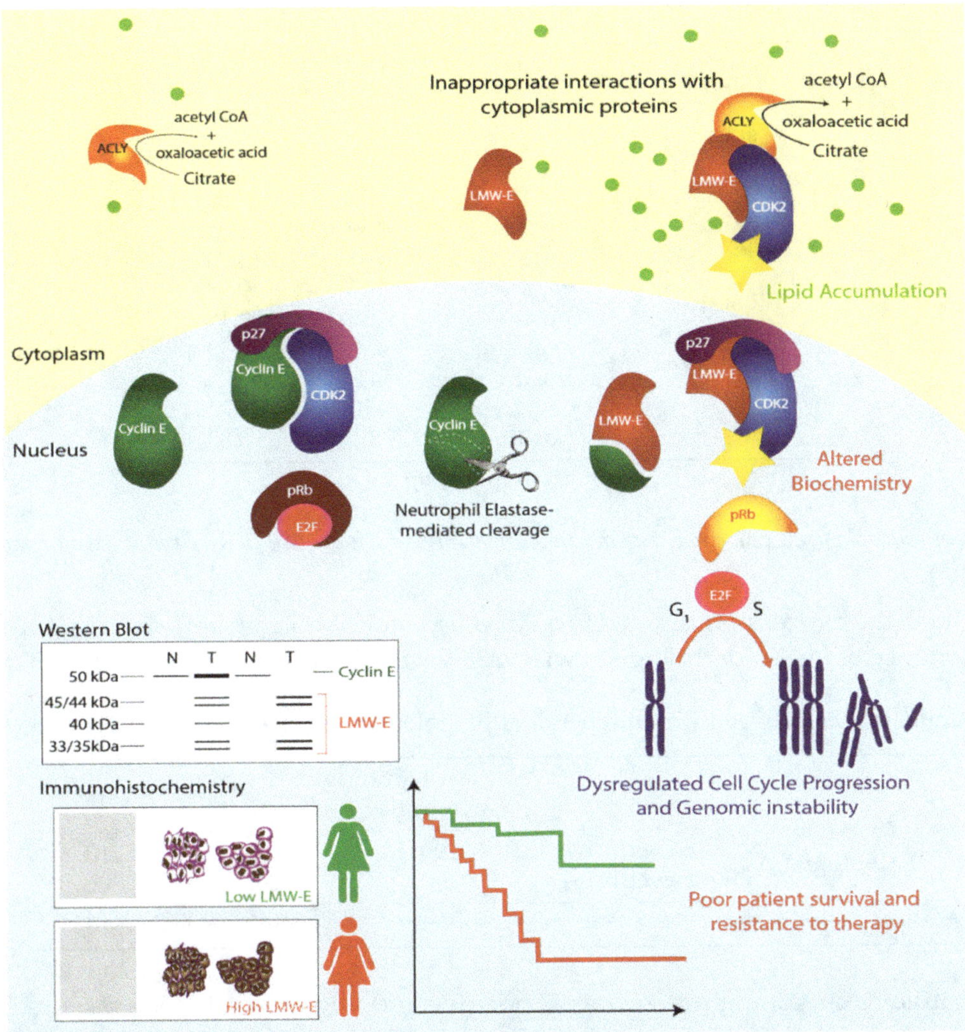

Figure 1. Model: Low molecular weight cyclin E (LMW-E) isoforms are generated by neutrophil elastase-mediated proteolytic cleavage, removing the N-terminal nuclear localization signal. LMW-E isoforms accumulate in the cytoplasm where they inappropriately interact with cytoplasmic proteins, such as ACLY. The altered biochemistry of LMW-E results in hyperactivation of CDK2, resistance to endogenous CDK-inhibitors (p21CIP1 and p27KIP1) and altered substrate interactions, which results in enhanced cell cycle progression, genomic instability and other pro-tumorigenic features. Evaluation of LMW-E by Western blot (protein size) or immunohistochemistry (cytoplasmic localization) is prognostic of poor prognosis and predicts failure of standard treatment modalities.

2. Results

Patient clinicopathological characteristics are summarized in Table 1. Median follow-up was 6.3 years (95% CI, 6.1–7.1 years).

Table 1. Summary of patient characteristics ($n = 517$).

Variable	Group	n	%
age	70 to <75 yrs	206	39.8%
	75 to <80 yrs	202	39.1%
	80 to <85 yrs	83	16.1%
	≥85 yrs	26	5.0%
tumor size	<20 mm	153	31.7%
	≥20 mm	329	68.3%

Table 1. *Cont.*

Variable	Group	*n*	%
stage	1	183	57.5%
	2	98	30.8%
	3	37	11.6%
grade	1	51	12.0%
	2	169	39.8%
	3	205	48.2%
ER status	negative	143	29.9%
	positive	335	70.1%
HER2 status	negative	453	91.7%
	positive	41	8.3%
Metastasis [1]	negative	430	83.2%
	positive	87	16.8%

[1] at last follow-up.

2.1. *Expression of Cytoplasmic Cyclin E Associates with High-Grade, ER-/PR- Breast Tumors with High Ki67 Proliferative Index*

We examined the expression of c-cyclin E and a panel of biomarkers in breast tumors by IHC. Average concordance between pathologists was 93% for the Nottingham cohort (see Table 2).

Table 2. Concordance between two independent pathologists for the Nottingham cohort (n = 516).

		Pathologist B		Total
		c-cyclin E+	c-cyclin E−	
Pathologist A	c-cyclin E+	199	11	210
	c-cyclin E−	11	295	306
				516

Representative IHC staining for c-cyclin E positive and negative cases is presented in Figure 2.

To assess the potential clinical relevance of c-cyclin E, we first compared c-cyclin E expression with clinicopathological features at initial diagnosis (age, tumor size, stage and grade) and markers of disease biology in current clinical use, including ER, PR, HER2 and Ki67 status.

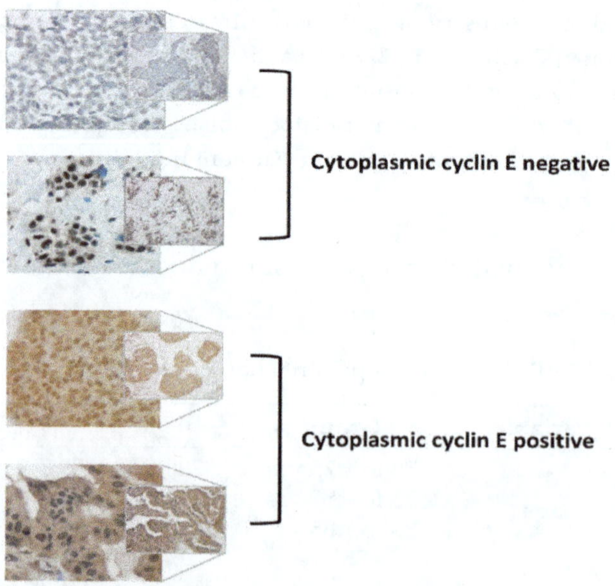

Figure 2. Representative images of positive and negative staining for cytoplasmic cyclin E using antibody C-19.

There was a strong association between c-cyclin E expression and higher grade ($p < 0.0005$, see Table 3). In contrast, there was no association between c-cyclin E and patient age, tumor size or stage. Cytoplasmic expression of cyclin E was significantly associated with negative ER and PR status ($p = 0.002$ and $p = 0.012$, respectively) and high Ki67 proliferative index ($p = 0.047$) (Table 3). No significant association was found between c-cyclin E and HER2 status.

Table 3. Association between tumor c-cyclin E status and clinicopathological factors.

Variable		c-Cyclin E−		c-Cyclin E+		p
age	70 to <80 yrs	170	(41.7%)	238	(58.3%)	0.743
	≥80 yrs	43	(39.4%)	66	(60.6%)	
size	<20 mm	64	(41.8%)	89	(58.2%)	0.921
	≥20 mm	135	(41.0%)	194	(59.0%)	
stage	1	83	(45.4%)	100	(54.6%)	0.350
	2	42	(42.9%)	56	(57.1%)	
	3	12	(32.4%)	25	(67.6%)	
grade	1	33	(64.7%)	18	(35.3%)	<0.0005 [1]
	2	87	(51.5%)	82	(48.5%)	
	3	64	(31.2%)	141	(68.8%)	
ER	negative	43	(30.1%)	100	(69.9%)	0.002 [1]
	positive	151	(45.1%)	184	(54.9%)	
PR	negative	74	(34.6%)	140	(65.4%)	0.012 [1]
	positive	122	(46.2%)	142	(53.8%)	
HER2	negative	187	(41.3%)	266	(58.7%)	0.869
	positive	16	(39.0%)	25	(61.0%)	
Ki67	negative	152	(44.3%)	191	(55.7%)	0.047 [1]
	positive	61	(35.1%)	113	(64.9%)	

[1] Statistical significance $p < 0.05$, by χ^2 test

Comparison of c-cyclin E status with other biomarkers revealed a positive association with VEGF ($p = 0.041$), and no other significant association.

2.2. *Cytoplasmic Cyclin E Expression Is Enriched in Basal Tumors*

We next assessed the association between tumor c-cyclin E expression and cellular phenotype as indicated by the expression of cytokeratin markers in the IHC protein panel.

Cytoplasmic cyclin E expression was associated with markers of basal disease (see Table 4). Basal cytokeratin markers significantly associated with c-cyclin E included CK5 and CK17 ($p = 0.001$ and $p = 0.036$, respectively). In contrast, there was no association between c-cyclin E and the luminal marker CK18.

Table 4. Association between tumor c-cyclin E status and clinicopathological factors.

Variable		c-Cyclin E−		c-Cyclin E+		p
CK5	negative	152	(45.5%)	182	(54.5%)	0.001 [1]
	positive	43	(29.5%)	103	(70.5%)	
CK5/6	negative	101	(43.3%)	132	(56.7%)	0.284
	positive	78	(37.9%)	128	(62.1%)	
CK14	negative	143	(43.7%)	184	(56.3%)	0.074
	positive	37	(33.9%)	72	(66.1%)	
CK17	negative	160	(43.1%)	211	(56.9%)	0.036 [1]
	positive	30	(31.3%)	66	(68.8%)	
CK18	negative	3	(21.4%)	11	(78.6%)	0.170
	positive	187	(41.9%)	259	(58.1%)	

[1] statistical significance $p < 0.05$, by χ^2 test. CK5, CK5/6 (antibody to both CK5 and CK6), CK14 and CK17 are basal markers; CK18 is a luminal marker.

2.3. Survival Analysis

Kaplan–Meier plots of breast cancer-specific survival (BCSS) and disease-free survival (DFS) as a function of c-cyclin E status are shown in Figure 3. Lack of c-cyclin E was associated with good prognosis in the patient cohort (BCSS and DFS both $p < 0.0005$ by logrank test). This was observed for luminal A/B (ER+ and/or PR+), HER2+ and triple negative breast cancer subtypes (see Figure 4).

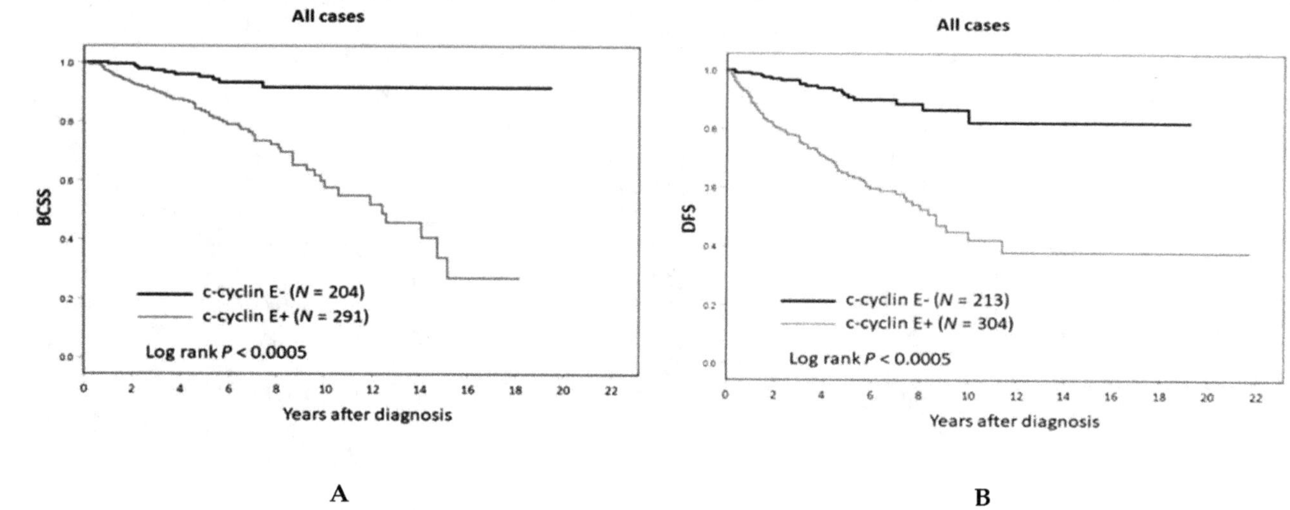

Figure 3. (**A**) Breast cancer-specific and (**B**) disease-free survival by cytoplasmic cyclin E status.

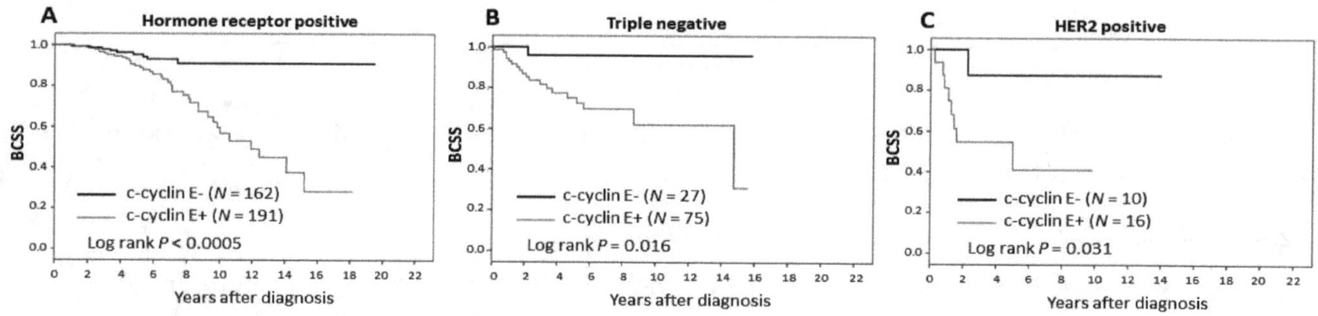

Figure 4. Breast cancer-specific survival by subtype: (**A**) hormone receptor (ER and/or PR) positive, (**B**) triple negative, (**C**) HER2 positive.

Survival analysis of c-cyclin E alongside the full panel of biomarkers was performed using data up to last follow-up. Due to the low proportion of low-grade tumors (grade 1, 12%), these were combined with intermediate-grade tumors (grade 2, 40%) and used as a statistical reference for comparison with high-grade tumors (grade 3, 48%). Multivariate analysis was performed on all clinicopathological factors and biomarkers significantly associated with BCSS in univariate testing.

Cytoplasmic expression of cyclin E was the only independent biomarker of BCSS and had a strong association in multivariate analysis (HR = 6.23, 95% CI 1.93–20.14; $p = 0.002$) (Figure 5). The only clinicopathological factor predictive of BCSS in the multivariate analysis was axillary nodal status (HR = 4.38, 95% CI 1.77–10.84; $p = 0.001$).

For the whole cohort of 517 patients, there was a strong positive association between c-cyclin E positivity and breast cancer-specific mortality at 5 years of follow-up ($p<0.0005$). Multivariate analysis demonstrates that c-cyclin E positivity is the strongest predictor of 5-year BCSS in this cohort (HR = 9.12, 95% CI 2.22–37.40; $p = 0.002$)—outperforming lymph node status (HR=4.49, 95% CI 1.66–12.15; $p = 0.003$) and all other biological disease markers.

At ten years of follow-up, BCSS for patients with c-cyclin E-negative tumors was 92% versus 58% for those with c-cyclin E-positive tumors (HR = 6.23, 95% CI 1.92–20.14; $p = 0.002$ in multivariate analysis). At completion of follow-up, the absolute difference in median overall survival (OS) by c-cyclin E status (positive versus negative) was 33 months (130 versus 97 months, $p = 0.01$ by logrank, Mantel–Cox) (see Figure 6).

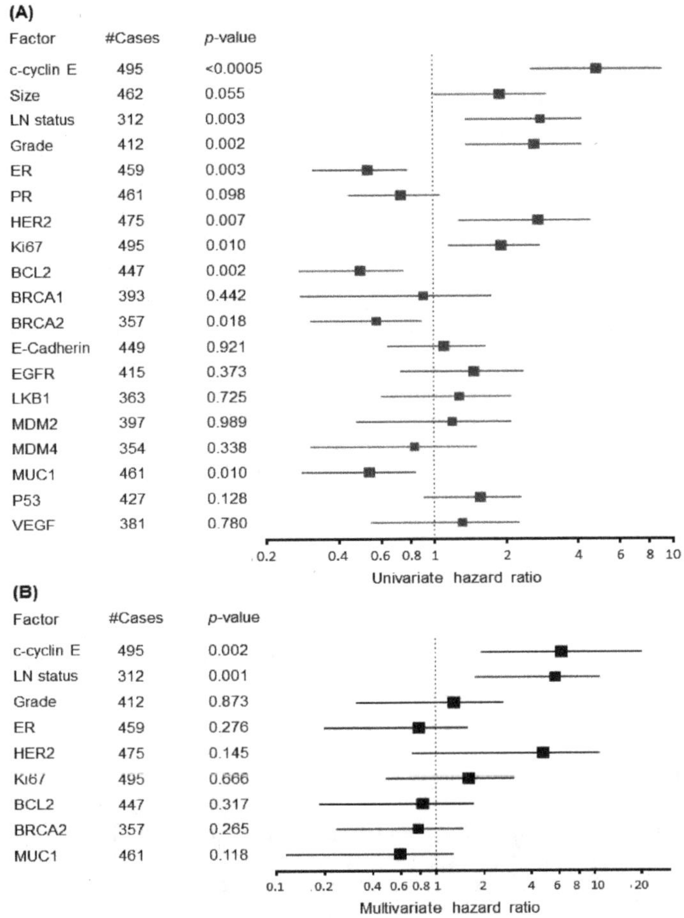

Figure 5. (**A**) Univariate and (**B**) multivariate analysis of c-cyclin E with clinicopathological and age-associated biomarkers.

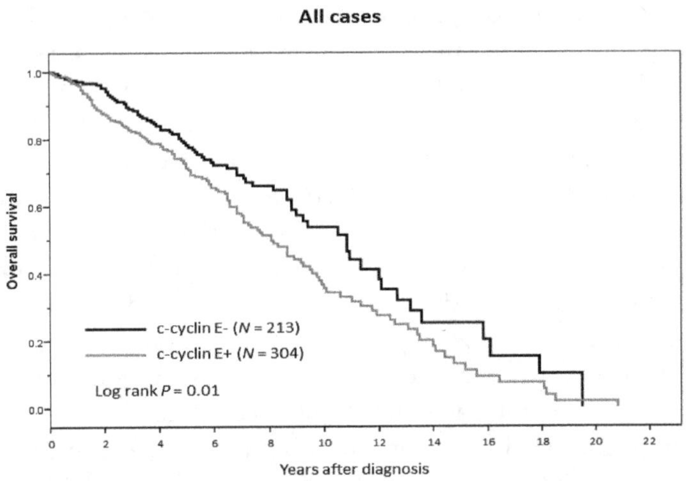

Figure 6. Overall survival (all cases) by cytoplasmic cyclin E status.

2.4. Prognostic Value of Cytoplasmic Cyclin E in Patients Treated with Endocrine Therapy

Patients with ER+ disease received up to 5 years of adjuvant endocrine therapy according to risk stratification by NPI (e.g., NPI > 2.4 or 3.4, according to best practice guidelines at the time of treatment). We next explored the prognostic value of c-cyclin E and its relationship to adjuvant endocrine therapy in patients with ER+ tumors.

In contrast to the whole cohort (where c-cyclin E was the strongest predictor of 5-year BCSS), in patients who received up to 5 years of adjuvant endocrine therapy ($n = 229$), c-cyclin E was not associated with 5-year BCSS ($p = 0.323$). After cessation of adjuvant endocrine therapy, c-cyclin E reached prognostic significance (positive association with breast cancer-specific mortality) at 10 years of follow-up ($p = 0.009$) (see Figure 7).

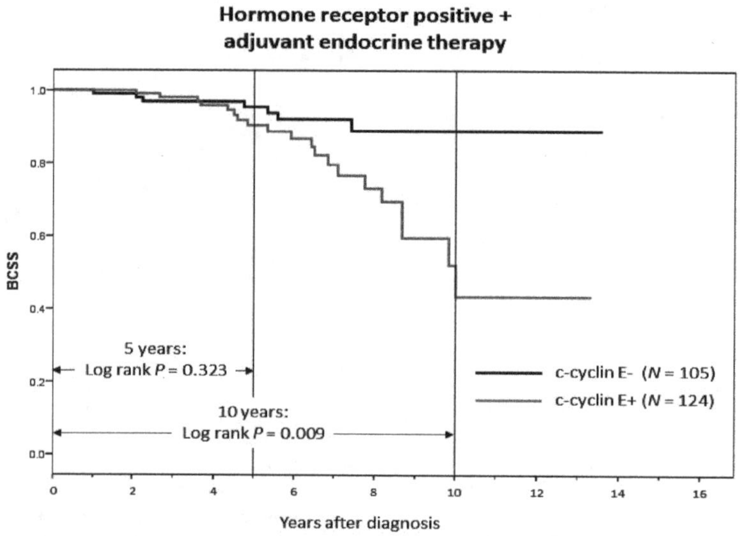

Figure 7. Adjuvant endocrine therapy negates the poor prognostic effect of c-cyclin E positivity, but only for as long as it is given (up to 5 years).

3. Discussion

In this study of 517 older women with primary breast cancer, c-cyclin E is the only independent biological marker of disease outcome. In terms of prognostic value, c-cyclin E status outperforms all standard clinical and age-associated biomarkers tested in this study.

For the older population, who more often present with complex comorbidities and psychosocial factors, considerations regarding competing causes of death are paramount in clinical decision-making [16]. The current study presents BCSS as a surrogate measure for the impact of tumor biology on patient mortality. Deaths due to non-breast cancer causes are excluded from the analysis. Unlike non-modifiable and time-dependent clinicopathological disease factors, such as tumor size and stage, those factors pertaining to tumor biology can be modified using systemic therapy.

Data from the current study supplement findings from an international study of four cohorts (including the Nottingham cohort) and add clinical context in older women [16]. In the combined analysis, freedom from recurrence (FFR), defined as the time between the date of diagnosis and the date of first locoregional or distant recurrence, was the primary endpoint. Unlike BCSS and DFS, FFR does not include death as an event, regardless of the cause of death.

In two of the other three cohorts in the combined analysis (MD Anderson (MDA) and National Cancer Institute (NCI)), c-cyclin E expression had the strongest effect on FFR. In the Nottingham cohort, c-cyclin E outperformed standard clinical biomarkers in terms of both FFR and BCSS.

Combined analysis of the two largest US clinical cohorts contributing to the multi-cohort study has also been reported (MDA and NCI) [14]. Data from the Nottingham cohort are consistent with the NCI and MDA cohorts. For example, there was 60% positive c-cyclin E staining in combined NCI/MDA analysis, compared to 59% in the Nottingham cohort. This demonstrates good reproducibility of IHC measurement of cytoplasmic expression of cyclin E—an important factor when considering the potential application of c-cyclin E status as a clinical biomarker.

In line with the Nottingham cohort, expression of c-cyclin E in the combined analysis of the NCI and MDA cohorts was associated with tumor markers, such as grade, ER and PR, and was associated with poor patient outcome. However, in the NCI/MDA analysis, c-cyclin E was only an independent marker of recurrence-free and overall survival when combined with the downstream kinase, cyclin-dependent kinase 2. In the NCI/MDA analysis, histological grade was also an independent prognostic factor.

Analysis of the Nottingham cohort of older women, in contrast, found that c-cyclin E was the only independent prognostic biomarker, outperforming even tumor grade in terms of prognostic value. Although c-cyclin E was not associated with age in any of the cohorts, overall findings from the older Nottingham cohort suggest a greater biological effect of high c-cyclin E expression in the older population. Breast cancer biology in the older population is considered more indolent, with less aggressive phenotypic features and enrichment for ER expression. This suggests that c-cyclin E has greater potential clinical utility in the older population and is better able to distinguish more aggressive tumors that are likely to lead to death from breast cancer.

Findings from the current study support c-cyclin E as a robust and reproducible biomarker of an aggressive disease course. The findings suggest that clinical outcomes of older women with primary breast cancer can be predicted from the biology of their tumor using c-cyclin E alone. Older patients with c-cyclin E-negative tumors are unlikely to die of their breast cancer. At ten years, only 8 patients out of 100 will die of their breast cancer if their tumor is c-cyclin E-negative. For many older patients, this finding will directly impact clinical decision-making.

Alongside existing clinical decision-making tools such as comprehensive geriatric assessment scales and biomarkers of treatment response such as ER expression, there is clear potential to utilize tumor c-cyclin E expression in the clinic. For example, c-cyclin E positivity may indicate a requirement for an aggressive initial treatment strategy, in terms of surgical management of the primary tumor and axillary lymph nodes, and the need for adjuvant therapy.

Although the clinical setting of the current study is patients selected to undergo initial surgery, who are more likely to have ER-negative tumors, it may be possible to extrapolate its findings on the value of c-cyclin E as a marker of aggressive disease biology to other clinical scenarios.

For example, ER/PR+ primary tumors that do not express c-cyclin E may be adequately treated by primary endocrine therapy. Alongside comprehensive geriatric assessment, c-cyclin E may serve as a biomarker in this context for patients who, because of comorbidity, psychosocial factors or individual choice, would prefer not to undergo initial surgery. Given the high proportion of older patients already receiving primary endocrine therapy (up to 40% of UK patients in the previous decade), there is a compelling case to investigate this hypothesis in prospective clinical trials [17].

In adjuvant therapy decision-making, c-cyclin E could supplement or replace gene expression predictors of chemotherapy response (e.g., Oncotype Dx and MammaPrint). Additionally, as cyclin-dependent kinase 2-targeting treatments, e.g., dinaciclib, emerge from early phase clinical trials, there may be a role for these drugs in older patients in preference to chemotherapy [18,19].

It is reported that c-cyclin E mediates resistance to endocrine therapy with aromatase inhibitors (AIs) in breast cancer [20]. This study suggests that c-cyclin E may identify ER/PR+ tumors that are unresponsive to AIs, which do not induce a cytostatic effect.

For patients with ER+ disease, evidence from the current study suggests that adjuvant endocrine therapy negates the poor prognostic effect of c-cyclin E positivity. This implies that extending adjuvant therapy beyond 5 years would improve long-term outcomes and would be a priority for patients with c-cyclin E-positive tumors.

4. Materials and Methods

Over a 37-year period (1973–2010), 1758 older (≥70 years) women with stage I–II primary breast cancer were managed in a dedicated facility in Nottingham, as previously described [21]. Of these patients, 813 underwent primary surgery.

Good quality formalin-fixed, paraffin embedded tissue from 575 tumors was available, from which 517 were successfully incorporated into a tissue microarray (TMA), as previously described [22]. Briefly, representative 0.6mm diameter cores were implanted in the TMA block using Beecher's manual tissue microarray (MP06 Beecher Instruments Inc., Sun Prairie, WI, USA).

Clinical information was available from diagnosis to death or last follow-up. Patient clinicopathological characteristics are summarized in Table 1. Median follow-up was 6.3 years (95% CI, 6.1–7.1 years).

The TMA was used to test expression of a panel of biomarkers by IHC, using the StreptAvidin Biotin Complex and EnVision methods, which have been extensively described [4]. Biomarkers tested in Nottingham included ER, PR, HER2, Ki67, Bcl2, BRCA1, BRCA2, E-Cadherin, EGFR, LKB1, MDM2, MDM4, MUC1, p53, VEGF and cytokeratin markers CK5, CK5/6, CK14, CK17 and CK18.

Staining of the biomarker panel was assessed as previously reported [4]. Cytoplasmic staining for cyclin E was centrally assessed at MD Anderson Cancer Center as previously described, using Santa Cruz clone C-19 polyclonal antibody to cyclin E [15]. TMA results were interpreted by two independent pathologists blinded to clinical outcome and assigned according to percentage of cells stained and intensity of staining. Cut-off values for all biomarkers were as reported in our previous studies [4,14].

Conventional pathological parameters as part of standard reporting for surgical specimens at Nottingham were measured, including size, grade and axillary stage (regional lymph node involvement). The policy of axillary surgery evolved according to clinical evidence-based guidelines over the 37-year period of sample collection, as previously described [21].

The primary endpoint was breast cancer-specific survival (BCSS), defined as time from diagnosis to last follow-up or death from breast cancer (i.e., excluding death due to competing causes). Secondary endpoints included disease-free survival (DFS), defined as time from diagnosis to first recurrence, and overall survival (OS), defined as time from diagnosis to last follow-up or death from any cause.

The bioinformatics software X-Tile was used to define thresholds for biomarker positivity, as previously described [23]. Biomarker expression was compared between groups by χ^2 test. Kaplan–Meier survival analysis was performed using logrank and generalized Wilcoxon tests. Multivariate analysis of BCSS was performed using the Cox regression model. Statistical significance was defined as $p < 0.05$. Reporting adhered to reporting recommendations for tumor marker prognostic studies (REMARK) criteria [24].

This research was conducted in accordance with the Declaration of Helsinki. The study protocol was approved by the Institutional Review Boards of the University of Nottingham, Nottingham University Hospitals NHS Trust and the University of Texas MD Anderson Cancer Center (MDA ref.33).

5. Conclusions

This study highlights the clinical value of tumor c-cyclin E status as a strong predictor of the biological course of primary breast cancer in older patients. Those who present with c-cyclin E-negative tumors are unlikely to die of their breast cancer. Alongside existing tools such as geriatric assessment and biomarkers of treatment response such as ER positivity, c-cyclin E status may assist initial therapy decision-making in terms of intensity, duration and modality. These hypotheses warrant prospective clinical evaluation in the specific clinical context of primary breast cancer in older women.

Author Contributions: Conceptualization, S.J.J., K.K.H., C.K., K.K. and K.-L.C.; methodology, B.M.S., J.A.C., K.K.H., C.K., K.K. and K.-L.C.; formal analysis, S.J.J., B.M.S. and C.J.M.; resources, A.R.G., I.O.E., K.K.H., C.K., K.K. and K.-L.C.; data curation, B.M.S.; writing—original draft preparation, S.J.J.; writing—review and editing, R.M.P., C.J.M., A.R.G. and K.-L.C.; visualization, S.J.J., C.J.M. and J.A.C.; supervision, K.-L.C.; project administration,

B.M.S. and K.-L.C.; funding acquisition, B.M.S., K.-L.C., K.K. and K.K.H. All authors have read and agreed to the published version of the manuscript.

Acknowledgments: The authors thank the Nottingham Health Science Biobank and Breast Cancer Now Tissue Bank for the provision of tissue samples.

References

1. Haybittle, J.L.; Blamey, R.W.; Elston, C.W.; Johnson, J.; Doyle, P.J.; Campbell, F.C.; Nicholson, R.I.; Griffiths, K. A prognostic index in primary breast cancer. *Br. J. Cancer* **1982**, *45*, 361–366. [CrossRef] [PubMed]
2. Fleming, S.T.; Rastogi, A.; Dmitrienko, A.; Johnson, K.D. A comprehensive prognostic index to predict survival based on multiple comorbidities: A focus on breast cancer. *Med. Care* **1999**, *37*, 601–614. [CrossRef] [PubMed]
3. Yancik, R.; Wesley, M.N.; Ries, L.A.; Havlik, R.J.; Edwards, B.K.; Yates, J.W. Effect of age and comorbidity in postmenopausal breast cancer patients aged 55 years and older. *JAMA* **2001**, *285*, 885–892. [CrossRef] [PubMed]
4. Syed, B.M.; Green, A.R.; Paish, E.C.; Soria, D.; Garibaldi, J.; Morgan, L.; Morgan, D.A.; Ellis, I.O.; Cheung, K.L. Biology of primary breast cancer in older women treated by surgery: With correlation with long-term clinical outcome and comparison with their younger counterparts. *Br. J. Cancer* **2013**, *108*, 1042–1051. [CrossRef]
5. Cheung, K.L.; Wong, A.W.; Parker, H.; Li, V.W.; Winterbottom, L.; Morgan, D.A.; Ellis, I.O. Pathological features of primary breast cancer in the elderly based on needle core biopsies–a large series from a single centre. *Crit. Rev. Oncol. Hematol.* **2008**, *67*, 263–267. [CrossRef]
6. Sparano, J.A.; Gray, R.J.; Makower, D.F.; Pritchard, K.I.; Albain, K.S.; Hayes, D.F.; Geyer, C.E., Jr.; Dees, E.C.; Goetz, M.P.; Olson, J.A., Jr.; et al. Adjuvant Chemotherapy Guided by a 21-Gene Expression Assay in Breast Cancer. *N. Engl. J. Med.* **2018**, *379*, 111–121. [CrossRef]
7. Cardoso, F.; van't Veer, L.J.; Bogaerts, J.; Slaets, L.; Viale, G.; Delaloge, S.; Pierga, J.Y.; Brain, E.; Causeret, S.; DeLorenzi, M.; et al. 70-Gene Signature as an Aid to Treatment Decisions in Early-Stage Breast Cancer. *N. Engl. J. Med.* **2016**, *375*, 717–729. [CrossRef]
8. Dou, Q.P.; Levin, A.H.; Zhao, S.; Pardee, A.B. Cyclin E and cyclin A as candidates for the restriction point protein. *Cancer Res.* **1993**, *53*, 1493–1497.
9. Porter, D.C.; Zhang, N.; Danes, C.; McGahren, M.J.; Harwell, R.M.; Faruki, S.; Keyomarsi, K. Tumor-specific proteolytic processing of cyclin E generates hyperactive lower-molecular-weight forms. *Mol. Cell. Biol.* **2001**, *21*, 6254–6269. [CrossRef]
10. Keyomarsi, K.; Tucker, S.L.; Buchholz, T.A.; Callister, M.; Ding, Y.; Hortobagyi, G.N.; Bedrosian, I.; Knickerbocker, C.; Toyofuku, W.; Lowe, M.; et al. Cyclin E and survival in patients with breast cancer. *N. Engl. J. Med.* **2002**, *347*, 1566–1575. [CrossRef]
11. Donnellan, R.; Kleinschmidt, I.; Chetty, R. Cyclin E immunoexpression in breast ductal carcinoma: Pathologic correlations and prognostic implications. *Hum. Pathol.* **2001**, *32*, 89–94. [CrossRef] [PubMed]
12. Porter, P.L.; Malone, K.E.; Heagerty, P.J.; Alexander, G.M.; Gatti, L.A.; Firpo, E.J.; Daling, J.R.; Roberts, J.M. Expression of cell-cycle regulators p27Kip1 and cyclin E, alone and in combination, correlate with survival in young breast cancer patients. *Nat. Med.* **1997**, *3*, 222–225. [CrossRef] [PubMed]
13. Delk, N.A.; Hunt, K.K.; Keyomarsi, K. Altered subcellular localization of tumor-specific cyclin E isoforms affects cyclin-dependent kinase 2 complex formation and proteasomal regulation. *Cancer Res.* **2009**, *69*, 2817–2825. [CrossRef] [PubMed]
14. Karakas, C.; Biernacka, A.; Bui, T.; Sahin, A.A.; Yi, M.; Akli, S.; Schafer, J.; Alexander, A.; Adjapong, O.; Hunt, K.K.; et al. Cytoplasmic Cyclin E and Phospho-Cyclin-Dependent Kinase 2 Are Biomarkers of Aggressive Breast Cancer. *Am. J. Pathol.* **2016**, *186*, 1900–1912. [CrossRef] [PubMed]
15. Hunt, K.K.; Karakas, C.; Ha, M.J.; Biernacka, A.; Yi, M.; Sahin, A.A.; Adjapong, O.; Hortobagyi, G.N.; Bondy, M.; Thompson, P.; et al. Cytoplasmic Cyclin E Predicts Recurrence in Patients with Breast Cancer. *Clin. Cancer Res.* **2017**, *23*, 2991–3002. [CrossRef]
16. Johnston, S.J.; Cheung, K.L. The role of primary endocrine therapy in older women with operable breast cancer. *Future Oncol.* **2015**, *11*, 1555–1565. [CrossRef]

17. Wyld, L.; Garg, D.K.; Kumar, I.D.; Brown, H.; Reed, M.W. Stage and treatment variation with age in postmenopausal women with breast cancer: Compliance with guidelines. *Br. J. Cancer* **2004**, *90*, 1486–1491. [CrossRef]
18. Mitri, Z.; Karakas, C.; Wei, C.; Briones, B.; Simmons, H.; Ibrahim, N.; Alvarez, R.; Murray, J.L.; Keyomarsi, K.; Moulder, S. A phase 1 study with dose expansion of the CDK inhibitor dinaciclib (SCH 727965) in combination with epirubicin in patients with metastatic triple negative breast cancer. *Investig. New Drugs* **2015**, *33*, 890–894. [CrossRef]
19. Mita, M.M.; Joy, A.A.; Mita, A.; Sankhala, K.; Jou, Y.M.; Zhang, D.; Statkevich, P.; Zhu, Y.; Yao, S.L.; Small, K.; et al. Randomized phase II trial of the cyclin-dependent kinase inhibitor dinaciclib (MK-7965) versus capecitabine in patients with advanced breast cancer. *Clin. Breast Cancer* **2014**, *14*, 169–176. [CrossRef]
20. Doostan, I.; Karakas, C.; Kohansal, M.; Low, K.H.; Ellis, M.J.; Olson, J.A., Jr.; Suman, V.J.; Hunt, K.K.; Moulder, S.L.; Keyomarsi, K. Cytoplasmic Cyclin E Mediates Resistance to Aromatase Inhibitors in Breast Cancer. *Clin. Cancer Res.* **2017**, *23*, 7288–7300. [CrossRef]
21. Syed, B.M.; Johnston, S.J.; Wong, D.W.; Green, A.R.; Winterbottom, L.; Kennedy, H.; Simpson, N.; Morgan, D.A.; Ellis, I.O.; Cheung, K.L. Long-term (37 years) clinical outcome of older women with early operable primary breast cancer managed in a dedicated clinic. *Ann. Oncol.* **2012**, *23*, 1465–1471. [CrossRef] [PubMed]
22. Camp, R.L.; Charette, L.A.; Rimm, D.L. Validation of tissue microarray technology in breast carcinoma. *Lab. Investig.* **2000**, *80*, 1943–1949. [CrossRef]
23. Camp, R.L.; Dolled-Filhart, M.; Rimm, D.L. X-tile: A new bio-informatics tool for biomarker assessment and outcome-based cut-point optimization. *Clin. Cancer Res.* **2004**, *10*, 7252–7259. [CrossRef] [PubMed]
24. McShane, L.M.; Altman, D.G.; Sauerbrei, W.; Taube, S.E.; Gion, M.; Clark, G.M.; Statistics Subcommittee of the NCIEWGoCD. Reporting recommendations for tumor marker prognostic studies (REMARK). *J. Natl. Cancer Inst.* **2005**, *97*, 1180–1184. [CrossRef] [PubMed]

16

Why has Breast Cancer Screening Failed to Decrease the Incidence of de Novo Stage IV Disease?

Danielle R. Heller [1], Alexander S. Chiu [1], Kaitlin Farrell [2], Brigid K. Killelea [2] and Donald R. Lannin [2,*]

1 Department of Surgery, Yale School of Medicine, New Haven, CT 06520, USA; d.heller@yale.edu (D.R.H.); alex.chiu@yale.edu (A.S.C.)
2 The Breast Center/Section of Surgical Oncology, Department of Surgery, Yale School of Medicine, New Haven, CT 06520, USA; kaitlinfarrell10@gmail.com (K.F.); Brigid.killelea@yale.edu (B.K.K.)
* Correspondence: Donald.lannin@yale.edu

Abstract: *Background*: Despite screening mammography, the incidence of Stage IV breast cancer (BC) at diagnosis has not decreased over the past four decades. We previously found that many BCs are small due to favorable biology rather than early detection. This study compared the biology of Stage IV cancers with that of small cancers typically found by screening. *Methods*: Trends in the incidence of localized, regional, and distant female BC were compared using SEER*Stat. The National Cancer Database (NCDB) was then queried for invasive cancers from 2010 to 2015, and patient/disease variables were compared across stages. Biological variables including estrogen receptor (ER), progesterone receptor (PR), human epidermal growth factor receptor 2 (Her2), grade, and lymphovascular invasion were sorted into 48 combinations, from which three biological subtypes emerged: indolent, intermediate, and aggressive. The distributions of the subtypes were compared across disease stages. Multivariable regression assessed the association between Stage IV disease and biology. *Results*: SEER*Stat confirmed that the incidence of distant BC increased between 1973 and 2015 (annual percent change [APC] = 0.46). NCDB data on roughly 993,000 individuals showed that Stage IV disease at presentation is more common in young, black, uninsured women with low income/education and large, biologically aggressive tumors. The distribution of tumor biology varied by stage, with Stage IV disease including 37.6% aggressive and 6.0% indolent tumors, versus sub-centimeter Stage I disease that included 5.1% aggressive and 40.6% indolent tumors ($p < 0.001$). The odds of Stage IV disease presentation more than tripled for patients with aggressive tumors (OR3.2, 95% CI 3.0–3.5). *Conclusions*: Stage I and Stage IV breast cancers represent very different populations of biologic tumor types. This may explain why the incidence of Stage IV cancer has not decreased with screening.

Keywords: breast cancer; stage IV; incidence; tumor biology; NCDB; SEER

---

1. Introduction

Despite widespread breast cancer screening in the United States, the incidence of de novo Stage IV breast cancer has not decreased. Esserman and colleagues called attention to this irregularity in 2009, showing that localized breast cancer incidence surged with the introduction of disease screening in the 1980s, without a corresponding decrease in distant disease [1]. Works by Bleyer and colleagues have reinforced the conclusion that screening is not meaningfully lowering the incidence of advanced disease [2,3].

The reasons underlying this problem are still unknown. Esserman presciently cited tumor biological factors as likely determinants of disease screenability, calling for the incorporation of such factors into screening and treatment guidelines [1]. Recently, Lannin and Wang showed that small tumors—the majority of which are found on mammography screening—have a distinctly favorable biological profile that dictates an indolent growth pattern [4]. Along similar lines, we hypothesized that de novo Stage IV breast cancer may have a uniquely aggressive biology, granting it growth properties that allow it to escape detection by screening. The purpose of this study was to compare the tumor biology of de novo Stage IV breast cancer with that of small cancers typically detected by screening mammography.

2. Methods

2.1. Data and Patient Selection

Data for this study were drawn from both the Surveillance, Epidemiology, and End Results database (SEER, November 2017 submission) and the National Cancer Database (NCDB 2015 Participant User File, downloaded 15 December 2017). The original SEER 9 registry data, spanning 1973–2015, were used to analyze long-term population-based incidence trends of the various disease stages. SEER was chosen over NCDB for this analysis, since it contains many more years of incidence data and is population-based and age-adjusted.

NCDB data from 2010 to 2015 were used to explore patient and disease characteristics of Stage IV disease in a large modern population, as well as to compare the tumor biological profiles of Stages I–IV. NCDB was chosen over SEER for this analysis since it contains more robust data on disease characteristics and captures a larger population of breast cancer patients in the United States. The NCDB is a joint project of the Commission on Cancer of the American College of Surgeons and the American Cancer Society. The data used in this study were derived from a de-identified NCDB file. The American College of Surgeons and the Commission on Cancer have not verified and are not responsible for the analytic or statistical methodology employed nor for the conclusions drawn from these data by the investigators.

Included in this study were female patients with invasive breast cancer with known disease stage (in situ and American Joint Committee on Cancer [AJCC] Stage 0 excluded). The analyses of the incidence and patient/disease factors were conducted using targeted statistical methods and software, as outlined below.

2.2. Incidence

To identify long-term breast cancer incidence trends by disease stage, the SEER 9 registry data were queried for cases of localized, regional, and distant breast cancer (SEER Historic Stage A variable) from 1973 to 2015. The Historic Stage A variable is traditionally used for analyses prior to 1988, when recoding for AJCC stage was unavailable in SEER. Localized disease includes cancer confined to the breast. Regional disease refers to contiguous organ spread, including regional lymph nodes and the chest wall. Distant disease denotes remote organ metastasis detected at the time of diagnosis. SEER*Stat software (Version 8.3.5, accessed on 20 April 2018) was used to calculate population-based incidence rates and annual percent change (APC). The two-sided p-values were set at <0.05.

2.3. Patient and Tumor Characteristics

The NCDB was queried for cases from 2010 to 2015 of "NCDB Analytic Stages I–IV," which uses the AJCC 7th edition pathologic stage classification to collapse sub-stages into their broader designations. Stages I–III cases were consolidated and compared with Stage IV in the univariable analysis of patient characteristics, including race/ethnicity, age, insurance, median household income, and education level, as well as disease characteristics, including histology, tumor size, estrogen receptor (ER) status, progesterone receptor (PR) status, human epidermal growth factor receptor 2 status (Her2), grade, and lymphovascular invasion (LVI). Nodal status was not included in this analysis, as debate exists as to whether lymph node spread marks biological predisposition versus a tumor's natural history when left untreated. All patients with known disease stage, including those with other missing variables, were included in this analysis, totaling 992,687 patients. Chi-squared testing was used to detect differences in patient and disease variables between Stage IV and non-Stage IV cancer, with statistical significance set at $p < 0.05$.

Five markers of biological activity reported in the NCDB were found to be associated with Stage IV in the univariable analysis: ER, PR, Her2, grade, and LVI. Their values were recombined into 48 possible permutations, generating a spectrum of tumor biology across 740,246 patients for whom these data were available. The rates of Stage IV disease were calculated across the permutation groups, which were then ranked in order of increasing Stage IV percentage. We aimed to cluster these groups into three subtypes of increasing biological aggressiveness, with up to 25% at the extremes, and the remainder intermediately aggressive. After testing multiple Stage IV percentage cut points in sensitivity analyses, we ultimately classified 22.3% of patients as "indolent," 61.7% of patients as "intermediate," and 16.0% of patients as "aggressive." This process of classification is summarized in Table 1.

Table 1. Classification system of breast cancer biological subtypes. ER: estrogen receptor, PR: progesterone receptor, HER2: human epidermal growth factor receptor 2, LVI: lymphovascular invasion.

Group	*n*	ER	PR	HER2	Grade	LVI	Row % with Stage IV	N Subtype	Subtype
1	119	−	+	−	1	−	0	165,150	Indolent
2	7	−	+	−	1	+	0		
3	3	−	+	+	1	+	0		
4	146,900	+	+	−	1	−	0.006		
5	12,409	+	−	−	1	−	0.01		
6	3917	+	+	+	1	−	0.012		
7	1795	−	−	−	1	−	0.013		
8	204,447	+	+	−	2	−	0.014	456,894	Intermediate
9	726	+	−	+	1	−	0.018		
10	691	−	+	−	2	−	0.019		
11	21,860	+	−	−	2	−	0.022		
12	12,597	−	−	−	2	−	0.022		
13	52,160	−	−	−	3	−	0.022		
14	9908	+	+	−	1	+	0.022		
15	18,147	+	+	+	2	−	0.026		
16	48,280	+	+	−	3	−	0.026		
17	3123	−	+	−	3	−	0.026		
18	373	−	−	+	1	−	0.027		
19	754	+	−	−	1	+	0.027		
20	14,045	+	−	−	3	−	0.029		
21	98	+	−	+	1	+	0.031		
22	49,161	+	+	−	2	+	0.031		
23	15,296	+	+	+	3	−	0.033		
24	5228	+	−	+	2	−	0.034		

Table 1. *Cont.*

Group	*n*	ER	PR	HER2	Grade	LVI	Row % with Stage IV	N Subtype	Subtype
25	5224	−	−	+	2	−	0.038		
26	14,608	−	−	+	3	−	0.038		
27	6336	+	−	+	3	−	0.042		
28	23	−	+	+	1	−	0.043		
29	949	−	+	+	3	−	0.044		
30	2805	−	−	−	2	+	0.045		
31	411	+	+	+	1	+	0.046		
32	5502	+	+	+	2	+	0.046		
33	318	−	+	+	2	−	0.047		
34	4922	+	−	−	2	+	0.048		
35	28,757	+	+	−	3	+	0.051	118,202	Aggressive
36	17,799	−	−	−	3	+	0.056		
37	6178	+	−	−	3	+	0.059		
38	8808	+	+	+	3	+	0.059		
39	1031	−	+	−	3	+	0.065		
40	147	−	−	−	1	+	0.068		
41	1468	+	−	+	2	+	0.068		
42	473	−	+	+	3	+	0.068		
43	175	−	+	−	2	+	0.069		
44	3168	+	−	+	3	+	0.083		
45	7249	−	−	+	3	+	0.086		
46	1665	−	−	+	2	+	0.091		
47	72	−	−	+	1	+	0.097		
48	114	−	+	+	2	+	0.114		

Frequencies of the above biological subtypes were calculated for all the staged breast cancer cases with known biological data, and their distributions were compared across Stages I–IV. Stage I was divided into tumors measuring 0.1–1.0 cm and 1.1–2.0 cm, in order to compare the biology of tiny tumors almost exclusively found on screening mammography with Stage IV biology. Patients without known tumor size or other demographic or disease variables were excluded from the analysis, resulting in 718,118 patients included. Chi-squared testing was used to detect differences in tumor biology across Stages I–IV, with statistical significance set at $p < 0.05$.

Finally, multivariable logistic regression using backward elimination tested Stage IV cases for significant associations with the demographic variables, including race/ethnicity, age, insurance, and median household income, as well as with disease variables, including histology, size, and biological category. Only the patients with known demographic and disease variables were included, again totaling 718,118 patients. Type I error was set at $p = 0.05$. The analyses were performed using SPSS Statistics software (IBM Version 25, Armonk, NY, USA).

3. Results

3.1. Breast Cancer Incidence Trends, 1973–2015

Age-adjusted population-based incidence trends for localized, regional, and distant disease are depicted in Figure 1. Based on SEER 9 registry data, the overall incidence of invasive breast cancer increased between 1973 and 2015. The localized disease rate per 100,000 persons increased from 39.0 in 1973 to 85.9 in 2015, generating an APC of 1.20 (95% CI 0.87–1.53). The regional disease rate per 100,000 slightly decreased from 36.9 in 1973 to 34.7 in 2015, with a negative APC of −0.47 (95% CI −0.61 to −0.34). The distant disease rate per 100,000 was lowest but experienced an overall increase from 6.2 in 1973 to 8.7 in 2015, with an APC of 0.46 (95% CI 0.32–0.60).

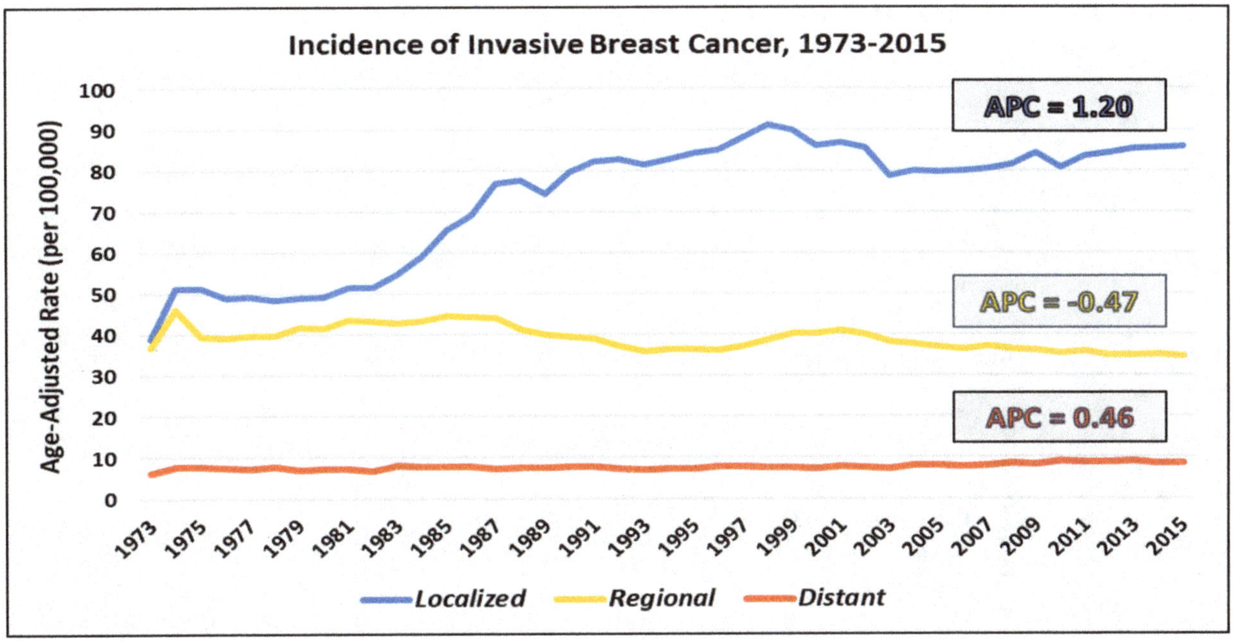

Figure 1. Age-adjusted incidence of localized, regional, and distant breast cancer in women, from 1973 to 2015 (SEER 9). APC: annual percent change.

3.2. Demographic and Disease Characteristics of Stage IV Patients

Between 2010 and 2015, there were 992,687 women in the NCDB with staged invasive breast cancer. Of these, 939,903 (94.7%) were Stages I–III, and 52,784 (5.3%) were Stage IV. Univariable analysis of the demographic and tumor characteristics is depicted in Table 2. Analysis of demographic data showed that women with Stage IV disease were more likely to be black, younger than 40 years of age, uninsured or on Medicaid, and living in zip codes where median household income was <$48,000, and where ≥13% of adult residents did not have a high school degree. Strikingly, Stage IV disease affected 8.0% of blacks, 8.8% of women under 30 years of age, and 14.2% of uninsured. Analysis of tumor data showed that women with Stage IV were more likely to have larger tumors, non-ductal or lobular undifferentiated histologies ("Other"), negative ER or PR status, positive Her2 status, LVI, and poorly differentiated grade. Conspicuously, Stage IV affected 19.0% of tumors > 5cm and 10.9% of tumors with undifferentiated histologies.

3.3. Tumor Biology Distribution by Stage

As mentioned in Methods, 740,264 patients had known tumor biology characteristics, including hormone receptor and Her2 status, LVI status, and grade. Of this cohort, 718,118 of patients had known tumor size and other demographic and disease characteristics, without missing data. These patients were included in the analysis of the tumor biological subtypes by stage.

Using the tumor biology classification shown in Table 1, a majority of the cohort, 61.7%, had intermediate biology, while 22.7% had indolent biology and 15.6% had aggressive biology. The distribution of biological categories varied tremendously by disease stage ($p < 0.001$ for all stages), as shown in Figure 2. Patients presenting with Stages III and IV disease had similar tumor biology and had over eight times the fraction of aggressive tumors and one-seventh the fraction of indolent tumors as patients with small Stage I tumors ≤1 cm.

Table 2. Univariable analysis of demographic and disease variables for American Joint Committee on Cancer Stages I–III and Stage IV. HS: high school.

Demographic/Disease Variables	Stages I–III N (Row%)	Stage IV N (Row%)	p-Value
Race/Ethnicity			
White	738,416 (95.1%)	38,453 (4.9%)	<0.001
Black	103,646 (92.0%)	8988 (8.0%)	
Asian	31,843 (95.6%)	1455 (4.4%)	
Hispanic	50,958 (94.5%)	2983 (5.5%)	
Missing	15,040 (94.3%)	905 (5.7%)	
Age			
<30	4594 (91.2%)	446 (8.8%)	<0.001
30–39	36,589 (93.5%)	2560 (6.5%)	
40–49	141,714 (95.6%)	6553 (4.4%)	
50–59	223,898 (94.6%)	12,803 (5.4%)	
60–69	259,993 (94.8%)	14,212 (5.2%)	
≥70	273,115 (94.4%)	16,210 (5.6%)	
Insurance			
None	17,883 (85.8%)	2961 (14.2%)	<0.001
Private	467,639 (95.9%)	20,062 (4.1%)	
Medicaid	59,468 (90.2%)	6476 (9.8%)	
Medicare	368,966 (94.5%)	21,609 (5.5%)	
Other Government	9705 (95.9%)	411 (4.1%)	
Unknown	16,242 (92.8%)	1265 (7.2%)	
Median Household Income			
≤$38,000	136,807 (93.2%)	9982 (6.8%)	<0.001
$38,000–$47,999	197,306 (94.3%)	11,842 (5.7%)	
$48,000–$62,999	251,060 (94.7%)	13,934 (5.3%)	
≥$63,000	351,943 (95.5%)	16,758 (4.5%)	
Missing	2787 (91.2%)	268 (8.8%)	
Median Education (No HS Diploma)			
≥21%	136,597 (93.3%)	9811 (6.7%)	<0.001
13–20.9%	221,484 (94.1%)	13,914 (5.9%)	
7–12.9%	309,839 (94.9%)	16,810 (5.1%)	
<7%	269,536 (95.7%)	12,002 (4.3%)	
Missing	2447 (90.8%)	247 (9.2%)	
Size (cm)			
0.1–2.0	606,385 (98.7%)	8052 (1.3%)	<0.001
2.1–5.0	268,290 (93.5%)	18,615 (6.5%)	
>5.0	56,294 (81.0%)	13,216 (19.0%)	
Missing	8934 (40.9%)	12,901 (59.1%)	
Histology			
Ductal	704,671 (95.5%)	33,525 (4.5%)	<0.001
Lobular	90,608 (94.2%)	5623 (5.8%)	
Mixed Ductal/ Lobular	49,264 (96.3%)	1912 (3.7%)	
Other	95,360 (89.1%)	11,724 (10.9%)	

Table 2. *Cont.*

Demographic/Disease Variables	Stages I–III N (Row%)	Stage IV N (Row%)	*p*-Value
ER			
Negative	155,062 (92.9%)	11,810 (7.1%)	<0.001
Positive	771,633 (95.5%)	36,720 (4.5%)	
Missing	13,208 (75.6%)	4254 (24.4%)	
PR			
Negative	243,415 (93.0%)	18,354 (7.0%)	<0.001
Positive	681,482 (95.8%)	29,586 (4.2%)	
Missing	15,006 (75.6%)	4844 (24.4%)	
Her2			
Negative	763,436 (91.5%)	33,677 (4.2%)	<0.001
Positive	119,352 (91.5%)	11,146 (8.5%)	
Missing	57,115 (87.8%)	7961 (12.2%)	
Grade			
Well-Differentiated	212,301 (98.6%)	3107 (1.4%)	<0.001
Moderately Differentiated	398,667 (96.1%)	16,333 (3.9%)	
Poorly Differentiated	270,103 (93.4%)	18,953 (6.6%)	
Missing	58,832 (80.3%)	14,391 (19.7%)	
LVI			
Negative	628,236 (98.1%)	12,155 (1.9%)	<0.001
Positive	154,951 (95.0%)	8237 (5.0%)	
Missing	156,716 (82.9%)	32,392 (17.1%)	

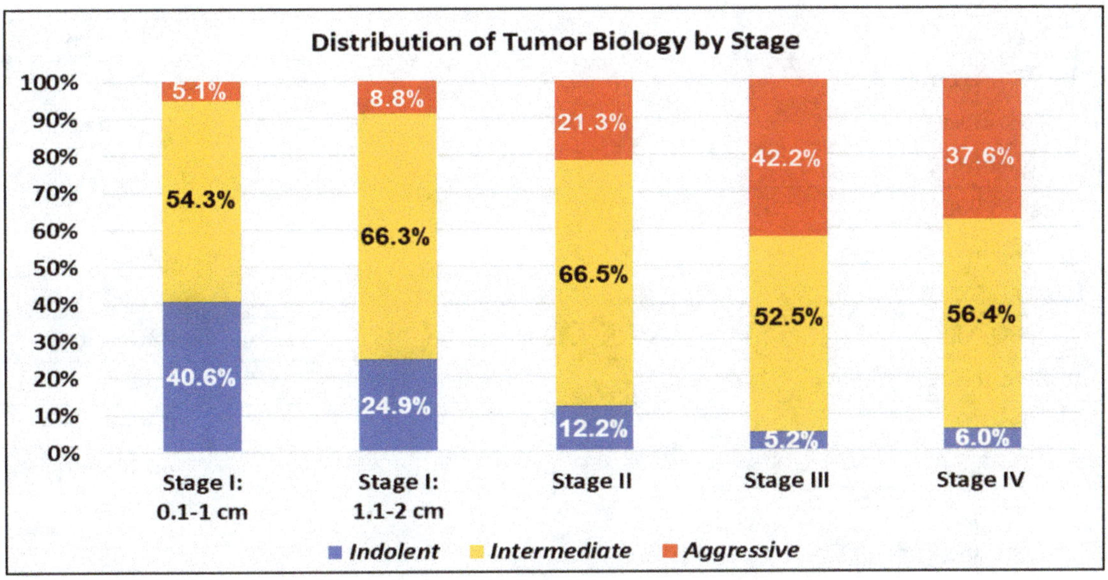

Figure 2. Tumor biology by AJCC 7th edition stage.

3.4. *Multivariable Analysis of Demographic and Disease Characteristics*

In the multivariable logistic regression model, many demographic and disease variables that were associated with Stage IV disease in univariable analysis remained significantly associated, as shown in Table 3. Large tumor size, aggressive biological subtype, and no insurance were the strongest predictors. Tumors with size >5 cm were more than 15 times as likely to predict Stage IV disease as tumors with size ≤2 cm (OR 15.6, 95% CI 14.9–16.5), and tumors with aggressive biology were more than 3 times as likely to present with Stage IV disease as indolent tumors (OR 3.22, 95% CI 2.99–3.47).

Race/ethnicity, age, household income, and histology remained significant in the model, but their effects were fairly minor.

Table 3. Multivariable logistic regression demonstrating the strength of association between Stage IV disease and demographic and disease factors.

Demographic/Disease Factors	Stage IV (De Novo) Odds Ratio	95% Confidence Interval
Race/Ethnicity		
White	Reference	Reference
Black	1.09	1.04–1.15
Asian	0.78	0.71–0.86
Hispanic	0.71	0.66–0.77
Age		
<30	1.38	1.17–1.63
30–39	1.08	0.99–1.18
40–49	0.87	0.81–0.93
50–59	1.07	1.01–1.14
60–69	1.06	1.01–1.12
≥70	Reference	Reference
Insurance		
None	Reference	Reference
Private	0.43	0.39–0.46
Medicaid	0.74	0.67–0.81
Medicare	0.51	0.47–0.56
Other Government	0.41	0.34–0.50
Unknown	0.57	0.49–0.68
Median Household Income		
≤$38,000	1.12	1.06–1.18
$38,000–$47,999	1.09	1.04–1.14
$48,000–$62,999	1.04	0.99–1.08
≥$63,000	Reference	Reference
Size (cm)		
0.1–2.0	Reference	Reference
2.1–5.0	4.40	4.21–4.60
>5.0	15.6	14.9–16.5
Histology		
Ductal	Reference	Reference
Lobular	0.83	0.78–0.88
Mixed Ductal/Lobular	0.82	0.75–0.88
Other	0.84	0.79–0.89
Biological Subtype		
Indolent	Reference	Reference
Intermediate	2.05	1.91–2.20
Aggressive	3.22	2.99–3.47

4. Discussion

Multiple studies have shown that, despite widespread screening programs in the United States, the incidence of Stage IV breast cancer has remained stable or increased over time [1–3,5,6]. In this study, we analyzed the most recent and comprehensive population-based SEER data and showed that the incidence of Stage IV disease has indeed been gradually increasing in recent decades.

Esserman and colleagues elegantly delineated this issue in 2009, contrasting the expected stage-based incidence of a theoretically effective disease-screening program with the actual breast cancer incidence trends since the rise of screening in the early 1980s. They highlighted that, while successful screening programs are able to downstage incident cancers over time, breast cancer screening has generated more localized disease diagnoses without congruently diminishing the incidence of advanced cancer [1].

Welch and colleagues pointed out that since the advent of widespread mammography screening, small cancers under 2 cm have increased in incidence over three times more than large tumors over 2 cm have decreased [7]. The clear implication is that not all small cancers are destined to become large cancers, and this leads to overdiagnosis. Lannin and Wang provided an explanation for this by comparing the biology of small and large cancers [4,8]. They found that many breast cancers are small, not because they are detected early, but because they have favorable biology. The current study is an extension of that work and shows that cancers presenting with distant metastases are a distinct subpopulation with a biology much more aggressive than that of the small tumors found by screening mammography. Only a small fraction of the tumors found by screening mammography have the biological profile that puts them at risk for de novo Stage IV disease.

Of course, there are other possible explanations for increasing Stage IV incidence. One contributing factor could be stage migration, the phenomenon whereby the use of high-resolution imaging, including positron emission/computed tomography scans and magnetic resonance imaging, leads to more frequent discovery of distant disease [9–11]. It seems unlikely, however, that this would precisely counterbalance a decline in advanced cancer diagnoses that might otherwise be seen from early mammographic detection.

Our data complement the body of literature suggesting that Stage IV cancers arise in unscreened and underprivileged populations, including the very young, the very old, and the disadvantaged with respect to healthcare access and quality. In our analyses, women younger than 40 years and older than 70 years of age had higher rates of Stage IV disease when compared to women aged 40–69 years, who are known to have the highest rates of disease screening [12]. Black women, known to suffer disparate breast cancer outcomes, had significantly higher rates of Stage IV disease than white women [13,14]. Those without health insurance and with Medicaid, as well as from regions in the lowest brackets for income and education—all of which imply low resource settings—also disproportionately presented with Stage IV disease [15–17]. These statistics must be interpreted cautiously, however, as NCDB data are not population-based and thus do not differentiate between higher incidence of Stage IV disease versus relatively lower incidence of Stages I–III disease. In fact, Welch and colleagues used population-based SEER data to show that poorer counties with less mammographic screening have lower overall breast cancer incidence but similar Stage IV disease incidence and cancer mortality compared with wealthier counties [18,19].

Even when adjusting for demographic and socioeconomic factors, our data support the concept that Stage IV tumors represent a unique subpopulation and are biologically distinct from the small, indolent tumors usually detected by mammography. Other studies have postulated that breast cancer presenting at an advanced stage may be innately endowed with biologic machinery that promotes swift growth and spread during the 12–24 months interval between mammograms [1,20,21]. Our findings give credence to this theory by highlighting the uniquely aggressive features of Stage IV disease.

In a previous study, Lannin used ER, PR, and grade to stratify patients into three prognostic groups based on breast cancer-specific survival, terming the groups "favorable", "intermediate", and "unfavorable". In this study, we added two additional variables to the model—Her2 and LVI—and used de novo Stage IV disease as the target outcome. These five tumor characteristics were specifically chosen to reflect the biological behavior that predicts distant metastases, thus the group names were changed to "aggressive", "intermediate", and "indolent".

Her2 is a well-known marker for biological aggressiveness and was formerly associated with poor prognosis. With effective targeted therapy, it currently confers a better than average prognosis and yet it is strongly associated with Stage IV disease [22–26]. LVI similarly marks aggressive growth patterns [27,28]. Unfortunately, its status was missing in nearly 20% of the dataset and well over half of Stage IV cases. This may be explained by the fact that many patients with Stage IV disease undergo needle biopsy only, and pathologists are either unable or unmotivated to evaluate for LVI. Despite missing data, we included LVI in our model, as it was highly informative of biology when known. As shown in Table 1, 18 of 19 groups with the highest rate of Stage IV disease presentation were positive for LVI. All 24 groups included in the "aggressive" category were positive for either LVI or Her2. The most biologically unfavorable cancers from the earlier prognostic-based model—triple negative with grades 2 and 3—only cluster to the current "aggressive" category when positive for LVI.

Tumor biology is evolving to become a critical factor in estimating prognosis and guiding treatment. In the AJCC 8th edition disease staging system, anatomical features like tumor size and nodal status are considered insufficient to accurately inform the stage and treatment plan, particularly in the developed world where testing for biomarkers is ubiquitous. The variables used in this study are primitive measures of tumor biology compared to molecular and genomic assays such as OncotypeDx or Mammaprint [4,29–31]. However, they are readily available in large datasets like SEER and the NCDB for use in estimating population trends in tumor biology. Future studies will likely elucidate more sophisticated biological mechanisms responsible for aggressive Stage IV tumors. It seems likely that these differing biological characteristics will explain why the incidence of Stage IV breast cancer has not decreased with screening mammography.

5. Conclusions

The incidence of de novo Stage IV breast cancer is increasing in the United States despite widespread mammography screening. This is likely related to the differing populations of biologic tumor types that comprise Stage IV tumors versus early-stage tumors commonly found on mammography. Our analysis demonstrates that aggressive tumor biology accounts for nearly 40% of advanced-stage tumors, versus only 5% of tiny early-stage tumors. Conversely, indolent biology is rarely associated with advanced disease. Aggressive biology resulting in insidious growth patterns may explain why the incidence of Stage IV cancer has not decreased with screening.

Author Contributions: Conceptualization, methodology, data curation, formal analysis, and preparation of the original draft of this study were performed by D.R.H. and D.R.L. A.S.C., K.F., and B.K.K. contributed to the data curation, formal analysis, and review and editing of the manuscript. B.K.K. and D.R.L. also supervised the study.

Abbreviations

SEER	Surveillance, Epidemiology, and End Results
NCDB	National Cancer Data Base
AJCC	American Joint Committee on Cancer
APC	Annual Percent Change
CI	Confidence Interval
ER	Estrogen Receptor
PR	Progesterone Receptor
Her2	Human Epidermal Growth Factor 2
LVI	Lymphovascular Invasion
OR	Odds Ratio

References

1. Esserman, L.; Shieh, Y.; Thompson, I. Rethinking screening for breast cancer and prostate cancer. *JAMA* **2009**, *302*, 1685–1692. [CrossRef] [PubMed]
2. Bleyer, A.; Welch, H.G. Effect of three decades of screening mammography on breast-cancer incidence. *N. Engl. J. Med.* **2012**, *367*, 1998–2005. [CrossRef] [PubMed]
3. Johnson, R.H.; Chien, F.L.; Bleyer, A. Incidence of breast cancer with distant involvement among women in the United States, 1976 to 2009. *JAMA* **2013**, *309*, 800–805. [CrossRef]
4. Lannin, D.R.; Wang, S. Are small breast cancers good because they are small or small because they are good? *N. Engl. J. Med.* **2017**, *376*, 2286–2291. [CrossRef] [PubMed]
5. Di Meglio, A.; Freedman, R.A.; Lin, N.U.; Barry, W.T.; Metzger-Filho, O.; Keating, N.L.; King, T.A.; Sertoli, M.R.; Boccardo, F.; Winer, E.P.; et al. Time trends in incidence rates and survival of newly diagnosed stage IV breast cancer by tumor histology: A population-based analysis. *Breast Cancer Res. Treat.* **2016**, *157*, 587–596. [PubMed]
6. Welch, H.G.; Gorski, D.H.; Albertsen, P.C. Trends in metastatic breast and prostate cancer-lessons in cancer dynamics. *N. Engl. J. Med.* **2015**, *373*, 1685–1687. [PubMed]
7. Welch, H.G.; Prorok, P.C.; O'Malley, A.J.; Kramer, B.S. Breast-cancer tumor size, overdiagnosis, and mammography screening effectiveness. *N. Engl. J. Med.* **2016**, *375*, 1438–1447. [CrossRef] [PubMed]
8. Lannin, D.R. Treatment intensity for mammographically detected tumors: An alternative viewpoint. *Ann. Surg. Oncol.* **2018**, *25*, 2502–2505. [CrossRef]
9. Feinstein, A.R.; Sosin, D.M.; Wells, C.K. The Will Rogers phenomenon—Stage migration and new diagnostic techniques as a source of misleading statistics for survival in cancer. *N. Engl. J. Med.* **1985**, *312*, 1604–1608. [CrossRef]
10. Polednak, A.P. Increase in distant stage breast cancer incidence rates in us women aged 25–49 years, 2000–2011: The stage migration hypothesis. *J. Cancer Epidemiol.* **2015**, *2015*, 710106. [CrossRef]
11. Chee, K.G.; Nguyen, D.V.; Brown, M.; Gandara, D.R.; Wun, T.; Lara, P.N. Jr. Positron emission tomography and improved survival in patients with lung cancer: The Will Rogers phenomenon revisited. *Arch. Intern. Med.* **2008**, *168*, 1541–1549. [CrossRef]
12. Centers for Disease Control and Prevention National Center for Health Statistics. Use of mammography among women aged 40 and over, by selected characteristics: United States, selected years 1987–2015. Available online: https://www.cdc.gov/nchs/hus/contents2016.htm#070 (accessed on 26 April 2018).
13. Taplin, S.H.; Ichikawa, L.; Yood, M.U.; Manos, M.M.; Geiger, A.M.; Weinmann, S.; Gilbert, J.; Mouchawar, J.; Leyden, W.A.; Altaras, R.; et al. Reason for late-stage breast cancer: Absence of screening or detection, or breakdown in follow-up? *J. Natl. Cancer Inst.* **2004**, *96*, 1518–1527. [CrossRef]
14. SEER Cancer Statistics Review, 1975–2015. Table 4.18. Cancer of the female breast (invasive): Age-adjusted rates and trends by race/ethnicity, 2011–2015. National Cancer Institute. Bethesda, MD. Available online: http://seer.cancer.gov/csr/1975_2015/ (accessed on 26 April 2018).
15. American Cancer Society. Cancer Prevention & Early Detection Facts & Figures, 2017–2018. Available online: https://www.cancer.org/content/dam/cancer-org/research/cancer-facts-and-statistics/cancer-prevention-and-early-detection-facts-and-figures/cancer-prevention-and-early-detection-facts-and-figures-2017.pdf (accessed on 26 April 2018).
16. Fayanju, O.M.; Kraenzle, S.; Drake, B.F.; Oka, M.; Goodman, M.S. Perceived barriers to mammography among underserved women in a Breast Health Center Outreach Program. *Am. J. Surg.* **2014**, *208*, 425–434. [CrossRef] [PubMed]
17. Ramachandran, A.; Snyder, F.R.; Katz, M.L.; Darnell, J.S.; Dudley, D.J.; Patierno, S.R.; Sanders, M.R.; Valverde, P.A.; Simon, M.A.; Warren-Mears, V.; et al. Barriers to health care contribute to delays in follow-up among women with abnormal cancer screening: Data from the Patient Navigation Research Program. *Cancer* **2015**, *121*, 4016–4024. [CrossRef] [PubMed]
18. Harding, C.; Pompei, F.; Burmistrov, D.; Welch, H.G.; Abebe, R.; Wilson, R. Breast cancer screening, incidence and mortality across US counties. *JAMA Intern. Med.* **2015**, *175*, 1483–1489. [CrossRef] [PubMed]
19. Welch, H.G.; Fisher, E.S. Income and cancer overdiagnosis—When too much care is harmful. *N. Engl. J. Med.* **2017**, *376*, 2208–2209. [CrossRef] [PubMed]

20. Lin, C.; Buxton, M.B.; Moore, D.; Krontiras, H.; Carey, L.; DeMichele, A.; Montgomery, L.; Tripathy, D.; Lehman, C.; Liu, M.; et al. Locally advanced breast cancers are more likely to present as Interval Cancers: Results from the I-SPY 1 TRIAL. *Breast Cancer Res. Treat.* **2012**, *132*, 871–879. [CrossRef] [PubMed]
21. Ikeda, D.M.; Andersson, I.; Wattsgard, C.; Janzon, L.; Linell, F. Interval carcinomas in the Malmo Mammographic Screening Trial. *Am. J. Roentgenol.* **1992**, *159*, 287–294. [CrossRef]
22. Wu, S.; Li, H.; Tang, L.; Sun, J.Y.; Zhang, W.W.; Li, F.Y.; Chen, Y.X.; He, Z.Y. The effect of distant metastases sites on survival in de novo Stage-IV breast cancer: A SEER database analysis. *Tumour Biol.* **2017**, *39*. [CrossRef]
23. Eccles, S.A. The role of c-erbB-2/HER2/neu in breast cancer progression and metastasis. *J. Mammary Gland Biol. Neoplasia* **2001**, *6*, 393–406. [CrossRef]
24. Piccart, M.; Lohrisch, C.; Di Leo, A.; Larsimont, D. The predictive value of HER2 in breast cancer. *Oncology* **2001**, *61*, 73–82. [CrossRef]
25. Yarden, Y. Biology of HER2 and its importance in breast cancer. *Oncology.* **2001**, *61*, 1–13. [CrossRef]
26. Rosenthal, S.I.; Depowski, P.L.; Sheehan, C.E.; Ross, J.S. Comparison of HER-2/neu oncogene amplification detected by fluorescence in situ hybridization in lobular and ductal breast cancer. *Appl. Immunohistochem. Mol. Morphol.* **2002**, *10*, 40–46. [CrossRef]
27. Zhang, S.; Zhang, D.; Yi, S.; Gong, M.; Lu, C.; Cai, Y.; Tang, X.; Zou, L. The relationship of lymphatic vessel density, lymphovascular invasion, and lymph node metastasis in breast cancer: A systematic review and meta-analysis. *Oncotarget* **2017**, *8*, 2863–2873. [CrossRef]
28. Rakha, E.A.; Martin, S.; Lee, A.H.S.; Morgan, D.; Pharoah, P.D.; Hodi, Z.; Macmillan, D.; Ellis, I.O. The prognostic significance of lymphovascular invasion in invasive breast carcinoma. *Cancer* **2012**, *118*, 3670–3680. [CrossRef]
29. AJCC 8th Edition Breast Cancer Staging System. The American College of Surgeons. Chicago, Illinois. Last updated 13 March 2018. Available online: https://cancerstaging.org/references-tools/deskreferences/Documents/AJCC%20Breast%20Cancer%20Staging%20System.pdf (accessed on 26 April 2018).
30. Braunstein, L.Z.; Niemierko, A.; Shenouda, M.N. Outcome following local-regional recurrence in women with early-stage breast cancer: Impact of biologic subtype. *Breast J.* **2015**, *21*, 161–167. [CrossRef]
31. Paik, S.; Shak, S.; Tang, G.; Kim, C.; Baker, J.; Cronin, M.; Baehner, F.L.; Walker, M.G.; Watson, D.; Park, T.; et al. A multigene assay to predict recurrence of tamoxifen-treated, node-negative breast cancer. *N. Engl. J. Med.* **2004**, *351*, 2817–2826. [CrossRef] [PubMed]

17

Cell-Free DNA Variant Sequencing Using CTC-Depleted Blood for Comprehensive Liquid Biopsy Testing in Metastatic Breast Cancer

Corinna Keup [1,*], Markus Storbeck [2], Siegfried Hauch [2], Peter Hahn [2], Markus Sprenger-Haussels [2], Mitra Tewes [3], Pawel Mach [1], Oliver Hoffmann [1], Rainer Kimmig [1] and Sabine Kasimir-Bauer [1]

1 Department of Gynecology and Obstetrics, University Hospital of Essen, 45122 Essen, Germany; pawel.mach@uk-essen.de (P.M.); Oliver.Hoffmann@uk-essen.de (O.H.); rainer.kimmig@uk-essen.de (R.K.); Sabine.Kasimir-bauer@uk-essen.de (S.K.-B.)

2 QIAGEN GmbH, 40724 Hilden, Germany; Markus.Storbeck@qiagen.com (M.S.); Siegfried.Hauch@qiagen.com (S.H.); Peter.Hahn@qiagen.com (P.H.); Markus.Sprenger-Haussels@qiagen.com (M.S.-H.)

3 Department of Medical Oncology, University Hospital of Essen, 45122 Essen, Germany; Mitra.Tewes@uk-essen.de

* Correspondence: Corinna.Keup@uk-essen.de

Abstract: Liquid biopsy analytes such as cell-free DNA (cfDNA) and circulating tumor cells (CTCs) exhibit great potential for personalized treatment. Since cfDNA and CTCs are considered to give additive information and blood specimens are limited, isolation of cfDNA and CTC in an "all from one tube" format is desired. We investigated whether cfDNA variant sequencing from CTC-depleted blood (CTC-depl. B; obtained after positive immunomagnetic isolation of CTCs (AdnaTest EMT-2/Stem Cell Select, QIAGEN)) impacts the results compared to cfDNA variant sequencing from matched whole blood (WB). Cell-free DNA was isolated using matched WB and CTC-depl. B from 17 hormone receptor positive/human epidermal growth factor receptor 2 negative (HR+/HER2−) metastatic breast cancer patients (QIAamp MinElute ccfDNA Kit, QIAGEN). Cell-free DNA libraries were constructed (customized QIAseq Targeted DNA Panel for Illumina, QIAGEN) with integrated unique molecular indices. Sequencing (on the NextSeq 550 platform, Illumina) and data analysis (Ingenuity Variant Analysis) were performed. RNA expression in CTCs was analyzed by multimarker quantitative PCR. Cell-free DNA concentration and size distribution in the matched plasma samples were not significantly different. Seventy percent of all variants were identical in matched WB and CTC-depl. B, but 115/125 variants were exclusively found in WB/CTC-depl. B. The number of detected variants per patient and the number of exclusively detected variants per patient in only one cfDNA source did not differ between the two matched cfDNA sources. Even the characteristics of the exclusively detected cfDNA variants in either WB or CTC-depl. B were comparable. Thus, cfDNA variants from matched WB and CTC-depl. B exhibited no relevant differences, and parallel isolation of cfDNA and CTCs from only 10 mL of blood in an "all from one tube" format was feasible. Matched cfDNA mutational and CTC transcriptional analyses might empower a comprehensive liquid biopsy analysis to enhance the identification of actionable targets for individual therapy strategies.

Keywords: metastatic breast cancer; liquid biopsy; cell-free DNA; next-generation sequencing; circulating tumor cells

1. Introduction

Liquid biopsies harbor great potential for personalized treatment strategies and real-time monitoring approaches. In oncology, cell-free DNA (cfDNA) and, specifically, cell-free tumor DNA (ctDNA), defined by the presence of variants [1], as well as circulating tumor cells (CTCs), are powerful tools to describe tumor heterogeneity and clonal evolution [2].

High levels of ctDNA were significantly correlated with decreased overall survival (OS) in breast cancer (BC) [2] and, more specifically, *ESR1* cfDNA variants were associated with a shorter duration of endocrine treatment effectiveness in metastatic BC (MBC) [3]. Since patients with *ESR1* variants were described to benefit from fulvestrant rather than from exemestane, compared to patients without this alteration, *ESR1* variants also have the potential to tailor treatment regiments [4]. For disease monitoring, cfDNA concentration was shown to indicate impending relapse of primary BC earlier than any other imaging or blood-based strategy [5] and can predate treatment response changes [6,7].

The prognostic value of CTCs was first introduced for MBC patients more than a decade ago [8]. A decreased CTC count after treatment was significantly associated with increased progression-free survival (PFS) and OS [9]. Consequently, CTC count dynamics were proposed to be more suitable for monitoring than radiological imaging [10]. In addition to CTC counts, the expression profiles of CTCs were correlated with response evaluation criteria in solid tumors (RECIST) [11,12]. Positive results for therapy decisions in BC based on the CTC count, dynamics, or molecular characteristics, however, have until now not been convincingly examined in large randomized blinded clinical studies, but great efforts are underway to prove the predictive value of CTCs [2].

CfDNA and CTCs isolated from the same liquid biopsy specimen can enable comprehensive results if seen as providing complementary, rather than competitive information. CtDNA, released mostly passively, might present dying and probably therapy-sensitive cells [5]. On the other hand, CTCs are viable cells actively migrating into the circulation as potential seeds of metastasis and, therefore, possibly indicating minimal residual disease. It is not only possible to conduct mutational analysis of cfDNA and transcriptional analysis of CTCs using both analytes in parallel, but it was already described for multiple myeloma that sequencing of cfDNA and CTCs uncovered more mutations than analysis of either analyte alone [13]. Therefore, one might assume that parallel cfDNA and CTC analysis is complementary rather than competitive or even redundant [14].

Practically, however, many studies comparing cfDNA and CTCs used the same patient inclusion criteria, but different large cohorts for either cfDNA or CTC analysis [15,16]. There were a few publications analyzing both cfDNA and CTCs from the same patients, but the cohort sizes were quite small and the two analytes were obtained from blood samples taken at different time points [15,16]. Even if the study design considered the same time points for withdrawal, different preservative blood tubes, e.g., Streck and/or CellSave tubes, were mostly used [7,15,17–19]. In contrast, EDTA blood enabled parallel analysis of cfDNA and CTC from the same blood sample [20–23], but different blood aliquots were needed for both analyses, such that the required blood volume was around 20 mL [24]. Consequently, for appropriate comparability and consistency, the usage of the same blood sample with minimized volume drawn and stored/shipped under the same conditions for isolation of both analytes to reach an unbiased comprehensive liquid biopsy in an "all from one tube" format would be desirable.

We here (1) compared the quantity and characteristics of cfDNA variants isolated from whole blood (WB) and blood after positive immunomagnetic selection of CTCs (CTC-depleted (depl.) B), and (2) studied the heterogeneity of cfDNA variants and CTC overexpression signals in an hormone receptor positive/human epidermal growth factor receptor 2 negative (HR+/HER2−) MBC cohort.

2. Results

2.1. Patient Characteristics

The cohort was specified to only consist of patients with MBC with HR+/HER2− primary tumors. The majority of patients were more than 50 years old, and the median follow-up time was 68 months (range: 12 to 322 months). Eleven of the seventeen patients were deceased at the time of analysis. At the time of blood draw, the majority of patients had secondary metastases, received more than three treatment lines, and exhibited progressive disease according to response evaluation criteria in solid tumors. All patient characteristics are listed in Table S1 (Supplementary Materials).

2.2. Cell-Free DNA Concentration and Fragmentation

The used volume of the matched plasma samples was identical and ranged from 2.8 mL to 6.0 mL (mean 4.4 mL). Cell-free DNA concentrations in the plasma of WB ranged from 4 ng/mL to 187 ng/mL (mean 58 ng/mL), while cfDNA concentration in plasma of CTC-depl. B ranged from 5 ng/mL to 153 ng/mL (mean 61 ng/mL). Wilcoxon signed-rank test considering all 17 matched samples revealed no significant difference of cfDNA concentration in the different plasma samples. However, in some matched samples, the cfDNA concentration differed greatly and, importantly, a high inter-individual variability was observed (Figure 1).

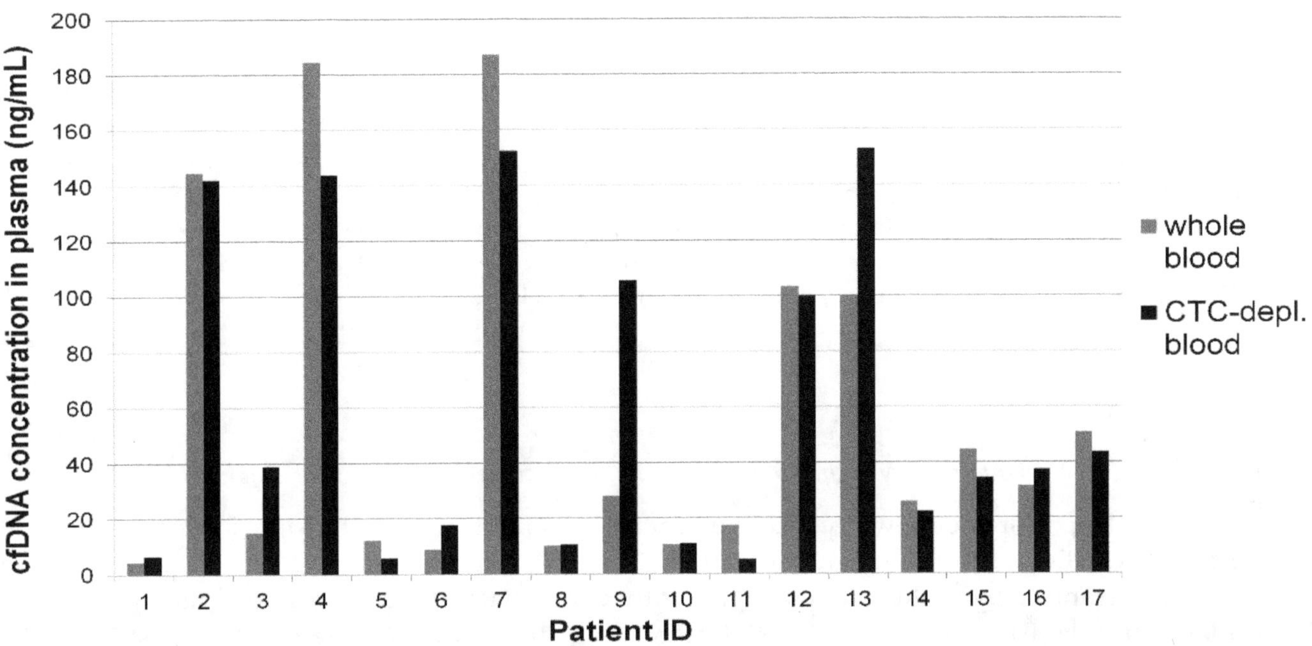

Figure 1. Inter-individual variability of cell-free DNA (cfDNA) concentration. Plasma from circulating tumor cell (CTC)-depleted (depl.)_blood (by AdnaTest EMT-2/StemCell Select) and matched plasma from whole blood were used in the same volume for cfDNA isolation with a QIAamp MinElute ccfDNA Kit, and cfDNA was quantified using an Agilent High Sensitivity Chip (fragments between 100–700 bp).

Capillary electrophoresis using the Agilent High Sensitivity DNA Chip resolved the fragment length of the cfDNA. The majority of isolated cfDNA of all patients consisted of mononucleosomal cfDNA fragments (100–280 bp), but cfDNA fragments with a length of 280–450 bp/450–700 bp (di- or trinucleosomal DNA) were also detectable. Size distribution was comparable in cfDNA samples from WB and CTC-depl. B, as depicted for two exemplary patients (Figure 2). There was no difference in high-molecular-weight DNA (700–10,000 bp) in cfDNA eluates of the two plasma sources.

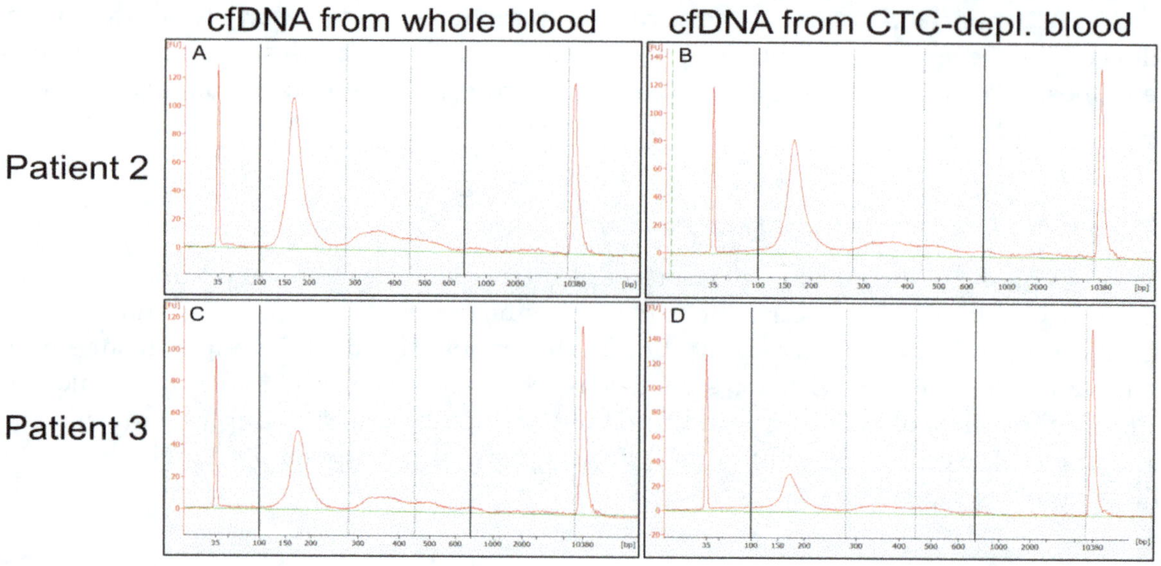

Figure 2. Size distribution of cfDNA. Matched cfDNA samples isolated from CTC-depl. blood (**B**,**D**; CTC isolation using AdnaTest EMT-2/StemCell Select) and from whole blood (**A**,**C**) of two exemplary patients (**A** + **B**; **C** + **D**) displayed a large mononucleosomal fraction and, in general, a similar size distribution without high-molecular-weight DNA (700–10,000 bp). Capillary electrophoresis was performed with an Agilent High Sensitivity Chip. (A) Cell-free DNA eluate from whole blood of patient 2, diluted 1:40; (**B**) cfDNA eluate from CTC-depl. blood of patient 2, diluted 1:40; (**C**) cfDNA eluate from whole blood of patient 3, diluted 1:5; (D) cfDNA eluate from CTC-depl. blood of patient 3, diluted 1:20.

2.3. Cell-Free DNA Variants from Matched Whole Blood and Circulating Tumor Cell-Depleted Blood

Targeted deep sequencing was conducted for all cfDNA libraries >4 nM, resulting in removal of two matched cfDNA samples from one patient (Table S2, Supplementary Materials). Sequencing quality was guaranteed by exclusion of samples with <5 or >100 million read fragments, <400 unique molecular indice (UMI) coverage, and if <95% of the target region was covered with at least 5% of the mean UMI coverage, causing four samples and their matched samples to be rejected from analysis. The mean read count of all remaining samples from twelve patients was 12.41 million, while we found a mean of 3.5 reads per UMI and an average of 99.58% of the target region was covered with a least 5% of the mean UMI coverage (of 2760) (Table S2, Supplementary Materials).

In total, 415 variants were detected by UMI verification and, after filtering with the Ingenuity software, in all 24 cfDNA samples from 12 MBC patients, 175 variants were identical in the cfDNA samples from both plasma sources, namely WB and CTC-depl. B (Figure 3A). Furthermore, 115 and 125 variants were exclusively found in WB and CTC-depl. B, respectively. Thus, the agreement was 70% with a κ-value of 0.355 (Figure 3B). Corresponding to the large overlap of identical variants found in both plasma sources depicted in the Venn diagram (Figure 3A), the number of detected variants per patient exhibited no significant difference between the two matched cfDNA sources (Figure 4A).

A

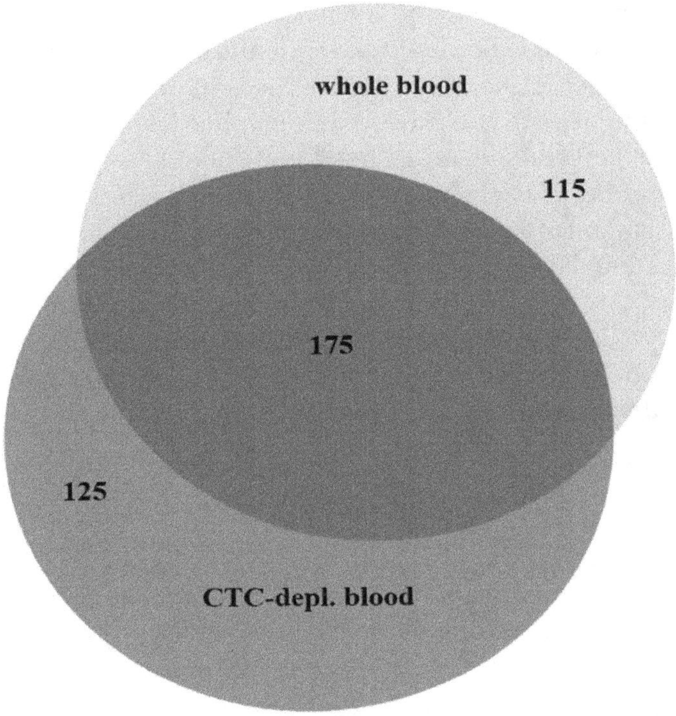

B

		whole blood	
		variants	no variants
CTC-depl. blood	variants	175	125
	no variants	115	383

agreement	70%
K-value	0.355

Figure 3. Venn diagram (**A**) and cross table (**B**) of matched cfDNA variants isolated from whole blood (light gray) and CTC-depleted blood (dark gray). Variants in all exonic regions of 17 genes were examined in 12 metastatic breast cancer (MBC) patients with hormone receptor positive/human epidermal growth factor receptor 2 negative (HR+/HER2−) primary tumor. Depletion of CTCs was conducted using AdnaTest EMT-2/StemCell Select. Variant calling by verification of unique molecular indices and filter of the Ingenuity Variant Analysis were described previously [25]. The proportional Venn diagram was computed using the tool BioVenn [26] and displays a great overlap of identical variants found in both cfDNA sources.

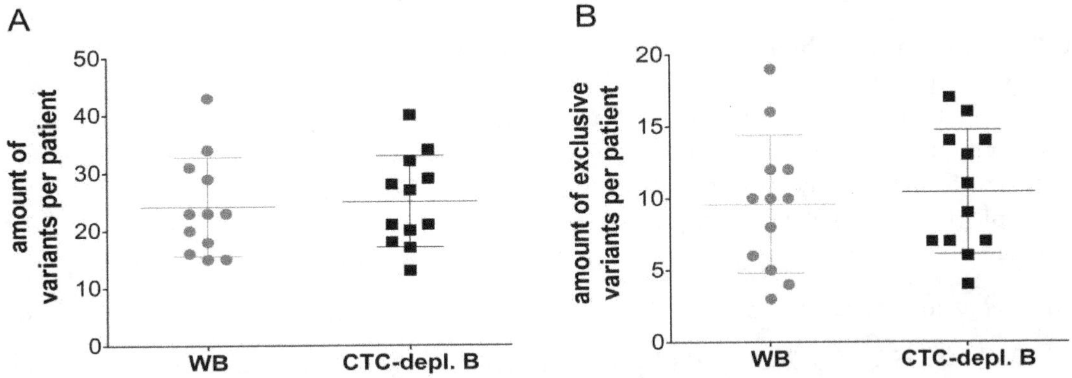

Figure 4. Boxplots describing the number of (**A**) detected cfDNA variants, and (**B**) the number of exclusively detected cfDNA variants per patient in whole blood (gray) and CTC-depleted blood (black, using AdnaTest EMT-2/StemCell Select). Means and standard deviations are also displayed, and the Wilcoxon signed-rank test indicated no significant difference between both cfDNA sources.

Additionally, the number of exclusively detected variants per patient in only one cfDNA source was also not significantly different (Figure 4B). Despite the similar quantity of variants found in only one of the two cfDNA sources, the characteristics of these variants might be different. Therefore, the number of variants per patient with the most common characteristics in the categories: translation impact, classification, gene, gene region, and allele frequency (AF) was compared in matched samples (Figure 5). The average number of exclusive frameshift variants, *BRCA2* variants, or variants with an allele frequency between 1% and 5% was slightly higher in the cfDNA samples isolated from CTC-depl. blood, but the Wilcoxon signed-rank test indicated no significant difference between the number of exclusive variants with specific characteristics (frameshift, pathogenic and likely pathogenic, uncertain significance, *AR*, *BRCA2*, *MUC16*, exonic, AF <1%, AF 1–5%) isolated from WB compared to variants isolated from CTC-depl. B. Therefore, we concluded that cfDNA variants from matched WB and CTC-depl. B harbor no differences.

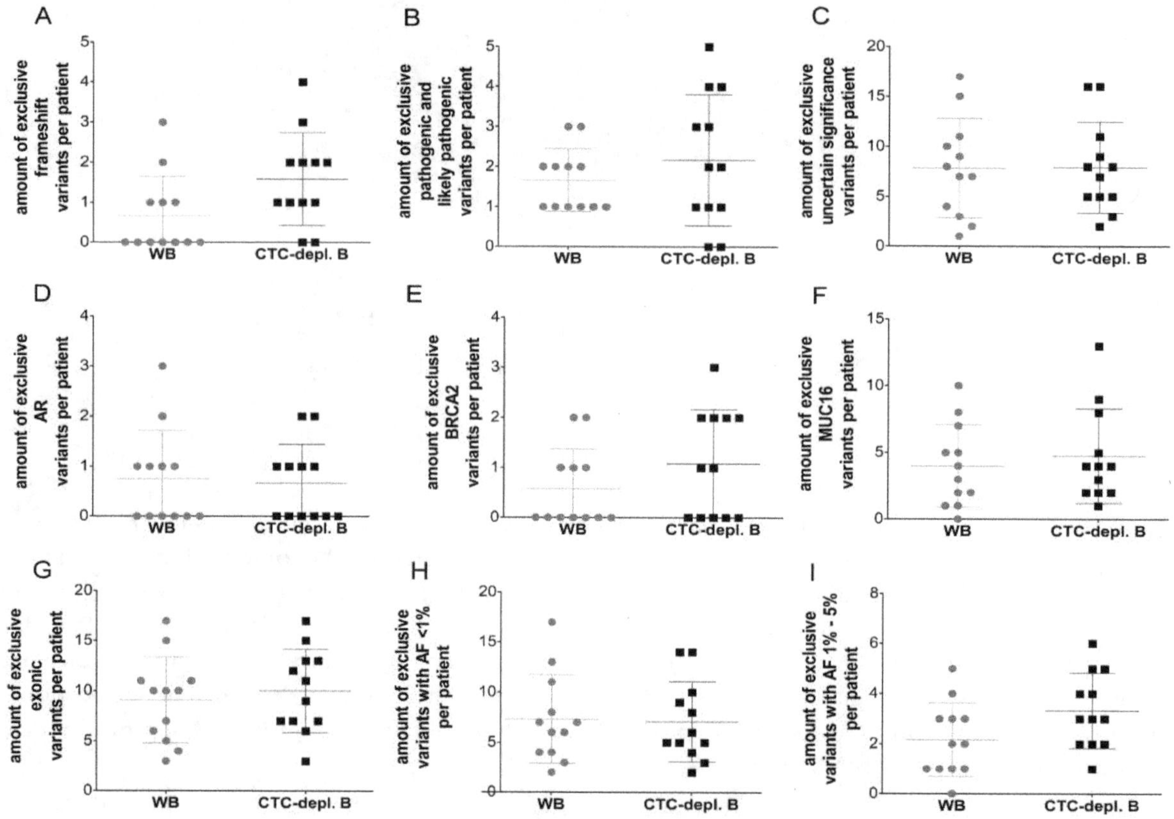

Figure 5. Boxplots describing the number of exclusively detected cfDNA variants per patient with specific characteristics in whole blood (gray) and CTC-depleted blood (black, using AdnaTest EMT-2/StemCell Select). The averages and standard deviations are indicated. Depicted characteristics are the major parameters of the categories: translation impact (frameshift (**A**)), classification (pathogenic and likely pathogenic (**B**), uncertain significance (**C**)), gene (*AR* (**D**), *BRCA2* (**E**), and *MUC16* (**F**)), gene region (exonic (**G**)), and allele frequency (<1% (**H**), 1–5% (**I**)). The Wilcoxon signed-rank test indicated no significant difference between the 12 matched cfDNA sources regarding any depicted characteristic.

2.4. Clinically Relevant Characteristics of Cell-Free DNA Variants and Circulating Tumor Cell Expression

In the cohort of HR+/HER2− MBC patients, 50.0% of detected variants were located in the *MUC16* gene irrespective of the cfDNA source (Figure 6A,E). In total, 21.7%/22.5% of all variants isolated from WB/CTC-depl. B were located in the *AR* gene, and the third most commonly altered gene found was *BRCA2* (Figure 6A,E). Furthermore, 54.1%/52.3% of all variants had an AF of <1%, and 39.7%/42.0% of all variants isolated from WB/CTC-depl. B appeared with an AF of between 1% and 5% (Figure 6B,F). Moreover, 75.2/73.0% of all variants were of uncertain significance, but 23.8/25%

of the variants isolated from WB/CTC-depl. B were already described to be either pathogenic or likely pathogenic (Figure 6C,G). Around 30% of these 69/75 pathogenic or likely pathogenic variants in WB/CTC-depl. B were located in the *AR* or *BRCA2* gene, followed by variants in *BRCA1* (Figure 6D,H). In summary, the distribution of cfDNA variants was similar in samples isolated from WB and CTC-depl. B with most variants having a low AF, being mostly of uncertain significance and being located in the *MUC16*, *AR*, or *BRCA2* gene.

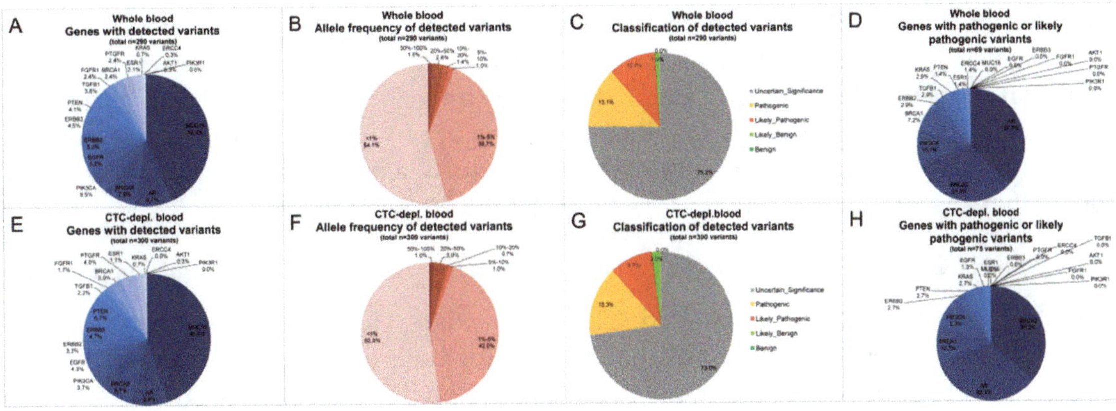

Figure 6. Distribution of called cfDNA variants isolated from whole blood (**A–D**) and CTC-depleted blood (**E–H**) of HR+/HER2− MBC patients (n = 12) according to their gene location (**A**,**D**,**E**,**H**), allele frequency (**B**,**F**), and classification (**C**,**G**). (**A**,**E**) Distribution of (exclusive (**D**,**H**)) variants according to their gene location. Most variants were found in the *MUC16* gene, while pathogenic or likely pathogenic variants were mostly located in the *AR* or *BRCA2* gene. (**B**,**F**) Allele frequency of all variants; 90% of all variants showed AFs <5%. (**C**,**G**) Classification of variants according to their known impact (benign, likely benign, uncertain significance, likely pathogenic and pathogenic) done by IVA. Nearly 25% of all variants are known to be likely pathogenic or pathogenic. No significant different distribution was detected for cfDNA variants from matched whole blood and CTC-depl. blood.

To confirm that CTC analysis is feasible in addition to cfDNA analysis from the same blood sample, overexpression was examined by quantitative PCR (qPCR) in lysates of pooled CTCs. *mTOR* was the most commonly overexpressed transcript in CTCs of the studied cohort (Figure S1, Supplementary Materials). *AKT2* was also commonly overexpressed with a frequency of 88% in the cohort. *ERBB2, ERBB3, ERCC1, AURKA,* and *SRC* transcripts were overexpressed in the CTCs of more than 50% of all patients (Figure S1, Supplementary Materials).

3. Discussion

We here demonstrate that direct comparison of cfDNA variants isolated from matched WB and CTC-depl. B revealed no significant differences. The cfDNA concentration and size distribution, as well as the number of detected variants, were similar for both cfDNA sources. Even the characteristics of the exclusively detected cfDNA variants in either WB or CTC-depl. B showed no significant differences.

3.1. Cell-Free DNA Sequencing from Circulating Tumor Cell-Depleted Blood Favored in the Future

The study was conducted to question the hypothesis that differences between WB and CTC-depl. B during cfDNA analysis occur, which were suspected to be caused by potential damage of CTCs and/or blood cells during CTC isolation, an influence of the immunomagnetic bead cocktail used for CTC enrichment, or an effect of additional 30-min incubation of WB at room temperature. However, since we found no differences in quantity and characteristics of the cfDNA variants isolated from WB versus CTC-depl. B, any systematic bias in sequencing cfDNA isolated from CTC-depl. B instead of WB can be excluded. Furthermore, we observed an unchanged sensitivity for cfDNA analysis using CTC-depl. B instead of WB. The blood supernatant remaining after positive immunomagnetic selection of CTCs using the AdnaTest EMT-2/StemCell Select procedure can, therefore, be used as source for an additional liquid biopsy analyte. Isolation of CTCs and subsequent cfDNA isolation from CTC-depl. B using the QIAamp MinElute cfDNA Kit, followed by UMI-confirmed sequence analysis in a combined workflow, provide the advantage of cfDNA mutation analysis in concert with a CTC molecular profiling from exactly the same blood sample. However, in contrast to the original AdnaTest protocol, 5 mL of WB turned out to be not enough to obtain a CTC-depl. B volume sufficient for the subsequent cfDNA analysis, because targeted PCR-based deep sequencing of cfDNA requires a high input amount of cfDNA. Consequently, the CTC isolation process was conducted in duplicate from 2 × 5 mL of WB to finally obtain minimally 4 mL of combined plasma from CTC-depl. B for cfDNA isolation with a yield >30 ng. Thus, we describe a workflow to isolate the two liquid biopsy analytes cfDNA and CTCs from a minimal blood volume of only 10 mL, resulting in reduction of the burden of blood-draw volume for the patient, while simultaneously empowering a comprehensive liquid biopsy analysis.

3.2. Additive Value of Cell-Free DNA Mutational and Circulating Tumor Cell Transcriptional Analyses

A few studies comparing cfDNA and CTC data exist. However, in contrast to our present approach, for these studies, the blood volume needed for both analyses was additive and, thus, an additional burden for patients. Moreover, most of the isolation protocols required different preservative blood tubes for cfDNA and/or CTC storage. It was examined in BC patients that both total cfDNA level and CTC count were correlated with OS [17], that cfDNA integrity was correlated with CTC presence [20], that *SOX17* promotor methylation and *ESR1* methylation were highly concordant in ctDNA and CTCs [19,23], and that cfDNA and CTCs showed overlapping mutation profiles [17]. Using cfDNA variant analysis and CTC expression analysis of the same 10 mL of blood material, we here described the high prevalence of pathogenic or likely pathogenic *AR* variants (33.3%), and 38% of all 12 patients displayed an *AR* overexpression signal in CTCs. We conclude that AR might be of importance in HR+/HER2− MBC patients, both on a mutational and transcriptional level, as previously described by us in both cfDNA and CTCs in larger HR+/HER2− MBC cohorts [12,27]. Moreover, this gene is of relevance, because targeted treatment against AR is available; however, at the moment, it is only approved for other indications [28]. Furthermore, AR was described as a potential target in triple-negative BC patients [29,30].

Despite the similar results and consequences that can be drawn from cfDNA and CTC analysis as described above, cfDNA and CTCs also exhibit additive value. We here showed the high prevalence of *ERBB3* (70%), *ERBB2* (55%), and *PIK3CA* (27%) transcript overexpression in CTCs, whereas the prevalence of cfDNA variants isolated from matched CTC-depl. B and located in *ERBB3*, *ERBB2*, and *PIK3CA* genes was low (*ERBB3* 1.7%, *ERBB2* 2.2%, and *PIK3CA* 4.8%). This further exemplifies the additive value of CTC expression in combination with the cfDNA analysis. The protein expression of HER2 (encoded by *ERBB2*) is routinely used as a predictive marker for targeted therapy in BC [31]; therefore, the frequent overexpression of *ERBB2* transcripts in CTCs of patients with HER2- primary tumors, in line with previous results [12,32], might be relevant for treatment management in the future. Compared to cfDNA, CTCs provide a unique opportunity to study DNA, RNA, and proteins, even on the single-cell level, while also providing an indicator for active metastasis [33]. In particular, the expression analysis in CTCs was shown to be relevant for prognosis [34–36], prediction [37–39], and monitoring [11,12].

In contrast to CTC counts, ctDNA in MBC patients exhibited a greater correlation with tumor burden, ctDNA was more frequently found, ctDNA showed a greater dynamic range, and ctDNA described the earliest indication of response to chemotherapies [7]. Moreover, it was shown in BC patients that sequencing of cfDNA revealed more mutations than sequencing of CTCs [17], *ESR1* variant detection was more sensitive in cfDNA compared to CTCs [40], and cfDNA was correlated in a great extent with PFS than CTC counts [18]. Here, the existence of 1.3/10.7% pathogenic or likely pathogenic *EGFR/BRCA1* cfDNA variants accompanied by 0/25% overexpression frequency of matched transcripts in CTCs also highlights the value of cfDNA in addition to CTC profiling. *EGFR* variant detection in cfDNA was the first liquid biopsy test to be approved by the USA Food and Drug Administration, as a companion diagnostic in non-small-cell lung cancer patients [41].

In multiple myeloma, it was shown that sequencing of both cfDNA and CTCs uncovered more mutations than in either analyte on its own, as in some cases a subclone was only detected in one analyte [13]. Thus, not only does the combined analysis of cfDNA variants and CTC transcriptional profiles provide additive information, but the mutational analysis of CTCs and cfDNA—from now on feasible using the same 10 mL of blood—is also assumed to be complementary rather than competitive [14].

4. Materials and Methods

4.1. Patient Population Characteristics and Eligibility Criteria

The study was conducted at the Department of Gynecology and Obstetrics, in collaboration with the Department of Medical Oncology (for specimen recruitment), both at the University Hospital Essen, Germany, and in collaboration with QIAGEN GmbH, Hilden, Germany (for library preparation and sequencing analysis). In accordance with the Declaration of Helsinki, written informed consent was obtained from all participants at enrolment, and specimens were collected using protocols approved in 2012 by the institutional review board that consists of medical doctors, nurses, psychologists, welfare workers, and a priest (12-5265-BO). In total, cfDNA from 17 MBC patients was studied between October 2015 and June 2018. All participants were $\geq$18 years, had Eastern Cooperative Oncology Group (ECOG) scores for performance status of 0–2, no severe, uncontrolled co-morbidities or medical conditions, and no second malignancies. Prior neoadjuvant and adjuvant treatment, radiation, all kinds of surgical intervention, or any other treatment of BC was permitted. Patients had estrogen (ER) and/or progesterone (PR) receptor-positive primary tumors (summarized as HR+) and no ERBB2 overamplification (n = 16). Patients with ER-positive and/or PR-positive and HER2-negative metastases were also included if their ER, PR, and HER2 status in the primary tumor was unknown (n = 1). Patient characteristics are listed in Table S1 (Supplementary Materials).

4.2. Sampling of Blood, Isolation of Circulating Tumor Cells and Processing of Plasma

Initially, 2 $\times$ 9 mL of EDTA blood was collected in S-Monovettes (Sarstedt AG & Co, Nuembrecht, Germany), stored at 4 °C, and processed within 4 h of blood draw. Five milliliters of whole blood were used in duplicate to isolate CTCs by positive immunomagnetic selection targeting EpCAM, EGFR, and HER2 (AdnaTest EMT-2/StemCell Select, QIAGEN, Hilden, Germany), as described in detail elsewhere [42]. The remaining matched whole blood not used for CTC isolation was centrifuged at 3000$\times$ g for 8 min, and plasma was frozen at $-$80 °C. This plasma sample isolated straight from whole blood was abbreviated as WB. The CTC-depleted blood remaining after positive immunomagnetic selection, abbreviated as CTC-depl. B, was centrifuged at 3000$\times$ g for 8 min, and plasma was frozen at $-$80 °C.

4.3. Isolation of Cell-Free DNA

Matched plasma samples from WB and CTC-depl. B were thawed, centrifuged at 16,000$\times$ g for 10 min at 4 °C, and passed through a 0.8-µm pore size syringe filter (Sartorius, Goettingen, Germany). Cell-free DNA was isolated from 2.8–6.0 mL (mean 4.4 mL; maximized plasma volume available) plasma by affinity-based binding to magnetic beads according to the manufacturer's instructions (QIAamp MinElute ccfDNA Kit, QIAGEN) and as described previously [25]. The same volume of plasma was used for isolation of matched cfDNA from WB and CTC-depl. B of the same patient. Cell-free DNA was eluted in 22 µL of ultraclean water and stored at $-$20 °C.

4.4. Cell-Free DNA Quantification

Diluted cfDNA (1:5 to 1:100) was applied to an Agilent Chip High Sensitivity DNA (Santa Clara, CA, USA). Concentrations of fragments with a length between 100 and 700 bp were summed using the 2100 expert software B02.08 (Agilent) to calculate the cfDNA yield.

4.5. Library Construction

The library was constructed with a customized QIAseq Targeted DNA Panel Kit (QIAGEN), as described in detail previously [25,27]. The input amount preferred for library preparation was in the range of 30–60 ng, but cfDNA samples with lower input were also included in the library preparation. The same cfDNA input amount of matched cfDNA samples from WB and CTC-depl. B was used for the library preparation, as listed in Table S2 (Supplementary Materials). Thus, the mean cfDNA input used across the cohort was 54.47 ng. We applied a 20 μL input volume in accordance with the protocol previously described [25]. Briefly, end-repair and A-addition was performed while the enzymatic fragmentation was inhibited. Subsequently, barcoded adapters including the UMI and sample-specific indices were ligated to the fragments. DNA was purified and free adapters were depleted by magnetic beads. The targeted enrichment was performed with a customized QIAGEN QIAseq Targeted DNA Panel primer designed to amplify all coding regions of the following genes: *AKT1, AR, BRCA1, BRCA2, EGFR, ERBB2, ERBB3, ERCC4, ESR1, KRAS, FGFR1, MUC16, PIK3CA, PIK3R1, PTEN, PTGFR*, and *TGFB1*. The universal PCR amplification was followed by a magnetic bead clean-up, and the final targeted enriched cfDNA library was eluted.

4.6. Sequencing

Libraries were quantified as published [25] by qPCR and the quality was checked using an Agilent Chip High Sensitivity DNA (Santa Clara). Libraries were diluted to 4 nM, and libraries with a lower yield (and matched libraries from the same patient; $n = 1$) were excluded. All pooled libraries were analyzed by paired-end sequencing on the Illumina NextSeq Sequencer with a NextSeq 550 System High-Output Kit, 2× 150-bp reads using a custom sequencing primer (QIAseq A Read1 Primer, QIAGEN).

4.7. Data Analysis/Bioinformatical Analysis

Data were initially analyzed using the QIAGEN GeneGlobe Data Analysis Center. Sufficient sequencing quality of all samples was guaranteed by exclusion of libraries with less than five million read fragments ($n = 1$), a UMI coverage lower than 400 ($n = 1$), and if less than 95% of the target region was covered with at least 5% of the mean UMI coverage ($n = 1$) [25,27]. Furthermore, libraries with >100 million read fragments were excluded to remove highly overrepresented libraries ($n = 1$). The matched libraries of the excluded ones were not analyzed to also guarantee comparison of only matched samples. The input amount, library yield, and sequencing quality parameter of each sample are summarized in Table S2 (Supplementary Materials). The QIAGEN Biomedical Genomics Workbench and the Ingenuity Variant Analysis plugin (IVA; QIAGEN) were used for further annotation, scoring, filtering (described previously [25]), and interpretation of variants detected in the UMI-based analysis. In detail, a consensus sequence was built from all fragments with the same UMI to exclude potential artefacts.

The IVA used five different filters for exclusion of called variants. The confidence filter excluded all variants with a call quality below 20. Moreover, the confidence filter only kept variants that were not located in the top 5% of the most exonically variable 100-base windows in healthy public genomes. Variants with a prevalence of >0.5% in the normal population (reference databases: (1) Allel Frequency Community (gnomAD&CGI), (2) 1000 Genomes Project, (3) ExAC, and (4) NHLBI ESP exomes) were excluded, unless the variant was already known to be a pathogenic common variant, to identify rare variants potentially associated with the evaluated condition of the tested cohort (common variant filter). The genetic analysis filter only kept variants that were associated with gain of function or with the following inheritance patterns: homozygous, compound heterozygous, haplosufficient, hemizygous, het-ambiguous, or heterozygous. Only variants located no more than 20 bases from the intron were included, as well as those described to be pathogenic and/or likely pathogenic from the American College of Medical Genetics and Genomics, or variants that are loss-of-function-associated, which induce frameshift, in-frame indel, start/stop changes, missense, intronic two-bp splice-site loss, or any splice-alteration predicted by MaxEntScan (predicted deleterious filter). The cancer driver variant filter kept only variants that were found in (1) cancer-associated mouse knockout phenotypes, (2) cancer-associated cellular processes with any directionality, (3) cancer-associated pathways with any directionality, (4) cancer therapeutic targets, (5) published cancer literature variants and gene level findings, (6) known or predicted cancer subnetwork regulatory sites, (7) COSMIC at a frequency greater than or equal to 0.01%, and (8) TCGA at a frequency greater than or equal to 0.01%.

Original raw sequencing data were uploaded as two fastq files plus MD5 checksum per sample, and are available at the European Nucleotide Archive with the study accession number PRJEB30449.

4.8. Messenger RNA Isolation and Quantitative PCR

Messenger RNA was isolated from the CTC lysates by oligo(dT)$_{25}$-coated magnetic beads and was reverse-transcribed (Adna-Test EMT-2/StemCell Detect, QIAGEN; [42]). The AdnaTest TNBC Panel prototype (QIAGEN), consisting of multimarker real-time (RT)-qPCR assays, was applied to the complementary DNA isolated from the CTCs for expression profiling of *AKT2, ALK, AR, AURKA, BRCA1, EGFR, ERCC1, ERBB2, ERBB3, KIT, KRT5, MET, MTOR, NOTCH1, PARP1, PIK3CA, SRC*, and *GAPDH*, in relation to the leukocyte-specific transcript *CD45* and healthy donor controls. Experimental set-up und data evaluation were described in detail previously [12].

4.9. Statistical analysis

Statistical analysis was performed using SPSS, version 11.5 (IBM, Armonk, NY, USA). The Wilcoxon signed-rank test was used to assess whether the matched samples differed. Diagrams were computed with GraphPad PRISM (GraphPad Software Inc., San Diego, CA, USA) and Microsoft Excel (Microsoft Corporation, Redmond, WA, USA). Box plots display individual values for each patient, as well as the mean and standard deviation. The Venn diagram was produced with the online tool BioVenn [26]. The kappa-value was calculated using the GraphPad QuickCalcs website [43].

5. Conclusions

In summary, cfDNA mutational and CTC transcriptional analyses can supplement each other. A comprehensive liquid biopsy, therefore, increases the chance for identification of actionable targets to direct therapy strategies. Thus, the isolation of both CTCs and cfDNA, in an "all from one tube" format without bias due to the initial CTC isolation process, as demonstrated in this research study, might be helpful in paving a way for individual treatment decision-making.

Author Contributions: Conceptualization, C.K., S.H., P.H., M.S.H., and S.K.B.; software, M.S.; formal analysis, C.K. and M.S.; investigation, C.K.; resources, M.T., P.M., O.H., and R.K.; data curation, C.K. and M.S.; writing—original draft preparation, C.K.; writing—review and editing, M.S., S.H., P.H., M.S.H., and S.K.B.; visualization, C.K.; supervision, S.H., P.H., M.S.H., and S.K.B. All authors finally approved the version to be published and agree to be accountable for all aspects of the work.

Acknowledgments: We highly appreciate the consent of all patients for their participation in this research study. We valuate the dedication of Ann-Kathrin Bittner for connecting clinical practice and research by diligent caring about the patients' medical needs and educating the patients about the presented research study. The authors thank all involved nurses and physicians from the Department of Gynecology and Obstetrics, University Hospital of Essen, Germany for their commitment in sampling and educating the patients. Karim Benyaa kindly supported the library construction. We are grateful for the spell check by Dominic O'Neil. We acknowledge support by the Open Access Publication Fund of the University of Duisburg-Essen.

References

1. Diaz, L.A.; Bardelli, A. Liquid biopsies: Genotyping circulating tumor DNA. *J. Clin. Oncol.* **2014**, *32*, 579–586. [CrossRef] [PubMed]
2. Krawczyk, N.; Fehm, T.; Banys-Paluchowski, M.; Janni, W.; Schramm, A. Liquid Biopsy in Metastasized Breast Cancer as Basis for Treatment Decisions. *Oncol. Res. Treat.* **2016**, *39*, 112–116. [CrossRef] [PubMed]
3. Takeshita, T.; Yamamoto, Y.; Yamamoto-Ibusuki, M.; Tomiguchi, M.; Sueta, A.; Murakami, K.; Omoto, Y.; Iwase, H. Analysis of *ESR1* and PIK3CA mutations in plasma cell-free DNA from ER-positive breast cancer patients. *Oncotarget* **2017**, *8*, 52142–52155. [CrossRef] [PubMed]
4. Fribbens, C.; O'Leary, B.; Kilburn, L.; Hrebien, S.; Garcia-Murillas, I.; Beaney, M.; Cristofanilli, M.; Andre, F.; Loi, S.; Loibl, S.; et al. Plasma *ESR1* Mutations and the Treatment of Estrogen Receptor-Positive Advanced Breast Cancer. *J. Clin. Oncol.* **2016**, *34*, 2961–2968. [CrossRef] [PubMed]
5. Wan, J.C.M.; Massie, C.; Garcia-Corbacho, J.; Mouliere, F.; Brenton, J.D.; Caldas, C.; Pacey, S.; Baird, R.; Rosenfeld, N. Liquid biopsies come of age: Towards implementation of circulating tumour DNA. *Nat. Rev. Cancer* **2017**, *17*, 223–238. [CrossRef] [PubMed]
6. Diehl, F.; Schmidt, K.; Choti, M.A.; Romans, K.; Goodman, S.; Li, M.; Thornton, K.; Agrawal, N.; Sokoll, L.; Szabo, S.A.; et al. Circulating mutant DNA to assess tumor dynamics. *Nat. Med.* **2008**, *14*, 985–990. [CrossRef] [PubMed]
7. Dawson, S.-J.; Tsui, D.W.Y.; Murtaza, M.; Biggs, H.; Rueda, O.M.; Chin, S.-F.; Dunning, M.J.; Gale, D.; Forshew, T.; Mahler-Araujo, B.; et al. Analysis of circulating tumor DNA to monitor metastatic breast cancer. *N. Engl. J. Med.* **2013**, *368*, 1199–1209. [CrossRef] [PubMed]
8. Cristofanilli, M.; Budd, G.T.; Ellis, M.J.; Stopeck, A.; Matera, J.; Miller, M.C.; Reuben, J.M.; Doyle, G.V.; Allard, W.J.; Terstappen, L.W.M.M.; et al. Circulating tumor cells, disease progression, and survival in metastatic breast cancer. *N. Engl. J. Med.* **2004**, *351*, 781–791. [CrossRef]
9. Hayes, D.F.; Cristofanilli, M.; Budd, G.T.; Ellis, M.J.; Stopeck, A.; Miller, M.C.; Matera, J.; Allard, W.J.; Doyle, G.V.; Terstappen, L.W.W.M. Circulating tumor cells at each follow-up time point during therapy of metastatic breast cancer patients predict progression-free and overall survival. *Clin. Cancer Res.* **2006**, *12*, 4218–4224. [CrossRef]
10. Budd, G.T.; Cristofanilli, M.; Ellis, M.J.; Stopeck, A.; Borden, E.; Miller, M.C.; Matera, J.; Repollet, M.; Doyle, G.V.; Terstappen, L.W.M.M.; et al. Circulating tumor cells versus imaging—Predicting overall survival in metastatic breast cancer. *Clin. Cancer Res.* **2006**, *12*, 6403–6409. [CrossRef]
11. Alix-Panabières, C.; Pantel, K. Circulating tumor cells: Liquid biopsy of cancer. *Clin. Chem.* **2013**, *59*, 110–118. [CrossRef]
12. Keup, C.; Mach, P.; Aktas, B.; Tewes, M.; Kolberg, H.-C.; Hauch, S.; Sprenger-Haussels, M.; Kimmig, R.; Kasimir-Bauer, S. RNA Profiles of Circulating Tumor Cells and Extracellular Vesicles for Therapy Stratification of Metastatic Breast Cancer Patients. *Clin. Chem.* **2018**. [CrossRef] [PubMed]
13. Manier, S.; Park, J.; Capelletti, M.; Bustoros, M.; Freeman, S.S.; Ha, G.; Rhoades, J.; Liu, C.J.; Huynh, D.; Reed, S.C.; et al. Whole-exome sequencing of cell-free DNA and circulating tumor cells in multiple myeloma. *Nat. Commun.* **2018**, *9*, 1691. [CrossRef] [PubMed]
14. Haber, D.A.; Velculescu, V.E. Blood-based analyses of cancer: Circulating tumor cells and circulating tumor DNA. *Cancer Discov.* **2014**, *4*, 650–661. [CrossRef]
15. Heidary, M.; Auer, M.; Ulz, P.; Heitzer, E.; Petru, E.; Gasch, C.; Riethdorf, S.; Mauermann, O.; Lafer, I.; Pristauz, G.; et al. The dynamic range of circulating tumor DNA in metastatic breast cancer. *Breast Cancer Res.* **2014**, *16*, 421. [CrossRef] [PubMed]
16. Delfau-Larue, M.-H.; van der Gucht, A.; Dupuis, J.; Jais, J.-P.; Nel, I.; Beldi-Ferchiou, A.; Hamdane, S.; Benmaad, I.; Laboure, G.; Verret, B.; et al. Total metabolic tumor volume, circulating tumor cells, cell-free DNA: Distinct prognostic value in follicular lymphoma. *Blood Adv.* **2018**, *2*, 807–816. [CrossRef] [PubMed]

17. Shaw, J.A.; Guttery, D.S.; Hills, A.; Fernandez-Garcia, D.; Page, K.; Rosales, B.M.; Goddard, K.S.; Hastings, R.K.; Luo, J.; Ogle, O.; et al. Mutation Analysis of Cell-Free DNA and Single Circulating Tumor Cells in Metastatic Breast Cancer Patients with High Circulating Tumor Cell Counts. *Clin. Cancer Res.* **2017**, *23*, 88–96. [CrossRef] [PubMed]
18. Rossi, G.; Mu, Z.; Rademaker, A.W.; Austin, L.K.; Strickland, K.S.; Costa, R.L.B.; Nagy, R.J.; Zagonel, V.; Taxter, T.J.; Behdad, A.; et al. Cell-Free DNA and Circulating Tumor Cells: Comprehensive Liquid Biopsy Analysis in Advanced Breast Cancer. *Clin. Cancer Res.* **2018**, *24*, 560–568. [CrossRef]
19. Mastoraki, S.; Strati, A.; Tzanikou, E.; Chimonidou, M.; Politaki, E.; Voutsina, A.; Psyrri, A.; Georgoulias, V.; Lianidou, E. *ESR1* Methylation: A Liquid Biopsy-Based Epigenetic Assay for the Follow-up of Patients with Metastatic Breast Cancer Receiving Endocrine Treatment. *Clin. Cancer Res.* **2018**, *24*, 1500–1510. [CrossRef]
20. Madhavan, D.; Wallwiener, M.; Bents, K.; Zucknick, M.; Nees, J.; Schott, S.; Cuk, K.; Riethdorf, S.; Trumpp, A.; Pantel, K.; et al. Plasma DNA integrity as a biomarker for primary and metastatic breast cancer and potential marker for early diagnosis. *Breast Cancer Res. Treat.* **2014**, *146*, 163–174. [CrossRef]
21. Coco, S.; Alama, A.; Vanni, I.; Fontana, V.; Genova, C.; Dal Bello, M.G.; Truini, A.; Rijavec, E.; Biello, F.; Sini, C.; et al. Circulating Cell-Free DNA and Circulating Tumor Cells as Prognostic and Predictive Biomarkers in Advanced Non-Small Cell Lung Cancer Patients Treated with First-Line Chemotherapy. *Int. J. Mol. Sci.* **2017**, *18*, 1035. [CrossRef] [PubMed]
22. Vo, J.H.; Nei, W.L.; Hu, M.; Phyo, W.M.; Wang, F.; Fong, K.W.; Tan, T.; Soong, Y.L.; Cheah, S.L.; Sommat, K.; et al. Comparison of Circulating Tumour Cells and Circulating Cell-Free Epstein-Barr Virus DNA in Patients with Nasopharyngeal Carcinoma Undergoing Radiotherapy. *Sci. Rep.* **2016**, *6*, 13. [CrossRef] [PubMed]
23. Chimonidou, M.; Strati, A.; Malamos, N.; Kouneli, S.; Georgoulias, V.; Lianidou, E. Direct comparison study of DNA methylation markers in EpCAM-positive circulating tumour cells, corresponding circulating tumour DNA, and paired primary tumours in breast cancer. *Oncotarget* **2017**, *8*, 72054–72068. [CrossRef] [PubMed]
24. Chimonidou, M.; Strati, A.; Malamos, N.; Georgoulias, V.; Lianidou, E.S. SOX17 promoter methylation in circulating tumor cells and matched cell-free DNA isolated from plasma of patients with breast cancer. *Clin. Chem.* **2013**, *59*, 270–279. [CrossRef] [PubMed]
25. Keup, C.; Hahn, P.; Hauch, S.; Sprenger-Haussels, M.; Tewes, M.; Mach, P.; Bittner, A.-K.; Kimmig, R.; Kasimir-Bauer, S.; Benyaa, K. Targeted PCR-based deep sequencing of cfDNA with unique molecular indices by a customized QIAseq Targeted DNA Panel. *Protocols* **2018**. [CrossRef]
26. Hulsen, T.; de Vlieg, J.; Alkema, W. BioVenn—A web application for the comparison and visualization of biological lists using area-proportional Venn diagrams. *BMC Genom.* **2008**, *9*, 488. [CrossRef] [PubMed]
27. Keup, C.; Benyaa, K.; Hauch, S.; Sprenger-Haussels, M.; Tewes, M.; Mach, P.; Bittner, A.-K.; Kimmig, R.; Hahn, P.; Kasimir-Bauer, S. Variants in cell-free DNA of hormone receptor positive, HER2 negative metastatic breast cancer assessed by targeted deep sequencing. *Cell. Mol. Life Sci.* **2018**, submitted.
28. Antonarakis, E.S.; Lu, C.; Luber, B.; Wang, H.; Chen, Y.; Zhu, Y.; Silberstein, J.L.; Taylor, M.N.; Maughan, B.L.; Denmeade, S.R.; et al. Clinical Significance of Androgen Receptor Splice Variant-7 mRNA Detection in Circulating Tumor Cells of Men with Metastatic Castration-Resistant Prostate Cancer Treated with First- and Second-Line Abiraterone and Enzalutamide. *J. Clin. Oncol.* **2017**, *35*, 2149–2156. [CrossRef] [PubMed]
29. Lehmann, B.D.; Bauer, J.A.; Schafer, J.M.; Pendleton, C.S.; Tang, L.; Johnson, K.C.; Chen, X.; Balko, J.M.; Gómez, H.; Arteaga, C.L.; et al. PIK3CA mutations in androgen receptor-positive triple negative breast cancer confer sensitivity to the combination of PI3K and androgen receptor inhibitors. *Breast Cancer Res.* **2014**, *16*, 406. [CrossRef] [PubMed]
30. Rahim, B.; O'Regan, R. AR Signaling in Breast Cancer. *Cancers* **2017**, *9*, 21. [CrossRef]
31. Wolff, A.C.; Hammond, M.E.H.; Hicks, D.G.; Dowsett, M.; McShane, L.M.; Allison, K.H.; Allred, D.C.; Bartlett, J.M.S.; Bilous, M.; Fitzgibbons, P.; et al. Recommendations for human epidermal growth factor receptor 2 testing in breast cancer: American Society of Clinical Oncology/College of American Pathologists clinical practice guideline update. *Arch. Pathol. Lab. Med.* **2014**, *138*, 241–256. [CrossRef] [PubMed]
32. Aktas, B.; Kasimir-Bauer, S.; Müller, V.; Janni, W.; Fehm, T.; Wallwiener, D.; Pantel, K.; Tewes, M. Comparison of the HER2, estrogen and progesterone receptor expression profile of primary tumor, metastases and circulating tumor cells in metastatic breast cancer patients. *BMC Cancer* **2016**, *16*, 522. [CrossRef] [PubMed]
33. Lianidou, E.; Pantel, K. Liquid Biopsies. *Genes Chromosomes Cancer* **2019**, *58*, 219–232. [CrossRef] [PubMed]

34. Bulfoni, M.; Gerratana, L.; Del Ben, F.; Marzinotto, S.; Sorrentino, M.; Turetta, M.; Scoles, G.; Toffoletto, B.; Isola, M.; Beltrami, C.A.; et al. In patients with metastatic breast cancer the identification of circulating tumor cells in epithelial-to-mesenchymal transition is associated with a poor prognosis. *Breast Cancer Res.* **2016**, *18*, 30. [CrossRef] [PubMed]
35. Spiliotaki, M.; Mavroudis, D.; Kapranou, K.; Markomanolaki, H.; Kallergi, G.; Koinis, F.; Kalbakis, K.; Georgoulias, V.; Agelaki, S. Evaluation of proliferation and apoptosis markers in circulating tumor cells of women with early breast cancer who are candidates for tumor dormancy. *Breast Cancer Res.* **2014**, *16*, 485. [CrossRef] [PubMed]
36. Adams, D.L.; Adams, D.K.; Stefansson, S.; Haudenschild, C.; Martin, S.S.; Charpentier, M.; Chumsri, S.; Cristofanilli, M.; Tang, C.-M.; Alpaugh, R.K. Mitosis in circulating tumor cells stratifies highly aggressive breast carcinomas. *Breast Cancer Res.* **2016**, *18*, 44. [CrossRef] [PubMed]
37. Antonarakis, E.S.; Lu, C.; Wang, H.; Luber, B.; Nakazawa, M.; Roeser, J.C.; Chen, Y.; Mohammad, T.A.; Chen, Y.; Fedor, H.L.; et al. AR-V7 and resistance to enzalutamide and abiraterone in prostate cancer. *N. Engl. J. Med.* **2014**, *371*, 1028–1038. [CrossRef] [PubMed]
38. Paolillo, C.; Mu, Z.; Rossi, G.; Schiewer, M.J.; Nguyen, T.; Austin, L.; Capoluongo, E.; Knudsen, K.E.; Cristofanilli, M.; Fortina, P. Detection of Activating Estrogen Receptor Gene (*ESR1*) Mutations in Single Circulating Tumor Cells. *Clin. Cancer Res.* **2017**, *23*, 6086–6093. [CrossRef] [PubMed]
39. Reijm, E.A.; Sieuwerts, A.M.; Smid, M.; Vries, J.B.-D.; Mostert, B.; Onstenk, W.; Peeters, D.; Dirix, L.Y.; Seynaeve, C.M.; Jager, A.; et al. An 8-gene mRNA expression profile in circulating tumor cells predicts response to aromatase inhibitors in metastatic breast cancer patients. *BMC Cancer* **2016**, *16*, 123. [CrossRef]
40. Beije, N.; Sieuwerts, A.M.; Kraan, J.; Van, N.M.; Onstenk, W.; Vitale, S.R.; van der Vlugt-Daane, M.; Dirix, L.Y.; Brouwer, A.; Hamberg, P.; et al. Estrogen receptor mutations and splice variants determined in liquid biopsies from metastatic breast cancer patients. *Mol. Oncol.* **2018**, *12*, 48–57. [CrossRef] [PubMed]
41. US Food & Drug Administration. Premarket Approval, P150044—Cobas EGFR MUTATION TEST V2. 2016. Available online: http://www.accessdata.fda.gov/scripts/cdrh/cfdocs/cfpma/pma.cfm?id=P150044 (accessed on 4 January 2019).
42. Bredemeier, M.; Edimiris, P.; Tewes, M.; Mach, P.; Aktas, B.; Schellbach, D.; Wagner, J.; Kimmig, R.; Kasimir-Bauer, S. Establishment of a multimarker qPCR panel for the molecular characterization of circulating tumor cells in blood samples of metastatic breast cancer patients during the course of palliative treatment. *Oncotarget* **2016**, *7*, 41677–41690. [CrossRef] [PubMed]
43. Quantify Agreement with Kappa. Available online: https://graphpad.com/quickcalcs/kappa1/\T1\textquotedblright (accessed on 18 December 2018).

Permissions

All chapters in this book were first published by MDPI; hereby published with permission under the Creative Commons Attribution License or equivalent. Every chapter published in this book has been scrutinized by our experts. Their significance has been extensively debated. The topics covered herein carry significant findings which will fuel the growth of the discipline. They may even be implemented as practical applications or may be referred to as a beginning point for another development.

The contributors of this book come from diverse backgrounds, making this book a truly international effort. This book will bring forth new frontiers with its revolutionizing research information and detailed analysis of the nascent developments around the world.

We would like to thank all the contributing authors for lending their expertise to make the book truly unique. They have played a crucial role in the development of this book. Without their invaluable contributions this book wouldn't have been possible. They have made vital efforts to compile up to date information on the varied aspects of this subject to make this book a valuable addition to the collection of many professionals and students.

This book was conceptualized with the vision of imparting up-to-date information and advanced data in this field. To ensure the same, a matchless editorial board was set up. Every individual on the board went through rigorous rounds of assessment to prove their worth. After which they invested a large part of their time researching and compiling the most relevant data for our readers.

The editorial board has been involved in producing this book since its inception. They have spent rigorous hours researching and exploring the diverse topics which have resulted in the successful publishing of this book. They have passed on their knowledge of decades through this book. To expedite this challenging task, the publisher supported the team at every step. A small team of assistant editors was also appointed to further simplify the editing procedure and attain best results for the readers.

Apart from the editorial board, the designing team has also invested a significant amount of their time in understanding the subject and creating the most relevant covers. They scrutinized every image to scout for the most suitable representation of the subject and create an appropriate cover for the book.

The publishing team has been an ardent support to the editorial, designing and production team. Their endless efforts to recruit the best for this project, has resulted in the accomplishment of this book. They are a veteran in the field of academics and their pool of knowledge is as vast as their experience in printing. Their expertise and guidance has proved useful at every step. Their uncompromising quality standards have made this book an exceptional effort. Their encouragement from time to time has been an inspiration for everyone.

The publisher and the editorial board hope that this book will prove to be a valuable piece of knowledge for researchers, students, practitioners and scholars across the globe.

List of Contributors

Cintia Rosa, Carla Nogueira, Suzane Lessa and Andrea Ramalho
Social Applied Nutrition Department, Micronutrients Research Center (NPqM), Federal University of Rio de Janeiro, Rio de Janeiro 21.941-902, Brazil

Carlos Franca
Social Applied Nutrition Department, Micronutrients Research Center (NPqM), Federal University of Rio de Janeiro, Rio de Janeiro 21.941-902, Brazil
Department of Radiation Oncology, Ingá Radiotherapy Clinic (CRI), Brazilian Institute of Oncology (IBO), Federal University of Rio de Janeiro, Niterói 24.210- 470, Brazil
Department of Radiation Oncology, Pontifical Catholic University of Rio de Janeiro, Rio de Janeiro 22.451-900, Brazil
Department of Radiology, Clementino Fraga Filho University Hospital, Federal University of Rio de Janeiro, Rio de Janeiro 21.941-902, Brazil

Sérgio Lanes Vieira and Antônio Penna
Department of Radiation Oncology, Ingá Radiotherapy Clinic (CRI), Brazilian Institute of Oncology (IBO), Federal University of Rio de Janeiro, Niterói 24.210-470, Brazil
Department of Radiation Oncology, Pontifical Catholic University of Rio de Janeiro, Rio de Janeiro 22.451-900, Brazil

Antônio Carvalho
Department of Radiology, Clementino Fraga Filho University Hospital, Federal University of Rio de Janeiro, Rio de Janeiro 21.941-902, Brazil

Clémence Dubois
Université Clermont Auvergne, INSERM, U1240, Imagerie Moléculaire et Stratégies Théranostiques, F-63000 Clermont Ferrand, France
Université Clermont Auvergne, Institut Universitaire de Technologie, INSERM, U1240, Imagerie Moléculaire et Stratégies Théranostiques, F-63000 Clermont Ferrand, France

Fanny Martin
Département de Radiothérapie, Centre Jean Perrin, F-63000 Clermont Ferrand, France

Chervin Hassel and Sylvie Guerder
Centre Hospitalier Universitaire Purpan, Centre de Physiopathologie de Toulouse Purpan, INSERM, UMR 1043/CNRS UMR 5282, Antigen Presenting Cells and CD4 T cell responses, F-31024 Toulouse, France

Florian Magnier
Service de Physique Médicale, Centre Jean Perrin, F-63000 Clermont Ferrand, France

Pierre Daumar, Emmanuelle Mounetou and Mahchid Bamdad
Université Clermont Auvergne, Institut Universitaire de Technologie, INSERM, U1240, Imagerie Moléculaire et Stratégies Théranostiques, F-63000 Clermont Ferrand, France

Corinne Aubel
Université Clermont Auvergne, Faculté de Médecine, INSERM, U1240, Imagerie Moléculaire et Stratégies Théranostiques, F-63000 Clermont Ferrand, France

Frédérique Penault-Lorca
Université Clermont Auvergne, INSERM, U1240, Imagerie Moléculaire et Stratégies Théranostiques, F-63000 Clermont Ferrand, France

Katarzyna Kulcenty, Igor Piotrowski and Wiktoria Maria Suchorska
Radiobiology Lab, Department of Medical Physics, Greater Poland Cancer, 61-866 Poznań, Poland
Department of Electroradiology, Poznan University of Medical Sciences, ul. Garbary 15, 61-866 Poznan, Poland

Joanna Patrycja Wróblewska
Department of Pathology, Poznan University of Medical Sciences and Greater Poland Cancer Center, ul. Garbary 15, 61-866 Poznan, Poland

Janusz Wasiewicz
Department of Breast Cancer Surgery, Greater Poland Cancer Centre, ul. Garbary 15, 61-866 Poznań, Poland

Anieta M. Sieuwerts and John W.M. Martens
Department of Medical Oncology and Erasmus MC Cancer Institute, 3015 GD Rotterdam, The Netherlands
Cancer Genomics Netherlands, Erasmus MC Cancer Institute, 3015 GD Rotterdam, The Netherlands

Shusma C. Doebar, Esther I. Verhoef, Marie C. Agahozo and Carolien H.M. van Deurzen
Department of Pathology, Erasmus MC Cancer Institute, 3015 GD Rotterdam, The Netherlands

Vanja de Weerd and Corine M. Beauford
Department of Medical Oncology and Erasmus MC Cancer Institute, 3015 GD Rotterdam, The Netherlands

Michael P. Lux, Naiba Nabieva, Bernhard Volz, Matthias W. Beckmann and Peter A. Fasching
Department of Gynecology and Obstetrics, Erlangen University Hospital, Comprehensive Cancer Center Erlangen-EMN, Friedrich-Alexander University of Erlangen–Nuremberg, Universitätsstrasse 21–23, 91054 Erlangen, Germany

Andreas D. Hartkopf, Florin-Andrei Taran, Diethelm Wallwiener and Sara Y. Brucker
Department of Obstetrics and Gynecology, University of Tübingen, 72076 Tübingen, Germany

Jens Huober and Wolfgang Janni
Department of Gynecology and Obstetrics, Ulm University Hospital, 89070 Ulm, Germany

Friedrich Overkamp
Oncologianova GmbH, 45657 Recklinghausen, Germany

Hans-Christian Kolberg
Marienhospital Bottrop, 46236 Bottrop, Germany

Peyman Hadji
Department of Bone Oncology, Nordwest Hospital, 60488 Frankfurt, Germany
Oncology Practice at Bethanien Hospital Frankfurt; 60389 Frankfurt, Germany

Lothar Häberle
Department of Gynecology and Obstetrics, Erlangen University Hospital, Comprehensive Cancer Center Erlangen-EMN, Friedrich-Alexander University of Erlangen–Nuremberg, Universitätsstrasse 21–23, 91054 Erlangen, Germany
Department of Gynecology and Obstetrics, Biostatistics Unit, Erlangen University Hospital, 91054 Erlangen, Germany

Johannes Ettl
Department of Obstetrics and Gynecology, Klinikum rechts der Isar, Technical University of Munich, 81675 Munich, Germany

Diana Lüftner
Charité University Hospital, Berlin, Campus Benjamin Franklin, Department of Hematology, Oncology and Tumour Immunology, 12203 Berlin, Germany

Markus Wallwiener
Department of Obstetrics and Gynecology, University of Heidelberg, 69120 Heidelberg, Germany

Volkmar Müller
Department of Gynecology, Hamburg-Eppendorf University Medical Center, 20246 Hamburg, Germany

Erik Belleville
ClinSol GmbH & Co KG, 97074 Würzburg, Germany

Pauline Wimberger
Department of Gynecology and Obstetrics, Dresden University Hospital, 01307 Dresden, Germany

Carsten Hielscher
gSUND Gynäkologie Kompetenzzentrum Stralsund, 18435 Stralsund, Germany

Matthias Geberth
Gynäkologische Praxisklinik am Rosengarten, 68165 Mannheim, Germany

Wolfgang Abenhardt
Medizinischen Versorgungszentrum Onkologie, Onkologie im Elisenhof, 80335 Munich, Germany

Christian Kurbacher
Department of Gynecology and Obstetrics, Medizinisches Zentrum Bonn Friedensplatz, 53111 Bonn, Germany

Rachel Wuerstlein
Department of Gynecology and Obstetrics, Breast Center and Comprehensive Cancer Center Munich, Munich University Hospital, 80337 Munich, Germany

Christoph Thomssen
Department of Gynecology, Martin Luther University of Halle-Wittenberg, 06120 Halle (Saale), Germany

Michael Untch
Department of Gynecology and Obstetrics, Helios Clinics Berlin Buch, 13125 Berlin, Germany

Tanja N. Fehm
Department of Gynecology and Obstetrics, Düsseldorf University Hospital, 40225 Düsseldorf, Germany

Andreas Schneeweiss
Department of Obstetrics and Gynecology, University of Heidelberg, 69120 Heidelberg, Germany
National Center for Tumor Diseases and Department of Gynecology and Obstetrics, Heidelberg University Hospital, 69120 Heidelberg, Germany

Victoria Teoh, Marios-Konstantinos Tasoulis and Gerald Gui
Department of Breast Surgery, Royal Marsden NHS Foundation Trust, Fulham Road, London SW36JJ, UK

Doris van Abbema
Department of Internal Medicine, GROW-School for Oncology and Developmental Biology, Maastricht University Medical Center, Peter Debyelaan 25, 6229 HX Maastricht, The Netherlands
ACHIEVE Centre of Applied Research, Faculty of Health, Amsterdam University of Applied Sciences, Tafelbergweg 51, 1105 BD Amsterdam, The Netherlands

Pauline Vissers
Department of Research, Netherlands Comprehensive Cancer Organisation (IKNL), Godebaldkwartier 419, 3511 DT Utrecht, The Netherlands

Judith de Vos-Geelen and Vivianne Tjan-Heijnen
Department of Internal Medicine, GROW-School for Oncology and Developmental Biology, Maastricht University Medical Center, Peter Debyelaan 25, 6229 HX Maastricht, The Netherlands

Valery Lemmens
Department of Research, Netherlands Comprehensive Cancer Organisation (IKNL), Godebaldkwartier 419, 3511 DT Utrecht, The Netherlands
Department of Public Health, Erasmus Medical Center, Wytemaweg 80, 3015 CN Rotterdam, The Netherlands

Maryska Janssen-Heijnen
Department of Clinical Epidemiology, VieCuri Medical Centre, Tegelseweg 210, 5912 BL Venlo, The Netherlands
Department of Epidemiology, GROW-School for Oncology and Developmental Biology, Maastricht University Medical Centre, Universiteitssingel 60, 6229 ER Maastricht, The Netherlands

Binafsha Manzoor Syed
Nottingham Breast Cancer Research Centre, School of Medicine, University of Nottingham Medical Research Centre, Liaquat University of Medical & Health Sciences, Jamshoro 71000, Pakistan

Andrew R. Green
Academic Pathology, Nottingham Breast Cancer Research Centre, Division of Cancer and Stem Cells, School of Medicine, University of Nottingham, Nottingham NG5 1PB, UK
Nottingham Breast Cancer Research Centre, School of Medicine, The University of Nottingham, Nottingham NG7 2RD, UK

Ian O Ellis and Kwok-Leung Cheung
Nottingham Breast Cancer Research Centre, School of Medicine, University of Nottingham

David A L Morgan
Department of Oncology, Nottingham University Hospitals, Nottingham NG5 1PB, UK

Patricia Gaule, Nupur Mukherjee, Brendan Corkery, Alex J. Eustace, Sandra Roche, Robert O'Connor, Naomi Walsh and Norma O'Donovan
Molecular Therapeutics for Cancer Ireland, National Institute for Cellular Biotechnology, Dublin City University, Dublin D09 NR58, Ireland

Kenneth J. O'Byrne
Institute of Health and Biomedical Innovation, Queensland University of Technology, Translational Research Institute, Woolloongabba QLD 4059, Australia

Michael J. Duffy
UCD School of Medicine, UCD Conway Institute of Biomolecular and Biomedical Research, University College Dublin, Dublin 4, Ireland
UCD Clinical Research Centre, St. Vincent's University Hospital, Dublin 4, Ireland

John Crown
Molecular Therapeutics for Cancer Ireland, National Institute for Cellular Biotechnology, Dublin City University, Dublin D09 NR58, Ireland

Kathy Gately
Trinity Translational Medicine Institute, St. James's Hospital Dublin, Dublin 8, Ireland

Sara S. Oltra, Juan Miguel Cejalvo, Marta Albanell, Ana Ferrer, Marta Nacher, Begoña Bermejo, Cristina Hernando, Isabel Chirivella, Maria Peña-Chilet and María Teresa Martinez
INCLIVA Biomedical Research Institute, Hospital Clínico Universitario Valencia, University of Valencia, 46010 Valencia, Spain

Eduardo Tormo, Pilar Eroles, Ana Lluch and Gloria Ribas
INCLIVA Biomedical Research Institute, Hospital Clínico Universitario Valencia, University of Valencia, 46010 Valencia, Spain Biomedical Research Centre Network in Cancer (CIBERONC), 46010 Valencia, Spain

Elisa Alonso and Octavio Burgués
Biomedical Research Centre Network in Cancer (CIBERONC), 46010 Valencia, Spain
Pathology Department, Hospital Clínico Universitario Valencia, University of Valencia, 46010 Valencia, Spain

Valentina Rossi and Leonardo Vigna
Breast Unit, S. Camillo-Forlanini Hospital of Rome, 00152 Rome, Italy

Paola Berchialla
Department of Clinical and Biological Sciences, University of Turin, 10124 Turin, Italy

Diana Giannarelli
Department of Medical Statistics, IRCCS Regina Elena National Cancer Institute, 00128 Rome, Italy

Cecilia Nisticò, Gianluigi Ferretti, Simona Gasparro, Michelangelo Russillo, Giovanna Catania and Alessandra Fabi
Division of Medical Oncology1, IRCCS Regina Elena National Cancer Institute, 00128 Rome, Italy

Rossella Letizia Mancusi
Department of Statistical Sciences, University Tor Vergata of Rome, 00133 Rome, Italy

Emilio Bria
Comprehensive Cancer Center, Fondazione Policlinico Universitario Agostino Gemelli IRCCS, 00168 Rome, Italy
Department of Medical Oncology, Università Cattolica del Sacro Cuore, 00168 Rome, Italy

Filippo Montemurro
Direzione Day Hospital Oncologico Multidisciplinare, Istituto di Candiolo, FPO-IRCCS, 10060 Candiolo, Italy

Francesco Cognetti
Università La Sapienza, 00185 Rome, Italy

Stefanie Corradini, Daniel Reitz, Montserrat Pazos, Stephan Schönecker, Maximilian Niyazi and Claus Belka
Department of Radiation Oncology, LMU University, 81377 Munich, Germany

Michael Braun
Department of Gynecology and Obstetrics, Red Cross Hospital, 80637 Munich, Germany

Nadia Harbeck
Breast Center, Department of Gynecology and Obstetrics, LMU University, 81377 Munich, Germany

Christiane Matuschek and Edwin Bölke
Department of Radiation Oncology, Heinrich Heine University, Medical faculty, 40225 Düsseldorf, Germany

Ute Ganswindt
Department of Radiation Oncology, Medical University, 6020 Innsbruck, Austria

Filippo Alongi
Department of Radiation Oncology, Sacro Cuore Don Calabria Hospital, 37024 Negrar-Verona, University of Brescia, 25121 Brescia, Italy

Jaeho Kim and Jin Hee Kim
Department of Radiation Oncology, Dongsan Medical Center, Keimyung University School of Medicine, Daegu 42601, Korea

Won Park and Doo Ho Choi
Department of Radiation Oncology, Samsung Medical Center, Sungkyunkwan University School of Medicine, Seoul 06351, Korea

Yeon-Joo Kim and Eun Sook Lee
Center for Breast Cancer, Research Institute and Hospital, National Cancer Center, Goyang 10408, Korea

Kyung Hwan Shin and Jin Ho Kim
Department of Radiation Oncology, Seoul National University College of Medicine, Seoul 03080, Korea

Kyubo Kim
Department of Radiation Oncology, Ewha Womans University Mokdong Hospital, Ewha Womans University School of Medicine, Seoul 07804, Korea

Yong Bae Kim
Department of Radiation Oncology, Yonsei Cancer Center, Yonsei University College of Medicine, Seoul 03722, Korea

Sung-Ja Ahn
Department of Radiation Oncology, Chonnam National University Medical School, Gwangju 61469, Korea

Jong Hoon Lee
Department of Radiation Oncology, St. Vincent's Hospital, The Catholic University of Korea College of Medicine, Seoul 06591, Korea

Mison Chun
Department of Radiation Oncology, Ajou University School of Medicine, Suwon 16499, Korea

Hyung-Sik Lee
Department of Radiation Oncology, Dong-A University Hospital, Dong-A University School of Medicine, Busan 49201, Korea

Jung Soo Kim
Department of Radiation Oncology, Chonbuk National University Medical School, Jeonju 54907, Korea

Jihye Cha
Department of Radiation Oncology, Wonju Severance Christian Hospital, Wonju 26426, Korea

Simon J. Johnston and Cíntia J. Monteiro
Nottingham Breast Cancer Research Centre, School of Medicine, The University of Nottingham, Nottingham NG7 2RD, UK
Gene Regulation Laboratory, School of Pharmacy, The University of Nottingham, Nottingham NG7 2RD, UK

Binafsha M. Syed
Nottingham Breast Cancer Research Centre, School of Medicine, The University of Nottingham, Nottingham NG7 2RD, UK
Medical Research Centre, Liaquat University of Medical and Health Sciences, Jamshoro 76080, Pakistan

Ruth M. Parks, Ian O. Ellis and Kwok-Leung Cheung
Nottingham Breast Cancer Research Centre, School of Medicine, The University of Nottingham, Nottingham NG7 2RD, UK

Joseph A. Caruso
Department of Pathology, University of California, San Francisco, CA 94143, USA

Kelly K. Hunt
Department of Breast Surgical Oncology, The University of Texas MD Anderson Cancer Center, Houston, TX 77030, USA

Cansu Karakas and Khandan Keyomarsi
Department of Experimental Radiation Oncology, The University of Texas MD Anderson Cancer Center, Houston, TX 77030, USA

Jean Ching-Yuan Fann
Department of Health Industry Management, College of Healthcare Management, Kainan University, Taoyuan 338, Taiwan

King-Jen Chang and Wen-Hung Kuo
Department of Surgery, National Taiwan University Hospital, Taipei 100, Taiwan

Chen-Yang Hsu
Graduate Institute of Epidemiology and Preventive Medicine, College of Public Health, National Taiwan University, Taipei 100, Taiwan

Amy Ming-Fang Yen and Sam Li-Sheng Chen
School of Oral Hygiene, College of Oral Medicine, Taipei Medical University, Taipei 110, Taiwan

Cheng-Ping Yu
Department of Pathology and Graduate Institute of Pathology and Parasitology, Tri-Service General Hospital, National Defense Medical Center, Taipei 114, Taiwan
Graduate Institute of Life Sciences, National Defense Medical Center, Taipei 114, Taiwan

László Tabár
Department of Mammography, Falun Central Hospital, 791823 Falun, Sweden

Hsiu-Hsi Chen
Graduate Institute of Epidemiology and Preventive Medicine, College of Public Health, National Taiwan University, Taipei 100, Taiwan

Danielle R. Heller and Alexander S. Chiu
Department of Surgery, Yale School of Medicine, New Haven, CT 06520, USA

Kaitlin Farrell, Brigid K. Killelea and Donald R. Lannin
The Breast Center/Section of Surgical Oncology, Department of Surgery, Yale School of Medicine, New Haven, CT 06520, USA

Corinna Keup, Pawel Mach, Oliver Hoffmann, Rainer Kimmig and Sabine Kasimir-Bauer
Department of Gynecology and Obstetrics, University Hospital of Essen, 45122 Essen, Germany

Markus Storbeck, Siegfried Hauch, Peter Hahn and Markus Sprenger-Haussels
QIAGEN GmbH, 40724 Hilden, Germany

Mitra Tewes
Department of Medical Oncology, University Hospital of Essen, 45122 Essen, Germany

Tarek M. A. Abdel-Fatah, Maaz Sadiq, Paul M. Moseley and Stephen Y. T. Chan
Department of Oncology, Nottingham University Hospitals, Nottingham NG5 1PB, UK

Reem Ali and Katia A. Mesquita
Translational Oncology, Nottingham Breast Cancer Research Centre, Division of Cancer and Stem Cells, School of Medicine, University of Nottingham, Nottingham NG5 1PB, UK

Graham Ball
School of Science and Technology, Nottingham Trent University, Clifton Campus, Nottingham NG11 8NS, UK

Emad A. Rakha
Academic Pathology, Nottingham Breast Cancer Research Centre, Division of Cancer and Stem Cells, School of Medicine, University of Nottingham, Nottingham NG5 1PB, UK

Srinivasan Madhusudan
Department of Oncology, Nottingham University Hospitals, Nottingham NG5 1PB, UK
Translational Oncology, Nottingham Breast Cancer Research Centre, Division of Cancer and Stem Cells, School of Medicine, University of Nottingham, Nottingham NG5 1PB, UK

Index

www.ingramcontent.com/pod-product-compliance
Lightning Source LLC
LaVergne TN
LVHW081027210926
848485LV00004B/966